Diseases of the Jaws

Isaäc van der Waal

Diseases of the Jaws
Diagnosis and treatment

Textbook & Atlas

Munksgaard

Diseases of the Jaws
Diagnosis and treatment

Copyright © 1991 Munksgaard, Copenhagen
All rights reserved

No part of this publication may be reproduced, stored in a retrieval system, or transmitted in any form or by any means, electronic, mechanical photocopying, recording or otherwise without prior permission by the copyright owner

Cover, layout and typesetting by Jens Lund Kirkegaard
Color reproduction by OR-2 Odense
Black and white reproduction by Grafikhuset, Copenhagen

Printed in Denmark 1991 by Lauersen AS, Tønder

ISBN 87-16-10618-0

Distributed in North America by Mosby-Year Book Inc., Chicago, Illinois

*To my children Charlotte and Rutger
and my wife Olga*

Foreword

In 1912 Charles L. Scudder published the first monograph "Tumor of the jaws". At that time it was a pioneering work. Since then, several books have appeared dealing not only with tumors but with all types of diseases of the jaws. The interest of the dental profession in diseases of the jaws reflects the modern concept of the role of the dentist: to be concerned not only with diseases of the teeth and periodontal structures but to have a genuine interest in adjacent structures, i.e. the oral mucosa, the salivary glands and the jaws, thus becoming what the World Health Organization has termed an "oral physician".

Professor Isaäc van der Waal's monograph on *Diseases of the Jaws* is a very comprehensive treatise on the subject, dealing with all aspects of jaw lesions ranging from congenital and developmental disturbances to inflammatory lesions, idiopathic conditions, all sorts of jaw tumors, systemic diseases and ending with disorders of the temporomandibular joint.

The book is structured in a systematic fashion providing overall information on each entity.

Professor Isaäc van der Waal is a world authority on oral pathology and is well-known for his clarity of style which is also found in the present book.

Dentists and everyone interested in diseases of the jaws will welcome this valuable contribution which certainly also could become of great utility to dental students.

Jens J. Pindborg

Preface

The jaws can be affected by a variety of lesions and disorders, being either of odontogenic or non-odontogenic origin, and arising primarily within the jaws or being of a generalized or metastatic nature. Lesions of the jaws can to a large extent be compared with lesions in other bones of the skull and the skeleton. However, there is a number of diseases that are more or less limited to the jaws, due to the presence of the dentition. As with all diseases, and even more so with diseases of bones, close cooperation between the clinician and pathologist, and in many instances also the radiologist, is essential to ensure proper management of the patient.

The references used in this text have largely been limited to the period from 1980, with a few exceptions of often-cited papers from earlier years. Furthermore, journals of various dental and medical disciplines have been covered in order to facilitate accessibility to the literature. For the same reason the references are not limited to the English language but include a number of German and French sources as well.

Even a single-authored text can not be the work of just one person. Many colleagues have unselfishly made pictures of their published cases available, permission also being granted by the respective journals. Quintessenz Publishing Co. has kindly given me permission to use the figures 2-3, 2-9, 6-5, 6-12, 6-16, 6-21, 7-3, 7-8, 10-3, 10-4, 10-8, 10-11, 10-12, 10-16, 10-32 which were published in I. van der Waal & W.A.M. van der Kwast: "Oral Pathology".

My sincere thanks and appreciation go to Prof.dr. W.A.M. van der Kwast, former head of the Department of Oral and Maxillofacial Surgery of the Free University, Amsterdam, who has always stimulated a close cooperation between the various dental and medical disciplines, as being reflected in this monograph. Furthermore, I am grateful to Prof.dr. J.J. Pindborg, head of the Department of Oral Pathology of the Royal Dental School, Copenhagen, for his encouragement and guidance in the preparation of the text.

Finally, I would like to thank Mrs. Dini Chevalking for her dedicated secretarial help, Mr. Willem W. de Jong for his technical assistance, Mr. G.J. Oskam and Mr. J.T. van Veldhuisen for their photographic help and my colleague and friend Dr. Willem F.B. de Jong for many inspiring discussions on the subject of diseases of the jaws.

Isaäc van der Waal

Contents

INTRODUCTION *15*

1. CONGENITAL AND DEVELOPMENTAL DISTURBANCES *17*

   Agnathia, micrognathia, and macrognathia *17*
   Cleidocranial dysostosis *18*
   Craniofacial dysostosis *20*
   Exostoses *20*
      Torus palatinus *20*
      Torus mandibularis *22*
      Multiple exostoses *24*
   Hemimaxillofacial dysplasia *24*
   Hyperostosis corticalis generalisata familiaris
     (Van Buchem's disease) *25*
   Infantile cortical hyperostosis (Caffey's disease) *26*
   Mandibulofacial dysostosis (Treacher Collins syndrome) *27*
   Osteogenesis imperfecta *27*
   Pycnodysostosis *28*

2. INFLAMMATORY LESIONS OF BONE *29*

   Alveolitis ("Dry socket") *29*
   Botryomycosis *30*
   Cholesterol granuloma *30*
   Mucormycosis *30*
   Osteomyelitis *31*
   Osteoradionecrosis *41*
   Periapical granuloma *45*
   Periodontal disease *48*

3. GIANT CELL LESIONS *51*

   Cherubism *51*
   Central giant cell granuloma *55*
   Giant cell tumor *60*

4. FIBROUS DYSPLASIA *61*

Fibrous dysplasia *61*
    Monostotic fibrous dysplasia *61*
    Polyostotic fibrous dysplasia *70*

5. NON-ODONTOGENIC CYSTS *71*

Aneurysmal bone cyst *71*
Dermoid cyst *73*
Globulomaxillary cyst *74*
Lingual cortical defect of the mandible *74*
Median mandibular cyst *76*
Median palatal cyst *77*
Nasolabial cyst *77*
Nasopalatine duct cyst *78*
Parasitic cyst *80*
Postoperative maxillary cyst *80*
Solitary bone cyst *82*

6. ODONTOGENIC CYSTS *85*

Developmental cysts *86*
    Dental lamina cyst of the newborn *86*
    Dentigerous cyst *88*
    Eruption cyst *92*
    Gingival cyst of the adult *95*
    Keratocyst *96*
    Lateral periodontal cyst (incl. Botryoid odontogenic cyst) *104*
    Primordial cyst *106*
    Sialo-odontogenic cyst (Glandular odontogenic cyst) *106*
Inflammatory cysts *107*
    Paradental cyst *107*
    Radicular cyst *108*
    Residual cyst *110*
    Mandibular infected buccal cyst *112*

7. NEOPLASMS OF PRIMARY BONE ORIGIN *113*

Benign neoplasms *113*
    Osteoma *113*
    Osteoblastoma (incl. Osteoid osteoma) *117*

Malignant neoplasms *119*
    Osteosarcoma *119*
    Ewing's sarcoma *129*

8. NEOPLASMS DERIVED FROM CARTILAGE *133*

    Benign neoplasms *133*
        Chondroma *133*
        Benign chondroblastoma *134*
    Malignant neoplasms *135*
        Chondrosarcoma *135*
        Mesenchymal chondrosarcoma *138*

9. NON-OSSEOUS, NON-CHONDROID NEOPLASMS *139*
(excl. odontogenic tumors)

    Chemodectoma *139*
    Chondromyxoid fibroma *139*
    Desmoplastic fibroma *142*
    Non-ossifying fibroma *144*
    Fibromatosis *146*
    Fibrosarcoma *148*
    Fibrous histiocytoma *149*
    Hemangioma *150*
    Angiosarcoma and hemangiopericytoma *154*
    Leiomyoma and leiomyosarcoma *155*
    Lipoma, lipoblastoma and liposarcoma *155*
    Lymphangioma *155*
    Lymphoreticular diseases *156*
        Malignant lymphoma (incl. Leukemia) *156*
        Burkitt's tumor (African jaw tumor) *160*
        Solitary plasma cell myeloma *162*
        Multiple myeloma (Kahler's disease) *163*
        Myelofibrosis *165*
        Waldenström's disease *165*
        Myelosarcoma (chloroma) *165*
    Melanotic neuroectodermal tumor of infancy *166*
    Metastatic tumors *168*
    Neuroblastoma *171*
    Neurofibroma and neurilemmoma *171*
    Ganglioneuroma *172*

Neurogenic sarcoma *172*
Rhabdomyosarcoma *173*
Salivary gland neoplasms *174*
Teratoma *176*

10. ODONTOGENIC TUMORS *177*

    Benign neoplasms *178*
       Benign ameloblastoma *178*
       Squamous odontogenic tumor *187*
       Calcifying epithelial odontogenic tumor (Pindborg tumor) *188*
       Ameloblastic fibroma *190*
       Ameloblastic fibro-dentinoma ("Dentinoma") *192*
       Ameloblastic fibro-odontoma *193*
       Odontoameloblastoma *194*
       Adenomatoid odontogenic tumor *194*
       Calcifying odontogenic cyst *196*
       Odontoma (compound; complex) *199*
       Fibroma (odontogenic), central and peripheral *202*
       Myxoma (odontogenic) *204*
       Cementum containing lesions *206*
    Malignant neoplasms *230*
       Odontogenic carcinomas *230*
       Odontogenic sarcomas *234*
       Odontogenic carcino-sarcoma *234*

11. SYSTEMIC DISEASES *235*

    Gaucher's disease *235*
    Histiocytosis X (Langerhans' cell granulomatosis) *236*
       Hand-Schüller-Christian disease *236*
       Letterer-Siwe disease *237*
       Eosinophilic granuloma *238*
    Osteopetrosis *241*
    Osteoporosis *243*
    Paget's disease *245*
    Renal osteodystrophy *248*
    Sarcoidosis *249*
    Scleroderma *249*
    Thalassemia *249*

12. MISCELLANEOUS LESIONS AND DISORDERS OF BONE 253

Atrophy of the alveolar ridges 253
Fibrous or sclerotic healing of extraction wounds 254
Focal osteoporotic bone marrow defect 255
Hemophilic pseudotumor of bone 258
Massive osteolysis 258
Overprojection of radiopaque structures 259
Squamous cell carcinoma 263
Uncontrolled growth of alveolar processes 263

13. DISORDERS OF THE TEMPOROMANDIBULAR JOINT 265

Introduction 265
Ankylosis 266
Arthrogryposis 266
Chondromatosis 267
Condylar changes in systemic disease 267
Cysts and neoplasms 267
Hyperplasia of the condyles (Bifid mandibular condyle) 268
Hypoplasia of the condyles 268
Hyperplasia of the coronoid process 268
Pain dysfunction syndrome (arthrosis deformans; osteoarthrosis) 269
(Sub)luxation 272
Trismus 273

REFERENCES 275

INDEX 301

Introduction

The mandible and the maxilla may be affected by both local and generalized diseases. The classification of bone lesions, as proposed by the World Health Organization in 1972[500], is only partly applicable to the jaw bones. Furthermore, a number of changes and additions have been proposed in the recent literature. The classification system used in this book is, therefore, somewhat arbitrary.

With regard to the diagnosis of a lesion or a disease of the jaw, the medical history and the clinical examination may already provide valuable information. In all instances radiographic examination is necessary and, in most cases, also a biopsy is required. In selected cases serologic studies are required.

In the radiographic examination of the toothbearing area, the intraoral periapical view usually provides the most detailed information. If necessary, an occlusal view can be taken. The panoramic view, now being frequently used, depicts the entire mandible and maxilla in one film and has been shown to be very valuable[14, 20, 45, 66, 614]. It should be stressed that the panoramic view is in most instances a supplement to, and not a substitute for the intraoral radiograph. In addition to periapical, occlusal and panoramic radiographs, radiographic examination of the jaws may include the use of conventional extraoral films, computer assisted tomography (CAT scan), xeroradiography[284], and scintigraphy, using radioisotopes[174, 253]. Limited experience is available yet with regard to the possible value of magnetic resonance imaging (MRI) in the diagnosis of lesions of the bone. When a vascular lesion is suspected, arteriography is indicated.

In radiolucent lesions of the jaws, fine needle aspiration biopsy may be a valuable technique[454].

For most lesions of the jaw, a biopsy can be carried out under local anesthesia via an intraoral approach. There is little chance of complications such as bleeding, damage to a nerve, or delayed wound healing. A biopsy specimen from the bone can be obtained using either a slowly rotating trepan bur or a regular bur, with or without the aid of a chisel. When rotating instruments are used, proper cooling is required to prevent damage to the biopsy specimen and the biopsy site as well. Whenever possible, the biopsy specimen should include both part of the normal and abnormal bone. Furthermore, it is important to take a biopsy of adequate size in order to enable the pathologist to embed the specimen in the proper direction. In general, it is not necessary to include the overlying periosteum or mucosa.

Several fixatives can be used. In the majority of cases formalin fixation is appropriate. The use of formic acid solution for the decalcification results in sections in which both the soft tissues and the (de)calcified structures can be adequately examined. The disadvantage of that solution is the rather long time-period required for decalcification. It is also possible to make use of undecalcified sections, embedded in plastic[152]. That technique is especially valuable for studying metabolic disorders.

Making the radiographs available to the pathologist may contribute considerably to a correct final diagnosis and is in many instances a "conditio sine qua non".

CHAPTER 1

Congenital and developmental disturbances

There are numerous congenital and developmental disorders in which the bones may be involved. In this chapter the emphasis is on the disorders that specifically affect the jaw bones or the bones of the skull.

Agnathia, micrognathia, and macrognathia

Agnathia

Agnathia, the complete congenital absence of the mandible or maxilla, is extremely rare[87]. In some cases just a part may be missing, e.g., half the mandible or one of the condyles.

Micrognathia

It is difficult to provide criteria for the proper size of the jaw and to define whether the jaw is too small (micrognathia) or too large (macrognathia). Even when the size is normal, the jaw may appear to be too small or too large if the position is abnormal.

The cause of micrognathia is unknown. Usually, it concerns the mandible, this being too small at birth. In some of these cases there are also abnormalities elsewhere in the skeleton. Occasionally, one is dealing with the Pierre Robin syndrome, consisting of micrognathia, cleft palate, and downward displacement of the tongue, sometimes causing breathing disturbances.

Furthermore, the size may be normal at birth but retardation may then occur in the growth of one or both jaws, again most often the mandible. The growth disturbance is almost always the result of a trauma or an infection in the region of one or both condyles.

As a result, ankylosis may take place, either of a bony or a fibrous nature.

The therapeutic possibilities are limited. With the exception of congenital micrognathia of the mandible, micrognathia generally does not appear to cause any functional disturbances, but problems may arise esthetically and psychologically. In such cases, good results can often be obtained by combined orthodontic and surgical treatment.

Macrognathia

Macrognathia refers to too large a mandible or maxilla (mandibular or maxillary prognathia). The term mandibular prognathia has been more or less replaced by progenia. The etiology is unknown. In some cases heredity seems to play a role. Macrognathia may also be the result of acromegaly, which usually involves the mandible. In the latter disease, resorption of roots as well as excessive hypercementosis have been reported.

Macrognathia may give rise to esthetic problems, especially in young adults, and may cause a disturbed chewing function or speech disturbances.

In many cases it is possible to reduce the enlarged maxilla or mandible surgically. A tongue reduction may be desirable at the same time.

Cleidocranial dysostosis

Cleidocranial dysostosis is a disorder of unknown etiology, characterized by abnormalities of the cranium, the clavicles, the teeth, the jaws, and sometimes also of the long bones[312]. In the past, cleidocranial dysostosis was thought only to affect bones that are being formed in an intramembranous way. In many cases there is autosomal dominant heredity. The syndrome is seen as often in men as in women.

In the skull there is a delayed closing of the fontanels. The frontal, parietal, and occipital bones are in general prominent. The paranasal sinuses remain small and underdeveloped. In the shoulder girdle one or both clavicles may be underdeveloped or partly absent (Fig. 1-1) and some patients can move their shoulders entirely forward or even bring them together.

Fig. 1-1. Chest film showing underdeveloped right clavicle in patient affected by cleidocranial dysostosis.

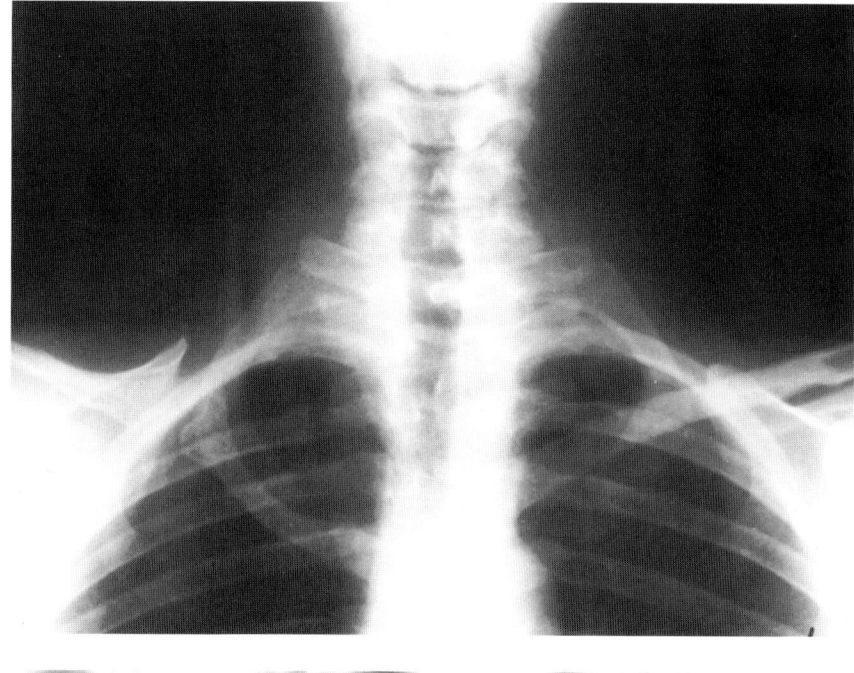

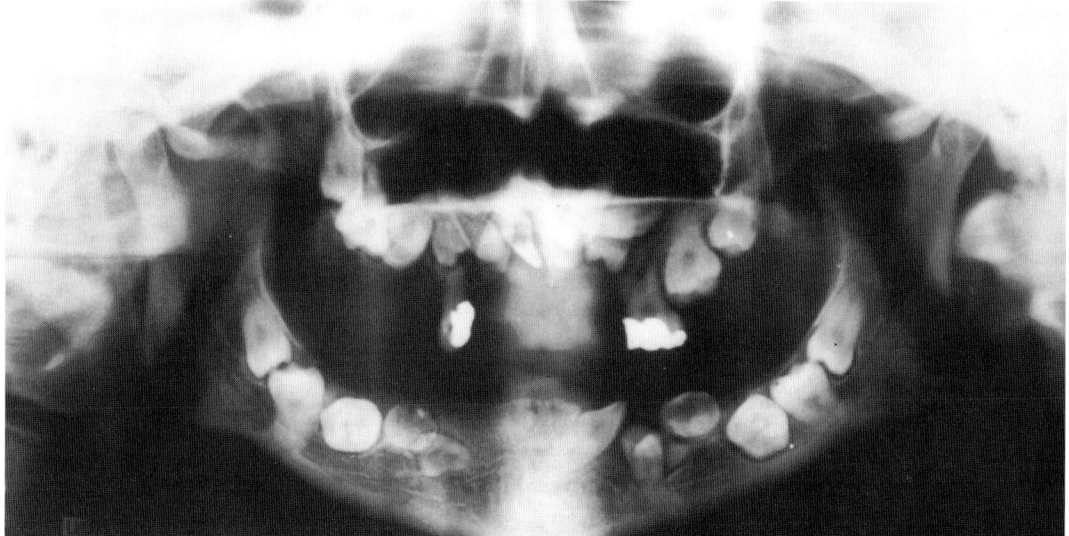

Fig. 1-2. Multiple impacted permanent teeth in patient shown in Fig. 1-1.

The oral abnormalities include a high, narrow palate. The maxilla is sometimes underdeveloped. There may be a true or submucous cleft present in the palate. The shedding of the teeth may be seriously delayed. There are often supernumerary permanent impacted teeth (Fig. 1-2). The supernumerary teeth are mainly found in the premolar and molar area. The roots of the erupted teeth may be shortened. There may be little or no cementum on the root surfaces[235]. Also hypocalcification of the enamel of the supernumerary teeth has been demonstrated[643].

No adequate treatment is available for this syndrome.

Craniofacial dysostosis

Craniofacial dysostosis, also called Crouzon's disease, is a disorder of unknown etiology. The abnormality is often inherited[227].

There is frontal bossing. Many patients show hypertelorism and exophthalmos. In some cases mental retardation has been observed. The maxilla is usually underdeveloped, the mandible remaining unaffected. The palate may be high and narrow and is sometimes clefted.

No treatment is available. The life expectancy for the patients is in general normal.

Exostoses

Torus palatinus

Definition and epidemiology

A torus palatinus is a slowly growing exostosis in the midline of the palate. The etiology is unknown. Possibly, heredity plays a role.

The protuberance is found in about 20% of the population, twice as often in women as in men. In Malays palatine tori were found in 22.6% and in Indians in only 5.5%[638]. The torus palatinus is mostly diagnosed after age 30. The number of torus cases increases in both men and women with age[440].

Clinical aspects

The size may vary from a few millimeters to a few centimeters. The shape can be flat, spindle, nodular or lobulated (Fig. 1-3). The patient is seldom aware of its presence.

The diagnosis can almost always be made on the basis of the clinical appearance. The most important aspect is its bony consistency at palpation, and the midline location. When the consistency is not clearly of a bony nature, a biopsy is indicated since various lesions, such as salivary gland neoplasms and nasal and paranasal neoplasms, may present themselves as a palatal swelling.

Fig. 1-3.
Torus palatinus.

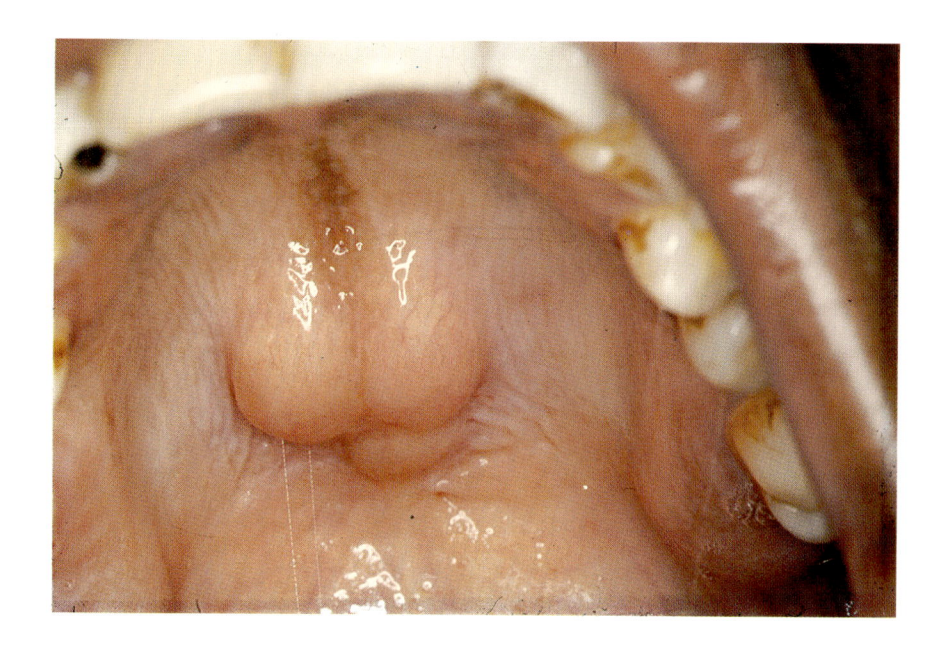

Radiographic aspects	Periapical, occlusal or panoramic radiographs are of little help in depicting a bony lesion at this specific site. For an occasional patient, planigrams or CT-scans may be indicated.
Histologic aspects	Microscopic examination will show normal, vital compact bone. Occasionally, cancellous bone may be encountered.
Treatment	Surgical correction is seldom indicated and should be considered only in case of problems in the preparation of a denture.

Torus mandibularis

Definition and epidemiology

The torus mandibularis is an often lobulated overgrowth or exostosis on the lingual aspect of the mandible, above the mylohyoid line, most often appearing symmetrically and usually in the premolar area (Fig. 1-4). As with the torus palatinus, the etiology is unknown. Possibly, heredity plays a role here as well.

There is no preference for either sex. The lesion is seen in about 2-7% of the population and is usually diagnosed after age 30. There is no correlation with the occurrence of the torus palatinus. In a survey of 2400 Malaysian patients the prevalence of mandibular tori was only 1.7%; none was found in male patients[638].

Clinical aspects

Sometimes a lingually impacted premolar may cause a bony swelling mimicking the features of a mandibular torus. In such a case, a radiograph will provide the correct diagnosis.

Radiographic aspects

In contrast to the torus palatinus, the mandibular torus may be visible as a well-circumscribed opacity on radiographs because there is little or no overprojection of other structures in the mandible (Fig. 1-5).

Histologic aspects

As with the torus palatinus, microscopic examination of bone removed from a mandibular torus will show vital, compact bone. In some cases hematopoietic marrow may be encountered.

Treatment

As with the torus palatinus, treatment is seldom indicated.

Exostoses • 23

Fig. 1-4. Torus mandibularis.

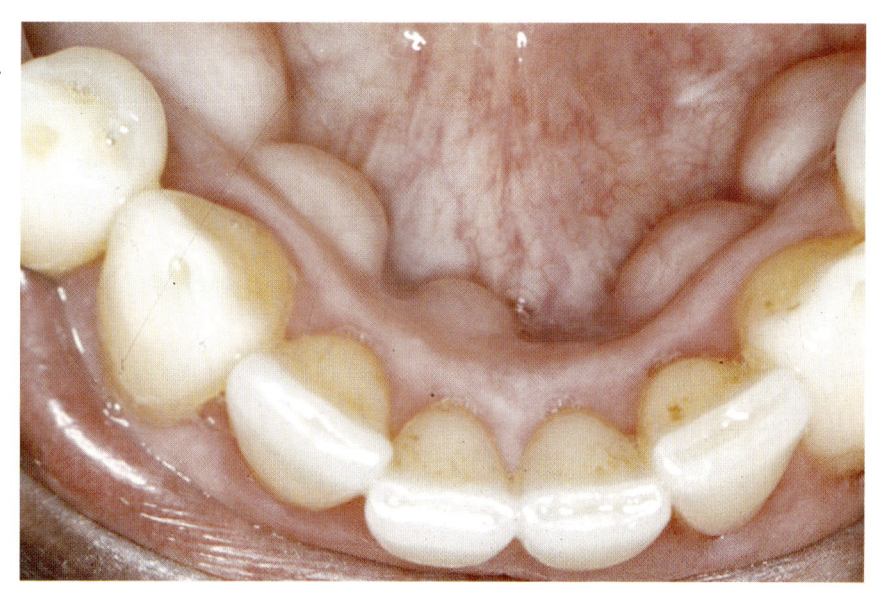

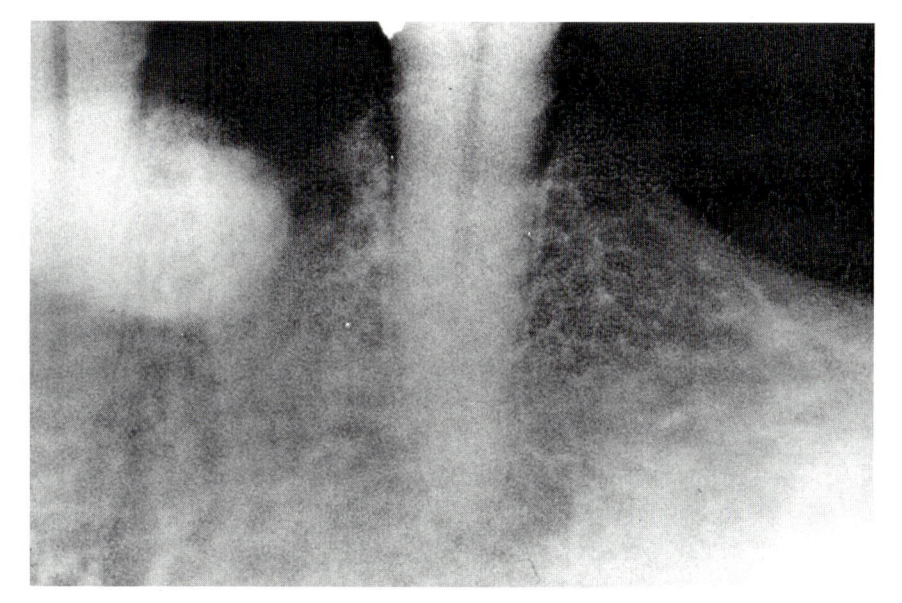

Fig. 1-5. Radiopacity caused by torus mandibularis.

Fig. 1-6. Multiple exostoses in the maxilla.

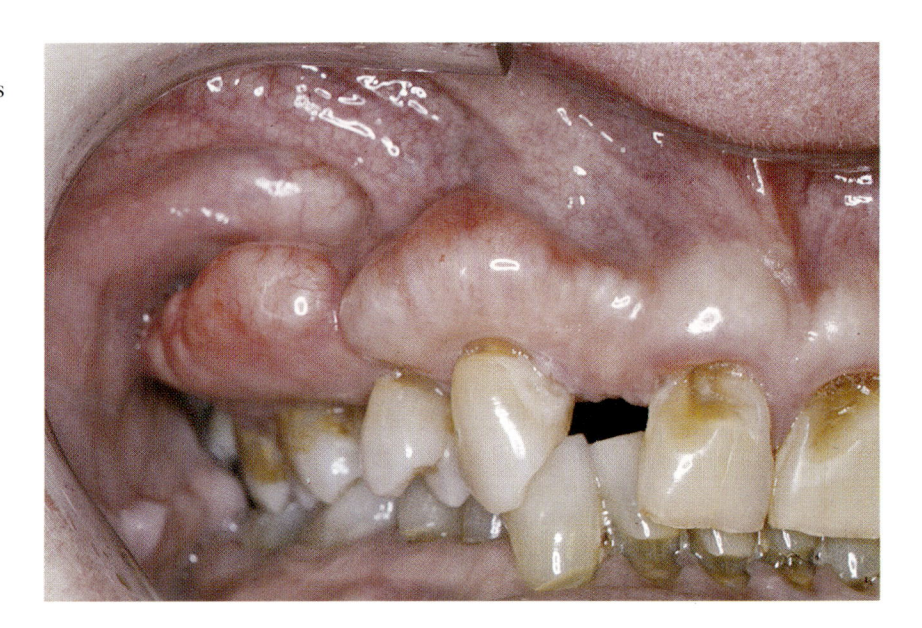

Multiple exostoses

Multiple bony swellings are sometimes observed on the buccal aspect of the maxilla and the mandible in adult and elderly patients (Fig. 1-6). There are no data available as to possible sex predilection.

The swellings are perhaps due to chronic irritation from the periodontal structures. Also bruxism has been mentioned as a possible cause. It is an asymptomatic, harmless phenomenon that needs correction only in case of preparation of a full denture[470].

Hemimaxillofacial dysplasia

Hemimaxillofacial dysplasia is a newly recognized disorder consisting of unilateral enlargement of the maxillary alveolar bone and the gingiva associated with hypoplastic teeth, facial asymmetry, and hypertrichosis of the facial skin on the ipsilateral side. The cause and pathogenesis are not well understood[377].

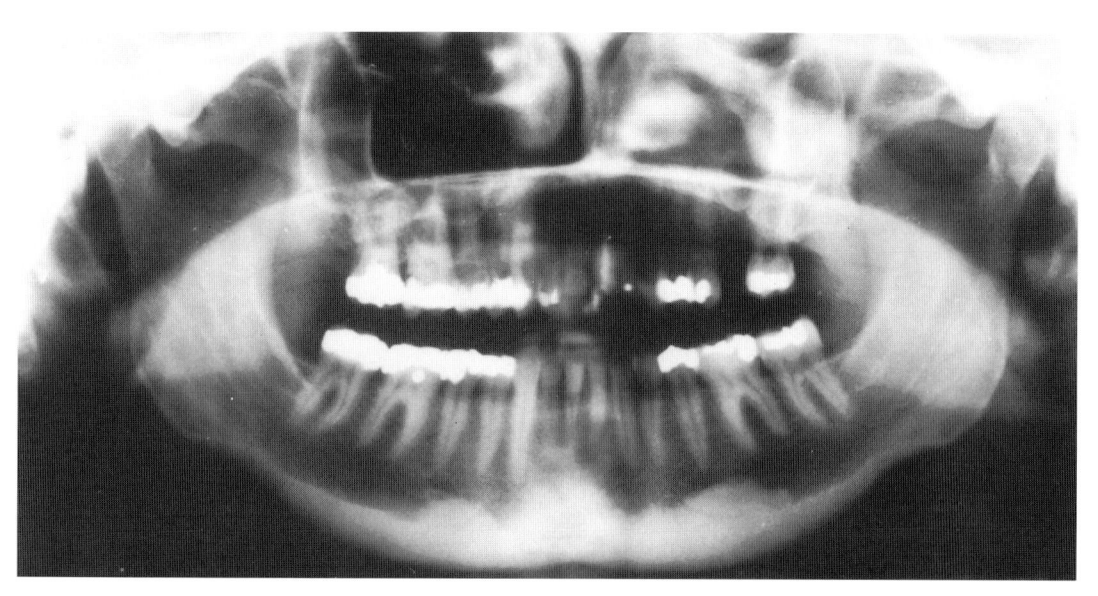

Fig. 1-7. Sclerosis of inferior mandibular border in an otherwise healthy patient, possibly representing a "forme fruste" of Van Buchem's disease.

Hyperostosis corticalis generalisata familiaris
(Van Buchem's disease)

Definition and epidemiology

Hyperostosis corticalis generalisata familiaris, also referred to as Van Buchem's disease, is a rare disorder characterized by a thickening and sclerosing of the bones, especially of the skull, jaws, clavicles and ribs. Due to the limited number of reported cases no statistics can be provided with regard to race, sex or age[158].

The disease can be inherited as an autosomal recessive or dominant trait. The basic defect seems to be excess deposition of endosteal bone together with irregular deposition of subperiosteal bone.

In rare instances only the inferior border of the mandible shows sclerosis, which is possibly to be regarded an expression of a "forme fruste" (Fig. 1-7).

Clinical aspects

Some patients are unaware of the condition. In other cases a dull aching pain has been mentioned. In severe cases the hyperostosis of the foramina of the base of the skull causes a deficit of vision or hearing. The dentition is usually normal.

Laboratory findings — The serum alkaline phosphatase may be increased, while all other findings, e.g. serum calcium and phosphorus, are within normal limits.

Radiographic aspects — Radiographically, a diffuse sclerosing and thickening of the mandible, usually anterior to the angles, is rather characteristic.

Histologic aspects — Histologically, excessive formation of lamellar bone can be observed within narrow or absent Haversian canals.

Treatment — The disease may progress slowly, the main threat being impingement of neural tissues due to the thickening of the skull bones. Pathological fractures are unusual in van Buchem's disease. Healing of bone lesions, e.g. after extraction of teeth, is normal[479]. A case has been reported in which resection of the lower border resulted in improved facial appearance[356].

Infantile cortical hyperostosis
(Caffey's disease)

Definition and epidemiology — Infantile cortical hyperostosis, also referred to as Caffey's disease or Caffey-Silverman syndrome, is a rare disease characterized by hyperostosis of the cortex of the affected bone, which is usually the mandible, clavicle and ulna. It affects infants in the first few months of life[300]. The etiology is unknown.

Clinical aspects — The disease generally begins as an acute febrile illness accompanied by painful swellings over one or more bones, with all the signs of inflammation.

Laboratory findings — The significant laboratory findings are an elevated sedimentation rate, an increased alkaline phosphatase, and a leukocytosis.

Radiographic aspects — It may take a few weeks before radiographic changes, consisting of hyperostosis, can be observed. It has been emphasized that the diagnosis is made from the characteristic laminated appearance of the new bone deposition as seen in roentgenograms and from the clinical history. Nevertheless, the radiographic differential diagnosis usually includes osteomyelitis and even osteogenic sarcoma.

Treatment   Treatment is most commonly restricted to analgesics and general supportive therapy. The value of the administration of steroids is debatable. The disease resolves spontaneously with few, if any, residual stigmata in the adult[664].

Mandibulofacial dysostosis
(Treacher Collins syndrome)

Mandibulofacial dysostosis, also called Treacher Collins syndrome, is a rare disorder. Heredity often plays a role in the etiology[441].

The syndrome is characterized by hypoplasia of the facial bones, particularly of the zygomatic bone and the mandible. There is malformation of the external ear and sometimes also of the middle and inner ears. Choanal atresia has also been reported to occur in patients affected by this syndrome. Macrostomia may be present. The palate is usually high and sometimes clefted. Occlusion disturbances are common as well.

On radiographic examination the zygomatic bone often appears to be underdeveloped on both sides. There is also underdevelopment of the paranasal sinuses. The mastoid is often sclerotic.

No treatment is available. The life expectancy for these patients is more or less normal.

Osteogenesis imperfecta

Osteogenesis imperfecta is a syndrome consisting of brittleness of the bones, blue sclerae, deafness, weakness of the articular ligaments, and often also dentinogenesis imperfecta[506]. There may be a strong tendency to capillary bleedings.

Several types of osteogenesis are distinguished, each having a specific hereditary pattern. The disorder is thought to be caused by a disturbance in the maturation of collagen. A number of children affected by osteogenesis imperfecta are stillborn or die shortly after birth.

No treatment is available.

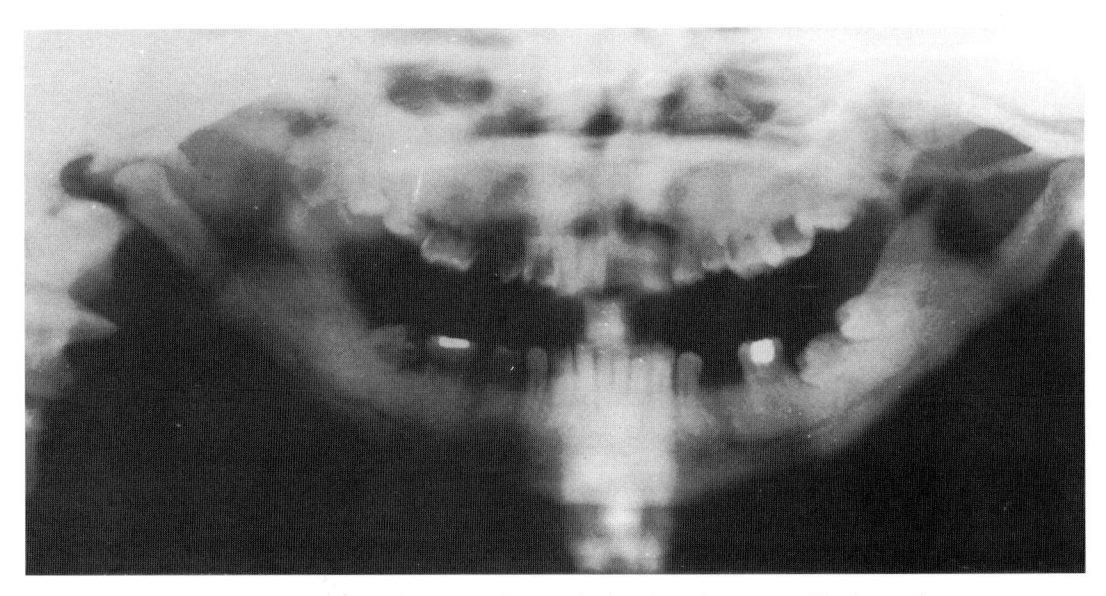

Fig. 1-8. Panoramic view of patient with pycnodysostosis showing obtuse mandibular angle.

Pycnodysostosis

Pycnodysostosis is a syndrome characterized by dwarfism, osteopetrosis, abbreviated terminal phalanges, cranial anomalies, such as persistence of fontanels and failure of closure of cranial sutures, and hypoplasia of the angle of the mandible (Fig. 1-8)[227]. Osteomyelitis of the jaws is a rather common complication[375].

CHAPTER 2

Inflammatory lesions of bone

Alveolitis ("Dry socket")

Definition and terminology

Alveolitis, also known as "dry socket", is a localized inflammatory condition of the alveolar bone that may arise a few days after extraction of a tooth. Some authors have simply defined dry socket as "a failure in the normal healing process of the extraction wound, regardless of the clinical presentation"[191]. Others have defined dry socket as "a painful socket which is increasing in severity 24 hours after the extraction"[477].

Epidemiology and etiology

Alveolitis occurs in 3-5% following all extractions, slightly more often in women than in men. It is an extremely painful condition that may take more than two weeks to heal, with or without supportive treatment.

The etiology is actually unknown. One of the hypotheses is that the blood clot in the alveolus undergoes disintegration for reasons as yet unknown. Anaerobic bacteria may play a role in the etiology as well[40]. There does not seem to be a correlation between general health and the occurrence of dry socket. Alveolitis is significantly more frequent after single extractions than after multiple extractions. There is a higher incidence of painful sockets in heavy smokers (20 of more cigarets per day) compared with non-smokers[371].

Clinical aspects

Alveolitis occurs much more frequently in the mandibular molar region than in any other site of the dentition. The disturbance in wound healing actually never occurs in extraction sites of deciduous teeth. The clinical impression is just that of an empty alveolus.

Radiographic aspects

Radiographic examination will not show any abnormality or irregularity. Nevertheless, a radiograph may be taken to rule out the presence of a root fragment or a foreign body, such as a fragment of a broken down metal restoration.

Diagnosis

The taking of a biopsy is indicated only in case of a questionable diagnosis. Otherwise, the diagnosis can be made with confidence based on the history of a recent tooth extraction and the clinical (and radiographic) finding of an empty, otherwise normal appearing alveolus.

Treatment

Many treatment modalities are available, varying from daily irrigation with luke salt water or 1.5% hydrogen peroxide, to the placement of iodine-containing gauzes, sulfathiazole cones, antibiotics etc., no one regimen being really superior to any other. Pre-operative irrigation of the gingival crevice and mouthrinsing with 0.2% chlorhexidine gluconate significantly reduces the chance of dry socket[190]. Also the prophylactic use of metronidazole has been shown to be effective[477].

Botryomycosis

Botryomycosis is an uncommon bacterial infection, capable of producing chronic granulomatous inflammation. It is characterized by the production of distinctive grains formed by the interaction of the infective bacteria with the host tissues[25].

Very few cases of botryomycosis involving the jaw bone have been reported[25].

Cholesterol granuloma

The literature contains a few cases of so-called cholesterol granulomas of the jaws that presented as a residual cyst[274]. The pathogenesis is poorly understood.

Histologically, the lesions consist of fibrous connective tissue without epithelial lining and are characterized by the presence of numerous cholesterol crystals, surrounded by multinucleated giant cells.

Treatment consists of enucleation.

Mucormycosis

Mucormycosis or phycomycosis, an infection due to fungi of the class Phycomycetes, is an uncommon disease. Most reported cases involve patients with diabetes mellitus, immunosuppression, or a debilitating disease of some type[93,478].

The saprophytic fungi are characterized by broad, nonseptate hyphae averaging 6 to 15μm in width and 100-200μm in length. The organism is found throughout the environment in soil, and is frequently found in the nasal passages and oral cavities of normal persons[93]. Although the nose is usually the portal of entry, any perforation of skin or mucosal lining may allow entrance of the organism. It invades the arteries, resulting in ischemic necrosis.

Maxillary involvement is common, while involvement of the mandible is rare. Treatment consists of wide surgical debridement and administration of amphotericin-B. Furthermore, the underlying predisposing disease should be taken care of, if possible.

Osteomyelitis

Terminology

Inflammation of the jaws usually has an odontogenic cause. The inflammation is often restricted to the apex of a tooth, resulting in a periapical granuloma. On theoretical grounds a periapical lesion can be regarded as a type of osteomyelitis. The same is true with regard to alveolitis and periodontitis. In practice, however, the term osteomyelitis is applied only when a more diffuse inflammatory change in the jaws, as demonstrated or supported by radiographic and/or scintigraphic findings, is present.

In most cases of osteomyelitis the inflammation spreads not only throughout the bone but also extends into the periosteum. Sometimes, the inflammation is more or less limited to the periosteum, without inflammatory signs or symptoms in the underlying bone, and may be designated as periostitis. Osteomyelitis of the jaws seldom gives rise to inflammation or formation of abscesses elsewhere in the body.

An animal model has been described which made it possible to establish osteomyelitis in rabbits without the use of considerable trauma to the bone[314].

Epidemiology

Osteomyelitis may occur at all ages, although it is rare in children[417].

In general, there is no distinct race or sex preference. Only the chronic diffuse sclerotic type is more common among women, especially in Negroes. In many parts of the world osteomyelitis has become rare, which is most likely due to better dental and medical care, including the availability of antibiotics.

Table 2-1.   Classification of osteomyelitis

> Acute (primary)
>
> Chronic (with or without proliferative periostitis)
>   suppurative (purulent)
>   sclerosing (sicca)
>   focal (condensing osteitis)
>   diffuse
>
> Chronic periostitis in denture wearers
>   (no or minimal involvement of the bone itself)
>
> (Osteoradionecrosis)

Etiology

Osteomyelitis of the jaws can be caused by a number of factors, such as a difficult extraction of a tooth or the presence of one or more non-vital teeth[268]. Less common causes are periodontal disease, a fracture of the jaws, extension of infection of the nasal and paranasal sinuses into the jawbone, i.e. the maxilla, the presence of a foreign body, e.g., metal wires or screws used in the treatment of a fracture, hematogenous infection from a focus elsewhere in the body[92] and, in patients reported from Nigeria, cancrum oris[9]. Furthermore, a slight trauma or an extraction of a tooth in irradiated bone may cause a severe type of osteomyelitis called osteoradionecrosis, to be discussed later. In edentulous patients food particles underneath the dentures may be pushed through the oral mucosa, resulting in a localized chronic periosteal reaction. Such food particles may perhaps also have been introduced through an extraction socket[381].

Other predisposing factors for the development of osteomyelitis are generalized bone diseases, such as osteopetrosis[133,238] and Paget's disease[77]. Otherwise, the general health of the patient seems hardly to play a role in the development of osteomyelitis, with the exception of sickle cell anemia[141,289]. Osteomyelitis, alveolar bone necrosis and tooth loss have been described in association with herpes zoster infection[391]. In some cases no locally demonstrable or apparent predisposing factors can be detected[317].

The immune status of patients with chronic sclerosing osteomyelitis has been studied, but no conclusions can be drawn yet[355].

Classification Like other inflammatory processes, osteomyelitis can be classified as either (primary) acute or chronic (Table 2-1). Chronic osteomyelitis can be subclassified in a suppurative (purulent) and a sclerosing (sicca) type. The sclerosing type can be further subdivided into a focal and a diffuse type. Focal chronic sclerosing osteomyelitis has also been called condensing osteitis.

Chronic osteomyelitis can be accompanied by proliferative periostitis, called by some periostitis ossificans or Garré's osteomyelitis[54,178]. Perhaps it is better not to use the term Garré's osteomyelitis at all[624].

Furthermore, there is chronic periostitis occurring in patients wearing dentures[333], with radiographically no or only minimal involvement of the underlying bone.

Although osteoradionecrosis can be considered a type of osteomyelitis, this subject will be dealt with as a separate entity (see p. 41).

Clinical aspects Osteomyelitis mainly occurs in the mandible. The preference for occurrence in the mandible is probably due to the dense bony structure and the limited vascular supply.

Primary acute osteomyelitis usually originates following an acute stage of periapical inflammation and may appear in both the maxilla and the mandible. Acute maxillary osteomyelitis has particularly been described in babies and small children[452]. Acute osteomyelitis is usually accompanied by pain and fever. The teeth in the involved area may show increased mobility. The lymph nodes in the neck may be swollen and painful.

The clinical symptoms of *chronic suppurative osteomyelitis* are the same as those of acute osteomyelitis, but in a milder form. Intra- or extraoral fistulas may arise at the same time. There may also be stages of acute exacerbations.

The *focal chronic sclerosing* type is seldom accompanied by complaints, does not produce expansion, and is usually discovered as an incidental finding on a radiograph.

The *diffuse chronic sclerosing* type is seen particularly in the elderly, usually in an edentulous area of the mandible. This type of osteomyelitis may proceed rather uncharacteristically or even asymptomatically, but may also exhibit painful exacerbations, sometimes accompanied by swelling and trismus[290]. The bone may be slightly expanded, with either a small or a large part of the mandible involved. The mandibular canal may serve as a pathway for

34 • Inflammatory lesions of bone

Fig. 2-1. Swelling of mucobuccal fold due to chronic periostitis.

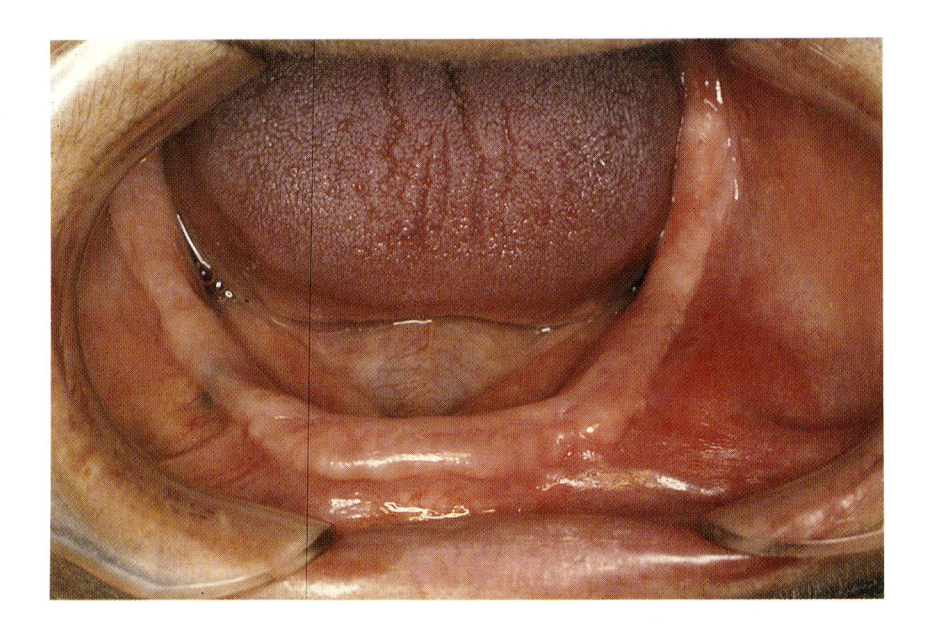

bacteria[603]. At the same time, one should realize that an infectious etiology of this type of osteomyelitis is somewhat questionable[376]. In the presence of proliferative periostitis, a hard swelling on the buccal, inferior, or lingual aspect of the mandible can be observed.

In patients wearing dentures the complaints associated with *chronic periostitis* with no or only minimal involvement of the underlying bone usually consist of pain and recurrent swelling. The mucosa of the alveolar ridges and the mucobuccal fold may have an erythematous appearance (Fig. 2-1).

Laboratory findings

The blood values are seldom abnormal. The erythrocyte sedimentation rate may be raised, but this is not a very specific finding. The values for calcium and phosphate remain unchanged.

Radiographic aspects

Radiographically, *primary acute* osteomyelitis, unlike an exacerbation of chronic osteomyelitis, is not at first abnormal. If not treated adequately the acute inflammation may turn into a more *chronic suppurative* one. Finally, necrotically changed fragments of bone, sequestra, may appear (Fig. 2-2). Furthermore, the radiologic features of proliferative periostitis, consisting of laminar periosteal new bone, effacement of follicular cortices of adjacent unerupted teeth, and maintenance of the radiographic shadow of the former mandibular cortex, may be present[408]. Somewhat similar periosteal reactions may be seen in infantile cortical hyperostosis (Caffey's

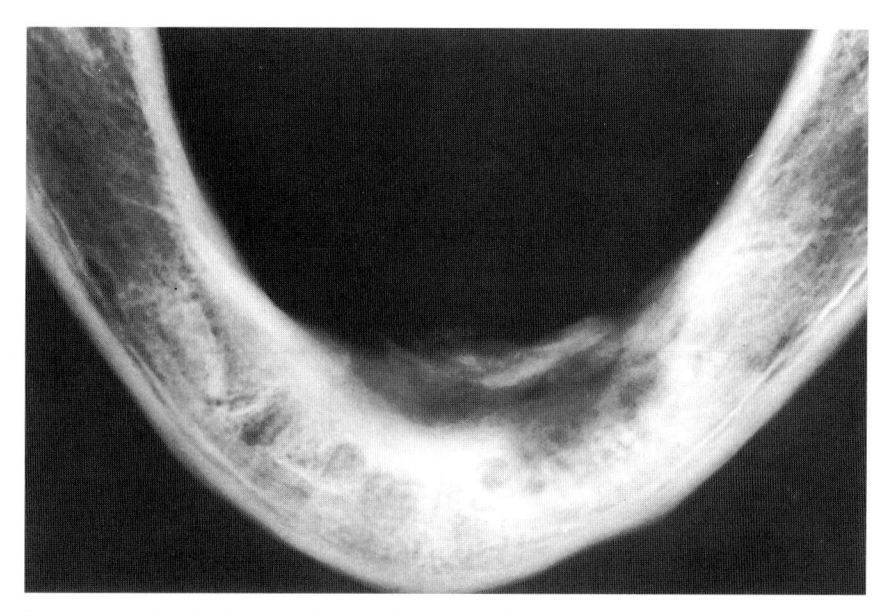

Fig. 2-2. Occlusal view showing the formation of a sequester at the lingual aspect of the mandible.

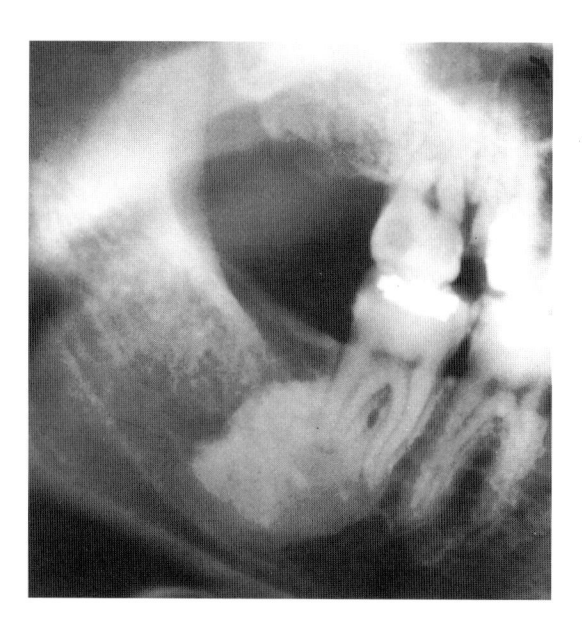

Fig. 2-3. Focal chronic sclerosing osteomyelitis at apex of 47.

disease), osteosarcoma, hypervitaminosis A, syphilis, leukemia, Ewing's sarcoma, and in metastatic tumors.

The radiographic aspect of *focal chronic sclerosing* osteomyelitis consists of a rather well-circumscribed radiopaque structure at the apex of a tooth. The original contour of the tooth remains visible, which is a characteristic feature in the distinction between focal chronic sclerosing osteomyelitis and hypercementosis (Fig. 2-3). There is no surrounding radiolucent zone as in a cementoblastoma (See chapter 10, p. 206). The suggestion has been made to make a distinction between focal sclerosing osteomyelitis (presence of a large carious lesion or deep restoration) and focal periapical osteopetrosis (presence of sound, nonrestored teeth or teeth with small restorations)[183].

In *diffuse chronic sclerosing* osteomyelitis opaque changes occur that are not clearly circumscribed (Fig. 2-4). Sometimes these changes are partly lucent as well, lacking the normal trabecular structure. This type, too, may be associated with radiologic signs of proliferative periostitis. Radiographically, the condition may mimic Paget's disease, fibrous dysplasia, eosinophilic granuloma, and malignant diseases such as osteosarcoma, malignant non-Hodgkin's lymphoma and metastatic lesions.

The radiograph of *chronic periostitis* in a patient wearing a denture usually shows no or only subtle changes. In a number of patients a cup-shaped defect or erosion of the alveolar crest may be observed (Fig. 2-5).

Scintigraphic aspects

Scintiscanning with Technetium 99m phosphate compounds will in most cases of osteomyelitis show a "hot spot"[293]. The value of such scanning is somewhat debatable due to occasional false-negative results. An additional Gallium 67 citrate scan may overcome this weakness[555]. Furthermore, the use of labelled leukocytes may be helpful in differentiating osteomyelitis from osteosarcoma[230].

Bacteriologic aspects

If discharge is present, the material should be examined bacteriologically. Usually Gram-positive, anaerobic staphylococci are involved. Sometimes, Gram-negative microorganisms such as Bacteroides melaninogenicus[609] seem to play a role. The literature also contains cases of tuberculous[629], syphilitic[655], actinomycotic[239], Alternaria[225], and blastomycotic osteomyelitis[596], as well as osteomyelitis due to Eikenella[550] or Pseudomonas aerigunosa[276]. However, it is questionable whether the presence of those microorganisms is in all instances of primary importance. Particularly in the chronic sclerosing type, culturing may not result in the finding of any pathogenic microorganisms.

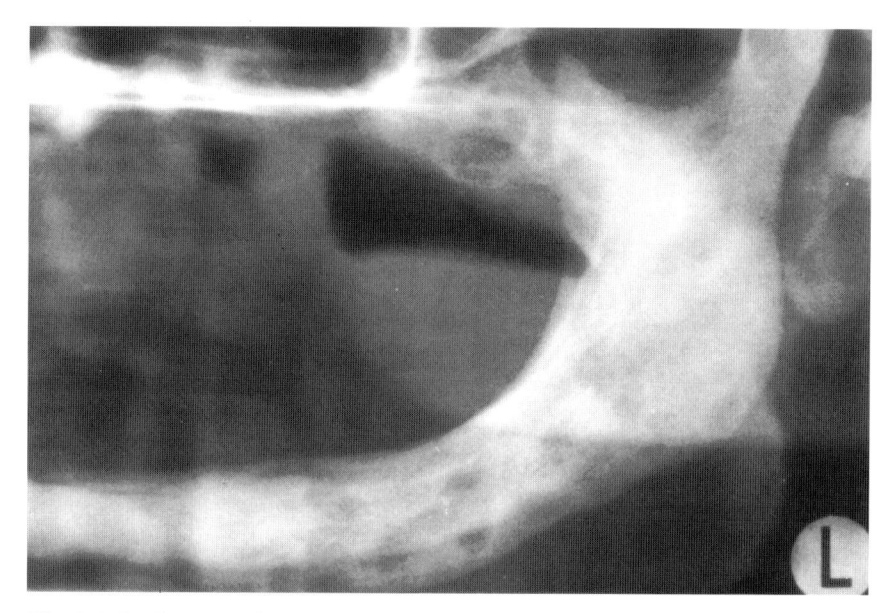

Fig. 2-4. Radiograph of diffuse chronic osteomyelitis of left mandible. Notice the "double" cortical layer at the inferior border as the result of proliferative periostitis.

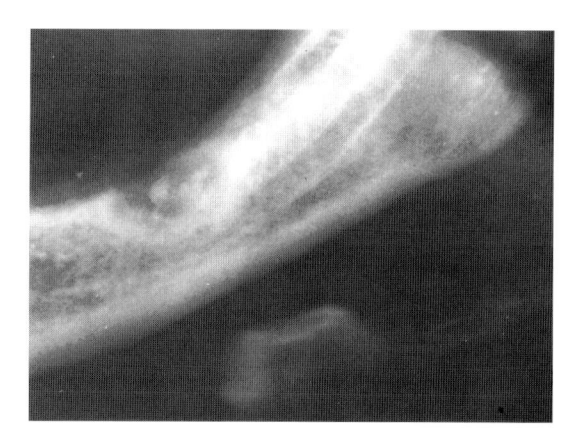

Fig. 2-5. Somewhat cup-shaped defect of alveolar crest caused by chronic periostitis.

Histologic aspects

Although histologic examination of inflamed bony tissue or of a sequestrum usually does not provide valuable information, the taking of a biopsy is a safe procedure to rule out the presence of other lesions, in particular primary or metastatic malignancies. On the other hand, reactive epithelial proliferation around sequesters may be misdiagnosed as a squamous cell carcinoma (Fig. 2-6). The combination of the history and the clinical and radiographic features will usually overcome this histologic pitfall.

In some cases cementum or cementum-like structures may be observed, mimicking to some extent the spectrum of fibrous dysplasia and cementum-containing lesions. In a study of patients with chronic sclerosing osteomyelitis of the mandible four different types of tissue reaction were found, varying from severely sclerotic bone tissue to granulation tissue without any hard tissue[291].

In osteomyelitis with proliferative periostitis a fibrous stroma is present with no or only limited numbers of inflammatory cells. Eversole et al. recognize three basic patterns of trabecular arrangement, being either parallel, retiform or fibrous dysplasia-like[178].

Histologic examination of tissue from chronic periostitis with no or only minimal changes of the underlying bone, as may occur in denture-wearing patients, may show hyaline changes of the blood vessels in a cellular stroma, formation of bone trabeculae, and multinucleated giant cells (Fig. 2-7). This foreign body reaction can, occasionally, also be observed in periapical granulomas and follicles of partly erupted teeth. Some authors interpret the histologic changes primarily as being of a vascular nature, using the term giant cell hyalin angiopathy[155]. Others consider the changes to be the result of chronic granulomatous inflammation with foreign body giant cells, as a reaction to vegetable particles, and apply the term "pulse granuloma"[381] or oral vegetable granuloma[254]. In an animal study it has, indeed, been possible to produce pulse granuloma-like lesions by implantation of homogenized cooked legumes into the orofacial region of rats[565]. McMillan et al. questioned both the term giant cell hyalin angiopathy and the term pulse granuloma and suggested describing the lesion as granulation tissue with giant cells and hyaline changes[370]. El-Labban and Kramer have described the ultrastructural findings of these hyaline structures[166].

An inflammation, diagnosed as periostitis on the basis of clinical and radiographic observation, may on microscopic examination appear to be a lipogranuloma caused by a foreign body introduced

Osteomyelitis • 39

Fig. 2-6. Sequesters surrounded by squamous epithelium, not to be mistaken for a carcinoma.

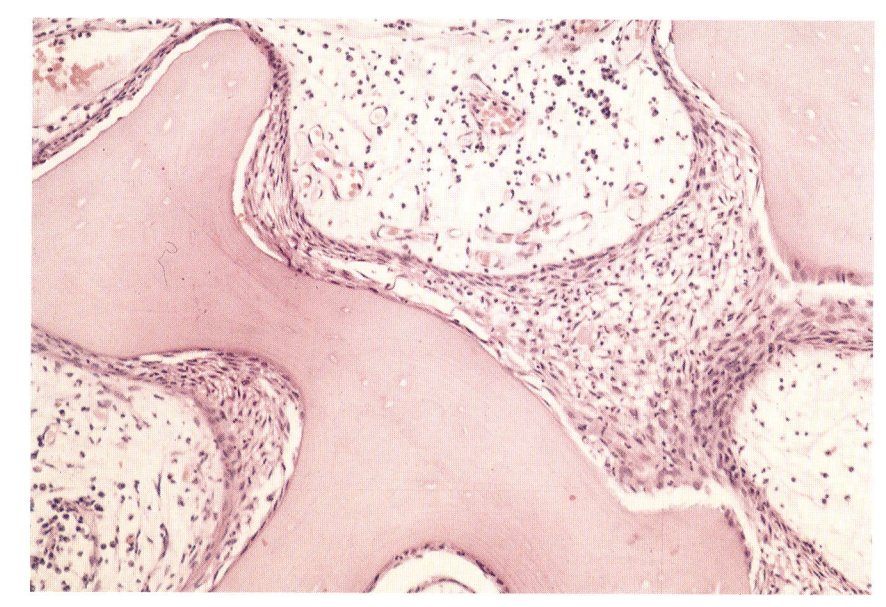

Fig. 2-7. Tissue from denture wearing patient with chronic periostitis. Notice the presence of multinucleated giant cells around vegetable particles.

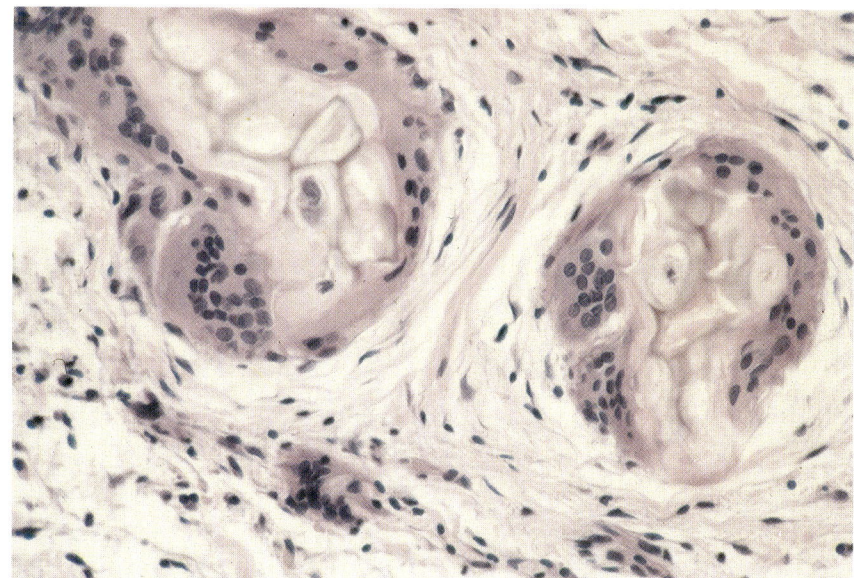

into the alveolus[231]. In fact, this is perhaps a lesion similar to the aforementioned pulse granuloma. Yet another granulomatous lesion that should be included in the histopathologic differential diagnosis is myospherulosis. Myospherulosis results from the action of lipid substances on extravasated erythrocytes. Petrolatum-based antibiotic ointments are the most frequent etiologic agents[53].

In rare instances the mandible is involved in systemic sarcoidosis. Therefore, sarcoid granulomas may occasionally be observed within the bone[587], as well as epithelioid cell granulomas caused by tuberculosis.

Treatment

Treatment of any type of inflammation is directed toward elimination of the presumed cause. This in itself is seldom sufficient to cure osteomyelitis of the jaws. Moreover, the causative factor or factors can often no longer be shown and the inflammation may behave as a more or less autonomous disease.

Acute types of osteomyelitis, either in the form of primary acute osteomyelitis or of an exacerbation of chronic osteomyelitis, can often be treated successfully with antibiotics. The choice, dosage, and route of administration should, if possible, be based on the results of the culture analysis, preferably in consultation with the bacteriologist. Administration of antibiotics for a period of two to three weeks may be better than limiting the treatment to only a few days and may lead to permanent success, especially in the primary acute type of osteomyelitis.

When clinical or radiographic signs of sequestration are present in chronic purulent osteomyelitis, the sequestra should be removed carefully. In longstanding cases it may be necessary to perform a more aggressive type of sequestrotomy, even to the extent of sacrificing the continuity of the mandible. The value of the administration of antibiotics in this type of osteomyelitis is questionable.

In general, treatment of focal sclerosing osteomyelitis is not required. In case of extraction of a tooth involved in focal sclerosing osteomyelitis the radiopacity at the apex will remain visible on the radiograph for many years, either unchanged or even increased in size. Antibiotics are of no use in this type of osteomyelitis.

For diffuse sclerosing osteomyelitis, treatment may consist of removal of the cortical bone plate and sometimes also of the inferior cortex of the mandible. The purpose of such decortication is the removal of badly vascularized or even necrotic bone that is heavily colonized with microorganisms. The results of decortication, carried out either via an intra- or extraoral approach, are not always encouraging. Therefore, some authors prefer a more radical surgical treatment, using bone grafts with or without hydroxylapatite for immediate reconstruction[72]. Another supplementary or supporting therapy for this type of osteomyelitis is the use of hyperbaric oxygen[374]. Yet another type of treatment consists of the systemic administration of corticosteroids[292] or the use of immunotherapy[35]. Supportive treatment with antibiotics can be given in various ways. Its value in this type of osteomyelitis is somewhat debatable. Some authors prefer the local placement of an antibiotic reservoir in the form of a chain[11]. Tooth extractions within the affected bone should be avoided and, if indicated, only be performed under antibiotic cover[290].

For chronic periostitis in a patient wearing a denture, it is sometimes sufficient to adjust the denture. Additional excision of the inflamed periosteum is often necessary. The extent of the excision is not easy to judge. It has been recommended not to approximate the sides of the wound, but to pack the wound open, allowing it to granulate[333]. The use of antibiotics is questionable.

Osteoradionecrosis

Pathogenesis In irradiated bone a severe and persistent inflammation, called osteoradionecrosis, may be provoked by dental extractions before, during and after irradiation, or by a slight irritating factor or just by mastication[358]. As a result of the irradiation the vascularization, and with it the regenerating capacity of the tissues, have been permanently reduced. Infection seems to play only a secondary role in the development of osteoradionecrosis[360].

In a study of 431 patients who have been irradiated for malignant tumors in the head and neck region, 21 developed osteoradionecrosis; risk factors for the development of radionecrosis were: advanced age, high radiation dose, superfractionation and the combination of tumor surgery and chemotherapy with traumatic tooth extraction[612].

42 • Inflammatory lesions of bone

Fig. 2-8a. Non-healing extraction wound two months after extraction of 47. The patient had been irradiated after the removal of a parotid gland tumor four years before. Unfortunately, no antibiotic prophylaxis had been used for the dental extraction.

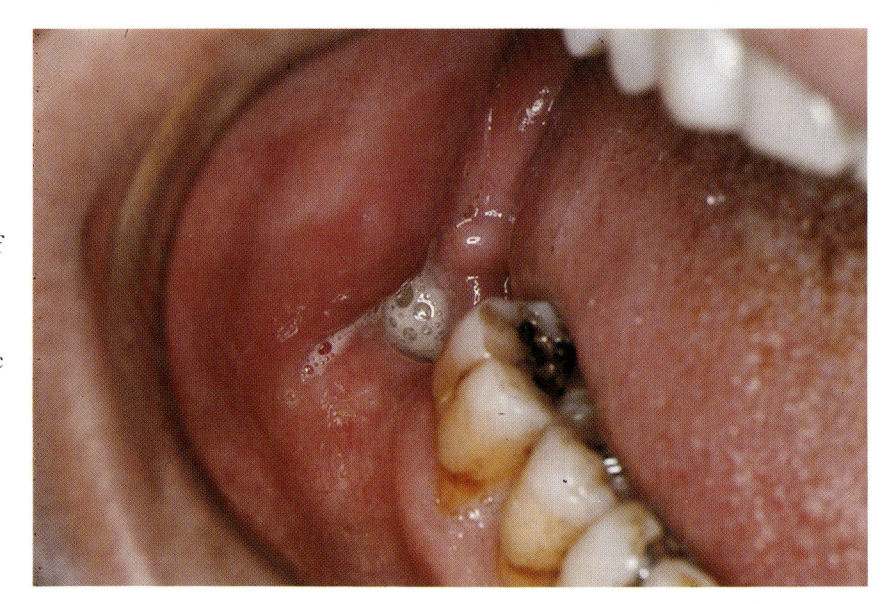

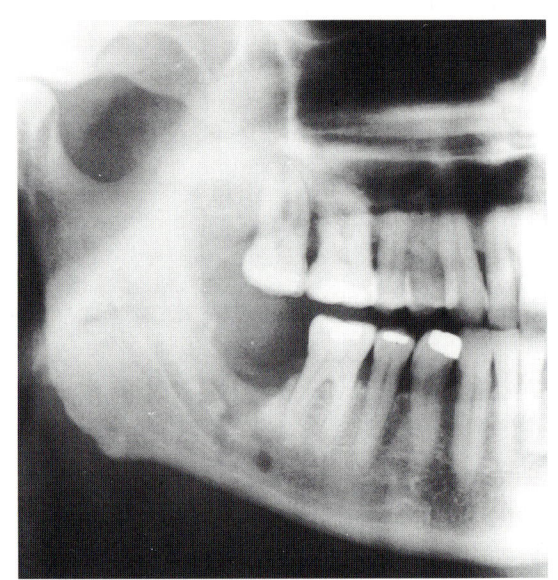

Fig. 2-8b. The radiograph shows some diffuse radiolucent changes.

Clinical aspects

The mandible is more often involved than the maxilla. In the latter site, extension into the skull base may take place[313].

Osteoradionecrosis may present as a lesion that heals spontaneously, as a slowly progressive disease, or as an actively progressive symptomatic disease[177]. Sequestration may or may not take

Osteoradionecrosis • 43

Fig. 2-8c.
After almost a year sequester formation appeared, resulting in an extraoral fistula.

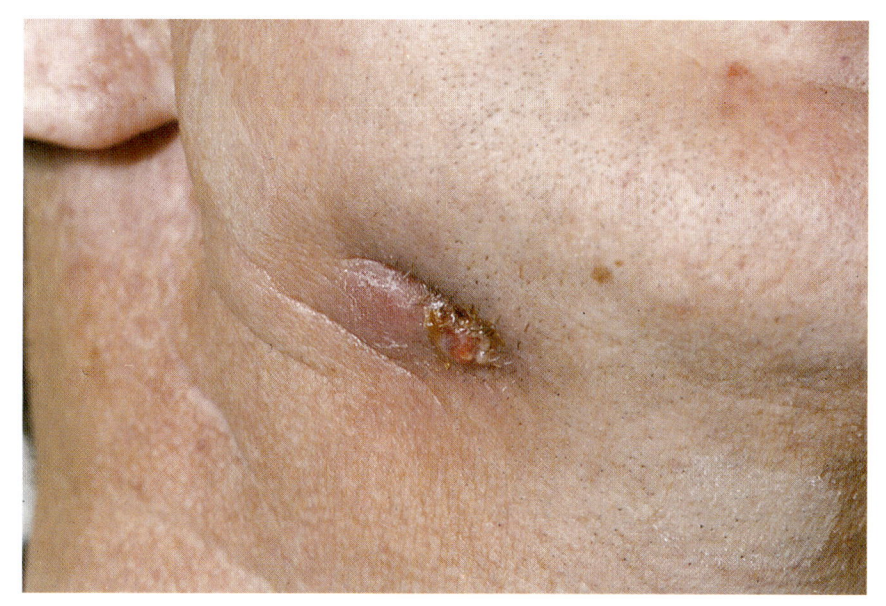

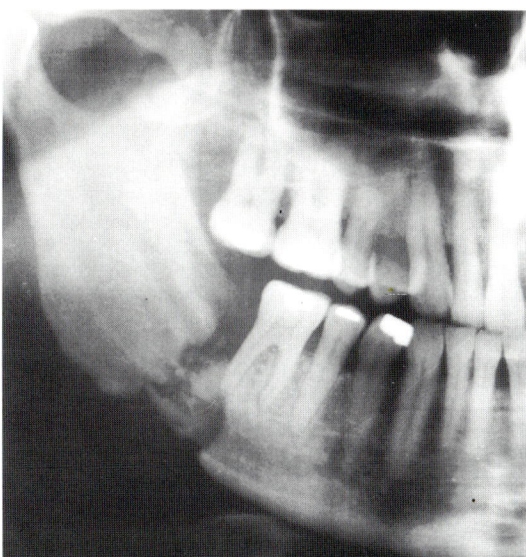

Fig. 2-8d.
Sequester formation due to osteoradionecrosis.

place, in some instances more than one year after the onset of the osteoradionecrosis (Fig. 2-8). In the absence of a pathologic fracture the condition is more or less asymptomatic, even when a large area of necrotic bone is exposed to the oral environment.

Radiographic aspects

The radiographic aspects of osteoradionecrosis may vary from minor osteolytic to marked osteosclerotic changes, with or without the appearance of sequesters.

Classification

Epstein et al. have proposed a clinical classification and treatment schedule for osteoradionecrosis[177]. Stages 1, 2 and 3 represent a resolved stage, a chronic (persistent, non-progressive) stage, and an active (progressive) stage, respectively. Each stage has been further subdivided with regard to the absence and the presence of a pathologic fracture.

Diagnosis

The clinico-radiographic features of a recurrent squamous cell carcinoma after irradiation may be mistaken for those of osteoradionecrosis. Therefore, one should not hesitate to take a biopsy in case of the slightest doubt. In this respect also the routine histopathologic examination of sequesters is recommended.

Treatment

In general, local wound care is essential. Otherwise, the treatment policy is more or less similar to that for chronic osteomyelitis. Supportive treatment with hyperbaric oxygen may be effective[65,359]. The use of antibiotics in the treatment of osteoradionecrosis seems questionable.

An overview of the management of osteoradionecrosis of the jaws has been presented by Morton and Simpson[389].

Prevention

The utmost care must be taken when treating the dentition of any patient who will be or who has been irradiated[394]. Extractions, foreseen in the near future, should be carried out before the irradiation is instituted. Otherwise, the teeth should be protected by local application of fluoride once or twice a week. That regimen should be continued for at least six months after completion of the irradiation. Of course, strict oral hygiene should be observed, if possible under the guidance of a dental hygienist.

In case of surgical dental procedures, including extraction of one or more teeth, the prophylactic use of antibiotics is required in every patient in whom the jaws have been exposed to irradiation, irrespective of the time lapse of such irradiation[65].

Fig. 2-9. Intraoral fistula caused by a periapical granuloma of one of the buccal apices of 26.

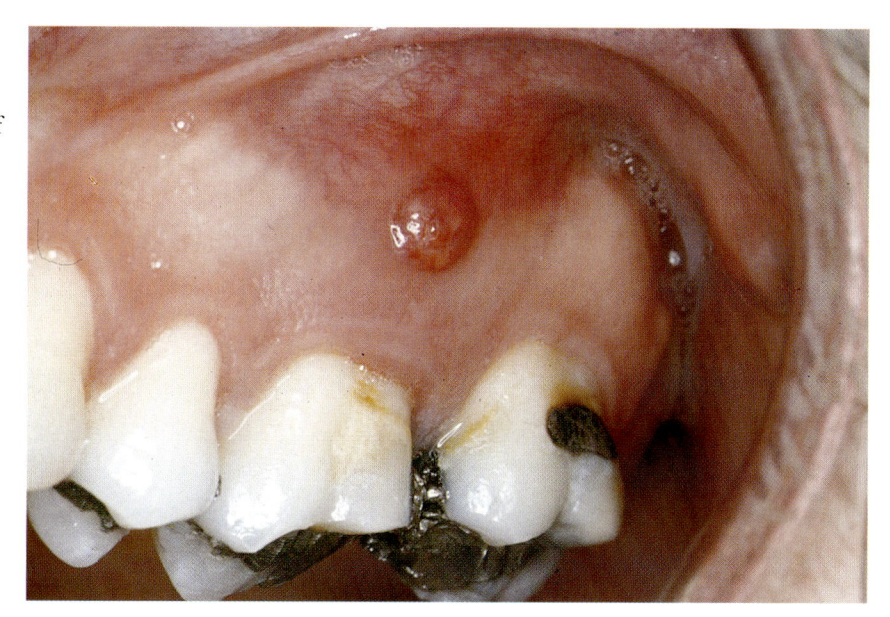

Periapical granuloma

The majority of periapical granulomas, being caused by a non-vital dental pulp, may remain asymptomatic. Some of the periapical granulomas lead to the formation of a cyst. A periapical granuloma or a periapical cyst (See chapter 6, p. 108), usually called radicular cyst, can be exacerbated and develop into an abscess. Finally, intraoral or extraoral sinus formation may occur (Figs. 2-9 to 2-12). Occasionally, a periapical inflammation spreads diffusely into the jaw bone, resulting in osteomyelitis.

Radiographically, a periapical granuloma is visible as a well or poorly circumscribed lucent change, varying in size from a few millimeters to several centimeters (Fig. 2-13). Occasionally, a periapical radiolucency represents the initial stage of a fibro-osseous cemental lesion or a metastatic process[380], leaving the vitality of the tooth at first intact. Therefore, a vitality test is advisable in all cases of a periapical radiolucency. In case of multirooted teeth, the pulp of one root may be vital, whereas the pulp of the other root may be non-vital, this being the cause of a periapical inflammation.

If a lucent lesion occurs at the apex of a central maxillary incisor, the possibility of a cyst of the nasopalatine duct should be considered. Overprojection of the mental foramen may mimic a periapical disorder of one of the mandibular premolars.

46 • Inflammatory lesions of bone

Fig. 2-10. Palatal abscess caused by non-vital 12. The radiograph is shown in Fig. 2-13.

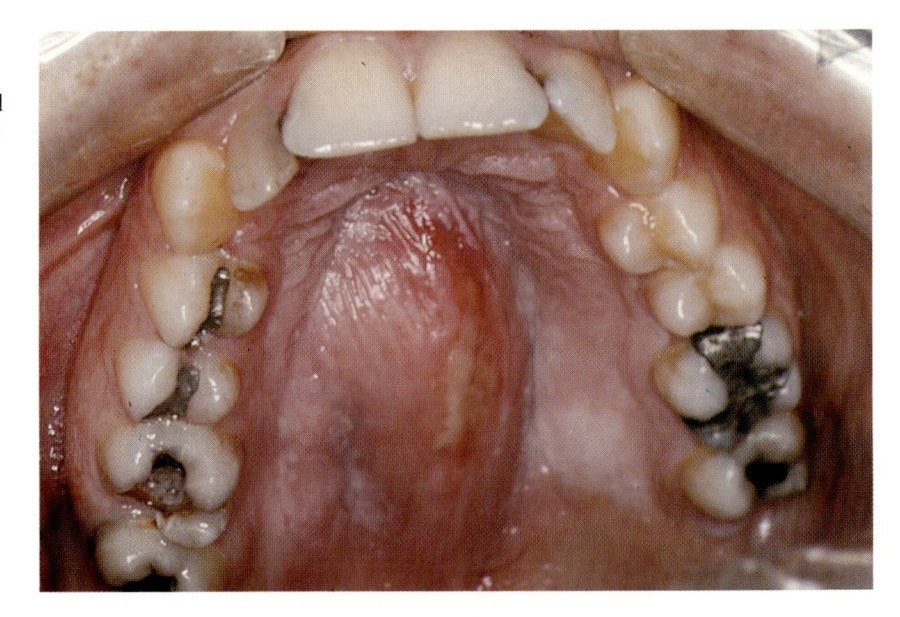

Fig. 2-11. Abscess of floor of mouth caused by non-vital 32.

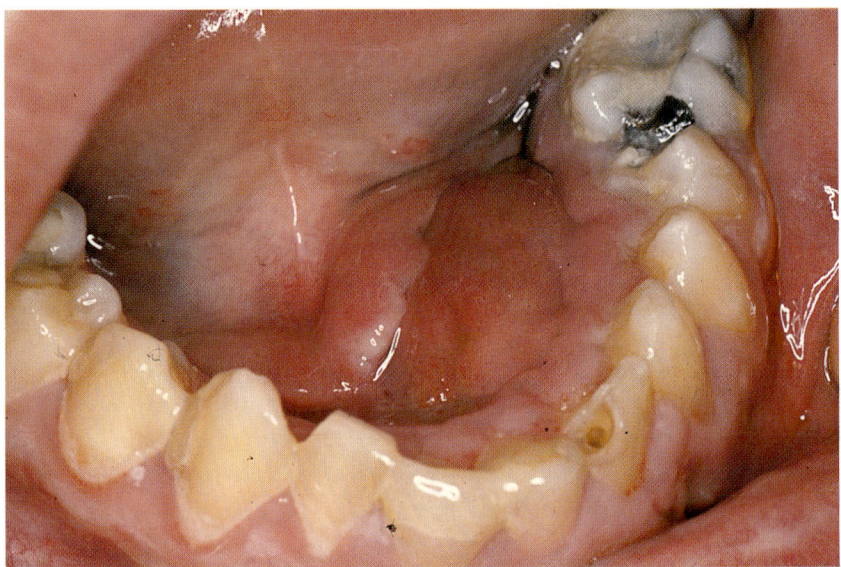

Histologically, a chronic, granulomatous reaction can be observed. Frequently, proliferation of squamous epithelium, derived from Malassez's epithelial rests, is encountered. A dense inflammatory infiltrate may be present in which plasma cells dominate, even to the extent of mimicking a plasmacytoma. In rare instances the

Periapical granuloma • 47

Fig. 2-12. Attempt of camouflage with make-up of a subcutaneous abscess caused by non-vital 14.

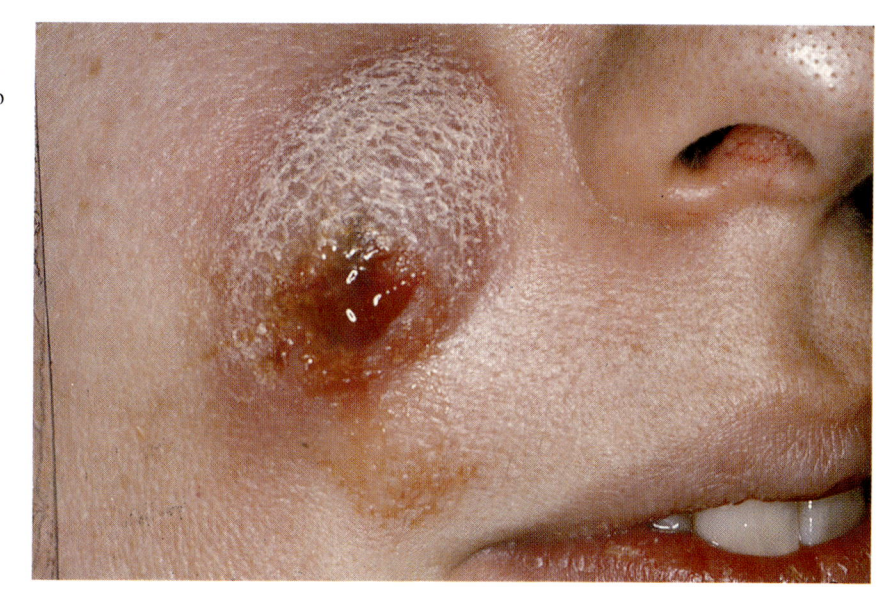

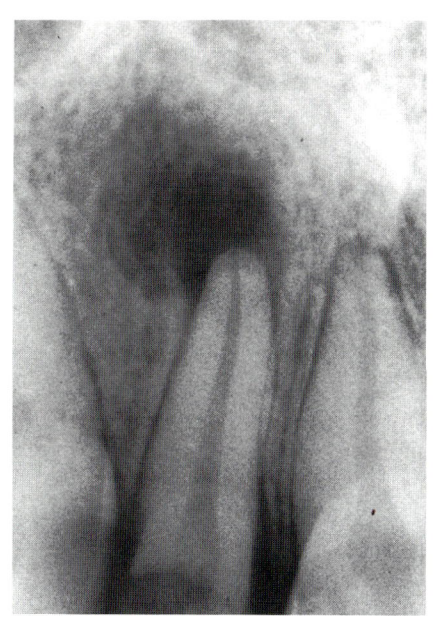

Fig. 2-13. Periapical radiolucency at apex of badly decayed, non-vital 12. The clinical aspect is shown in Fig. 2-10.

use of immunohistochemical techniques is needed to rule out monoclonality[633].

Treatment of periapical inflammation consists of root canal treatment, with or without apicoectomy, or extraction of the tooth. Healing is in most cases uneventful.

Periodontal disease

In periodontal disease, both in adults and in children, subtle or more extensive loss of alveolar bone may take place. It is beyond the scope of this text to deal with the epidemiology, pathogenesis and clinical aspects of this common dental disease.

On the radiograph several types of periodontal bone loss can be recognized, such as horizontal, vertical and angular bone loss. In most cases periodontal disease involves more than one, or even all teeth present. Occasionally, localized involvement may be observed, in some cases being the result of a trauma experienced many years previously (Fig. 2-14).

The diagnosis of periodontal disease can almost without exception be made based on the history and the clinical and radiographic findings. A biopsy is only rarely indicated. Culturing is only recommended in selected cases.

As a final remark it should be mentioned here that severe periodontal bone loss can be a manifestation of HIV-seropositivity, in some cases even being the first sign of that condition.

Fig. 2-14a. Localized periodontitis of 21. The patient had experienced a trauma some five years before.

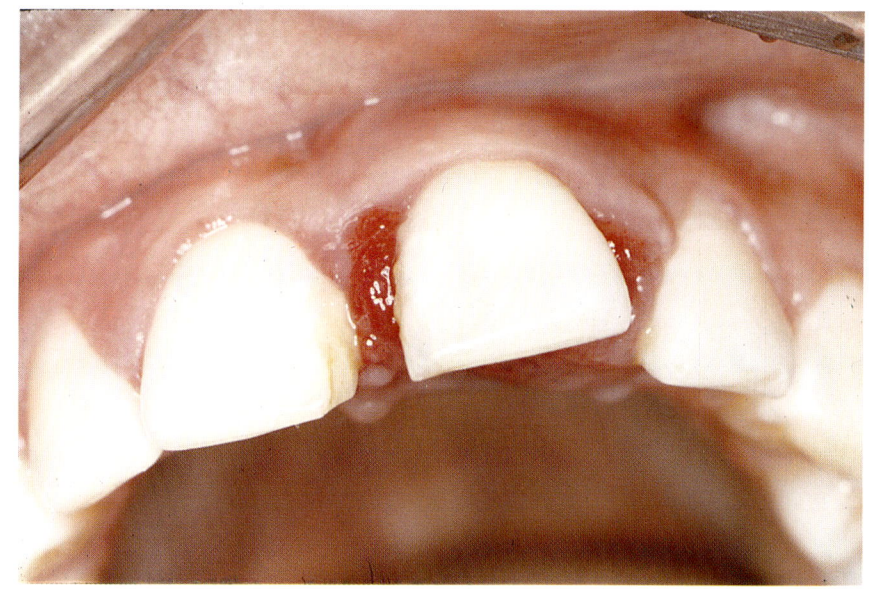

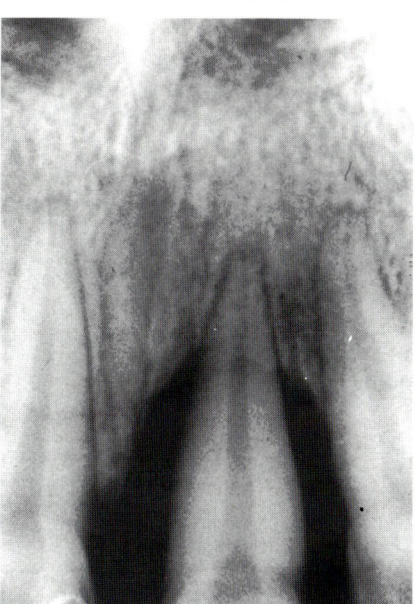

Fig. 2-14b. Localized periodontitis of 21.

CHAPTER 3

Giant cell lesions

There are numerous lesions of the jaw bones in which multinucleated giant cells may be encountered. The so-called pulse granuloma or giant cell hyalin angiopathy has been discussed already in chapter 2, as is, for instance, also the case with tuberculous osteomyelitis in which Langerhans' giant cells are a prominent feature. Fibrous dysplasia and osteoblastoma are other examples of lesions in which varying numbers of giant cells may be observed. Those lesions are discussed in chapters 4 and 7, respectively. In the present chapter only lesions and conditions of the bone will be dealt with in which giant cells are the "key cells".

Cherubism

Definition and epidemiology

Cherubism is a benign fibro-osseous disease of the jaws, which presents as a non-painful bilateral symmetrical enlargement of the mandible in early childhood. It is a hereditary disorder of an autosomal dominant gene with 100 % penetrance in males and variable expressivity. A study of 20 cases from one family has been reported[430]. From Paris, three children from the same Algerian family have been mentioned as suffering from cherubism[584]. The literature contains a similar report from Israel[669]. In some cases there is a lack of a familial history of the disease[234].

No racial variations have been noted. Males are affected about twice as frequently as females.

In the literature a few cases have been reported of the association of cherubism and the Noonan syndrome[157].

Clinical aspects

Clinically, cherubism is characterized by fullness of the cheeks and jaw bones that results in a round face with retraction of the lower eyelids and exposure of the sclera below the irises (Fig. 3-1); the "raised-to-heaven look" is suggestive of a cherub[451]. In some cases

52 • Giant cell lesions

Fig. 3-1a.
Five-year-old girl suffering from cherubism.

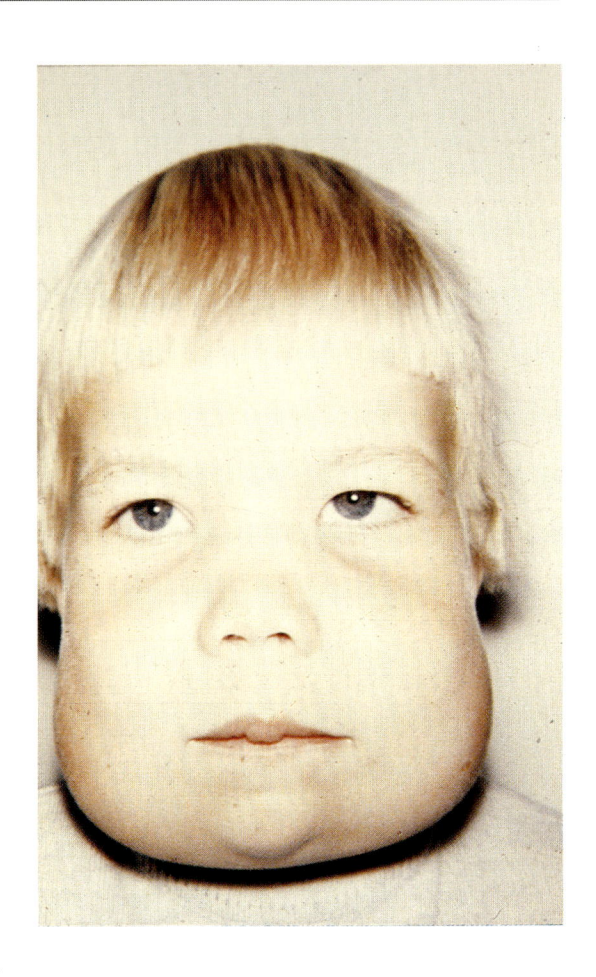

also the maxilla is involved. Occasionally, there is an initial unilateral presentation[458].

Laboratory findings Blood chemistry and electrolyte studies are usually within normal limits.

Radiographic aspects Radiographically, the lesions are multilocular ("soap bubble") appearance) with osseous expansion. The tooth germs present in the jaws may be considerably displaced. Abnormal scintigrams are found only in the regressive period with new bone formation[630].

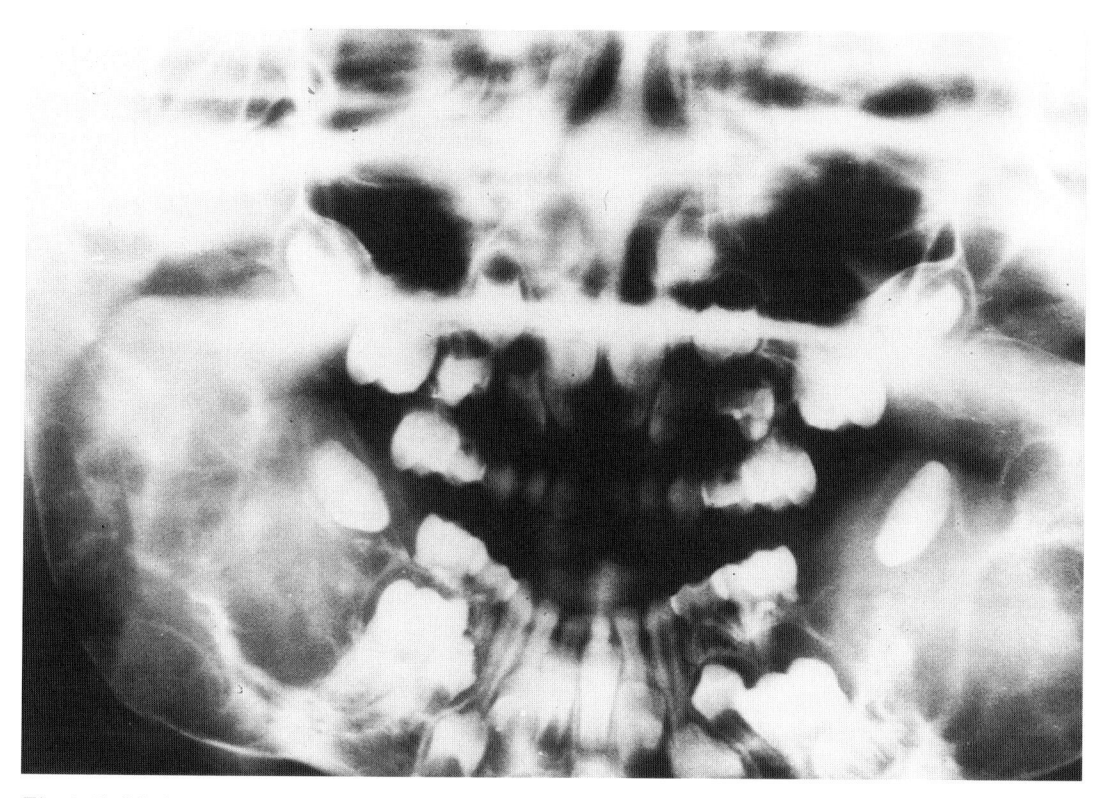

Fig. 3-1b. Notice the multilobular radiolucencies in the mandible and the displacement of several tooth germs. (Courtesy Prof.dr. P. Egeydi, The Netherlands).

Histologic aspects	Histologically, the lesion shows a fibrous stroma with multinucleated giant cells and prominent vascularity. Perivascular cuffing may be evident. The lesions resemble giant cell granuloma and are perhaps to some extent related to each other[99,110].
Treatment	The disease tends to regress after puberty, the maxillary lesions being the first to do so. Treatment, if necessary, consists of recontouring after the lesions have stabilized in size[319].

54 • Giant cell lesions

Fig. 3-2a.
Maxillary swelling due to central giant cell granuloma. All teeth were vital.

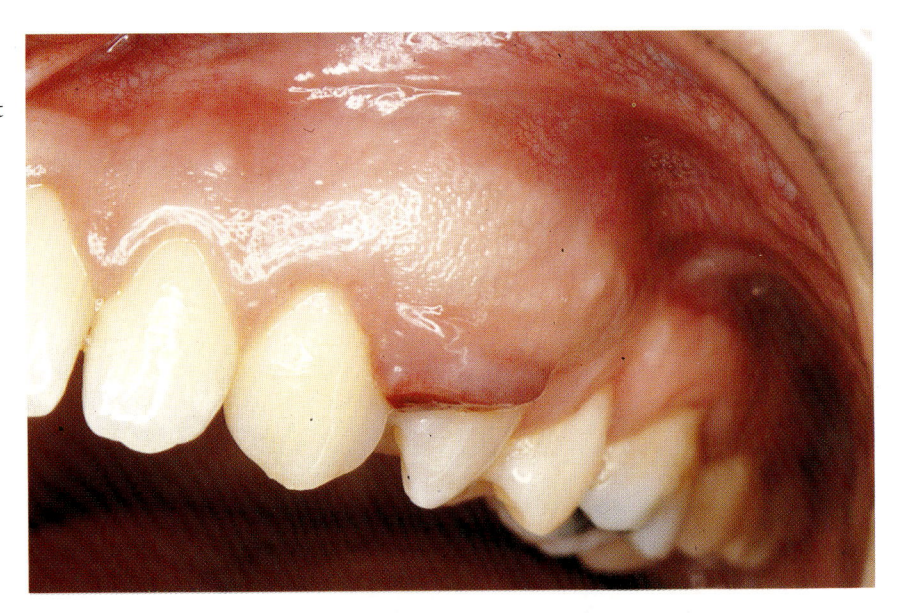

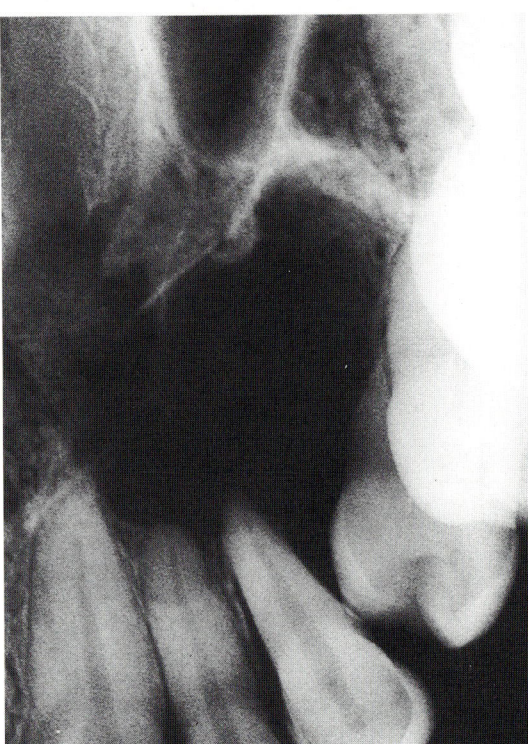

Fig. 3-2b.
The radiograph shows a large, somewhat circumscribed radiolucency.

Fig. 3-3.
Central giant cell granuloma in the mandible, to some extent mimicking the radiographic aspect of a solitary bone cyst. Both the 46 and 47 were vital. There is some apical resorption of 46.

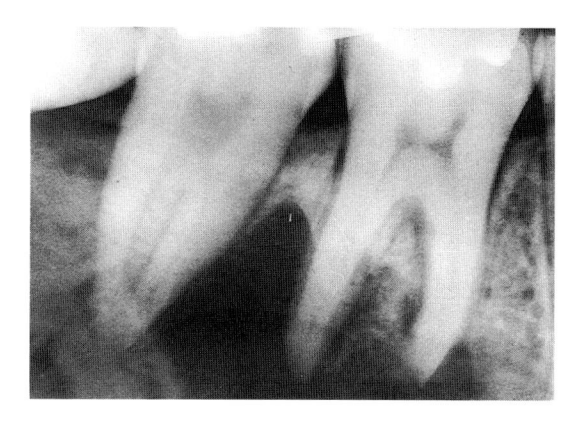

Central giant cell granuloma

Definition and epidemiology

Although the term granuloma indicates a reactive lesion, the true nature of the central giant cell granuloma is not fully understood. More or less empirically it has been shown that this lesion in the jaws almost never behaves as a true neoplasm. Nevertheless, central giant cell granuloma may cause extensive destruction of bone[500].

It is not always possible to make a sharp distinction between a central giant cell granuloma and a peripheral one that has caused secondary bone destruction. Central giant granulomas do not occur elsewhere in the skeleton, with the exception of the small bones of the hands and feet[435,620].

It has been suggested that central giant granulomas of the bones and giant cell tumors occurring elsewhere in the skeleton are varying expressions of the same disease (See also p. 60). Possibly, the multinucleated giant cells represent mononuclear phagocytic differentiation[423]. On the other hand, it has been suggested that the giant cells form and increase in size through fusion[123].

Central giant cell granuloma of the jaws has an estimated incidence of two per million population per year and appears mainly in children and adolescents. There is a slight preference for the female sex.

Clinical aspects

The mandible is affected more often than the maxilla, usually anterior to the first molars. Location outside the tooth-bearing area is exceptional. In rare instances the lesion occurs simultaneously in the mandible and the maxilla. Especially in the case of multiple occurrence, the possibility of cherubism should be taken into account, as well as hyperparathyroidism, although the latter disease may also cause solitary lesions[146].

The symptoms of a central giant cell granuloma may consist of slight swelling of the involved bone and sometimes an increased mobility of one or more teeth. The vitality of the teeth remains undisturbed (Fig. 3-2).

Laboratory findings

Laboratory values, especially of serum calcium and phosphorus levels, are within normal limits.

Radiographic aspects

The radiograph shows a more or less circumscribed lucency in which delicate bony septae may be seen. The cortical bone is often expanded and sometimes perforated as well. Migration and also resorption of teeth may take place (Fig. 3-3). The radiographic features are not diagnostic and may resemble, among other lesions, an ameloblastoma, an odontogenic myxoma, a solitary bone cyst, an aneurysmal bone cyst, an odontogenic keratocyst, and a so-called "brown tumor" caused by hyperparathyroidism.

Histologic aspects

On gross examination the tissue of a giant cell granuloma has a somewhat friable consistency and a red-brownish color. On microscopic examination connective tissue with proliferation of fibroblasts and capillaries can be seen. Vascularity may be abundant. There is no true encapsulation, although the lesion may be somewhat demarcated. Mitoses are not uncommon. The collagen fibers do not show a clear arrangement in bundles. Multinucleated giant cells are present in varying numbers (Fig. 3-4). Sometimes foci of new bone formation can be observed, particularly at the periphery of the lesion. On the ultrastructural level the presence of myofibroblasts has been demonstrated[167].

The histologic aspects of a central giant cell granuloma cannot reliably be distinguished from those of a skeletal lesion due to primary or secondary hyperparathyroidism ("brown tumor"), from changes in the bone in patients with cherubism, or from peripheral giant cell granuloma. The histologic features of a giant cell granuloma can also mimic those of an aneurysmal bone cyst and even of an osteosarcoma.

Some investigators have, rather unsuccessfully, tried to make a distinction, based on clinical, radiographic or histologic features, between a giant cell granuloma and a giant cell tumor[201]. For instance, it has been suggested that the giant cells in giant cell granulomas are less evenly distributed than those in giant cell tumors.

Fig. 3-4. Central giant cell granuloma. Notice the vascularity of the stroma.

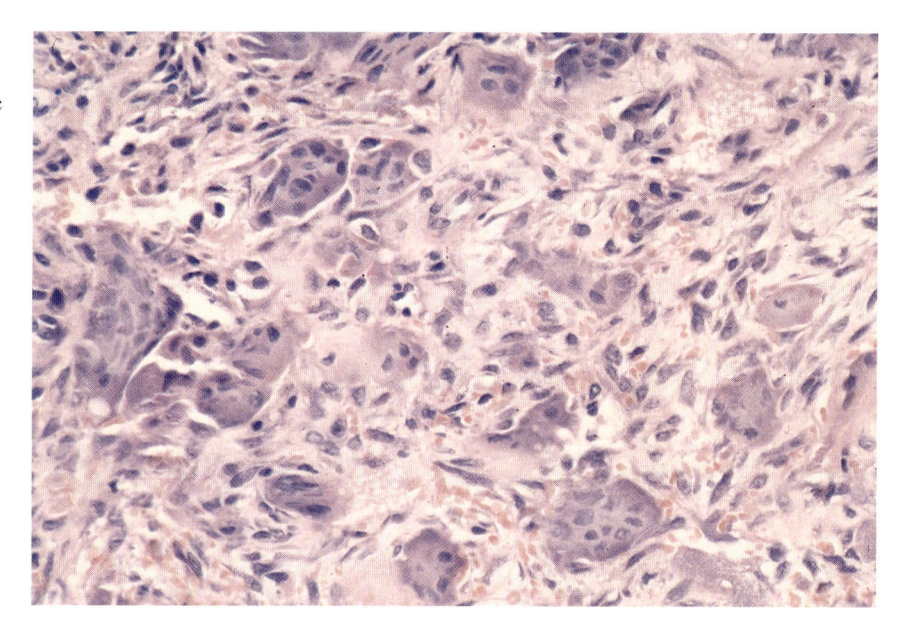

In one study the only statistically significant quantitative difference between the lesions was the greater number of nuclei in the giant cells of the giant cell tumor[39]. Also, determination of HLA-DR expression is apparently not helpful in discriminating between the various giant cell lesions[463].

It has been suggested that recurrent central giant cell granulomas have a higher relative size index of giant cells and a higher fractional surface area of giant cells per high-power field when compared with the nonrecurrent ones[118,188].

Treatment

Treatment of a central giant cell granuloma consists of thorough curettage, if possible followed by peripheral ostectomy using a rotary instrument. Before doing so, it is wise to do blood chemistry in order to rule out the presence of hyperparathyroidism, in spite of a low probability (Fig. 3-5).

In aggressive or recurrent lesions, combined curettage and cryosurgical treatment may be considered. Even in case of large and extensive lesions of the mandible it is usually possible to leave the continuity of the jaw intact. One should also aim at preservation of the inferior alveolar nerve. Occasionally, a recurrence is observed, in some cases many years after the first surgical procedure[529].

Only in an exceptional case may radiation therapy be considered[164].

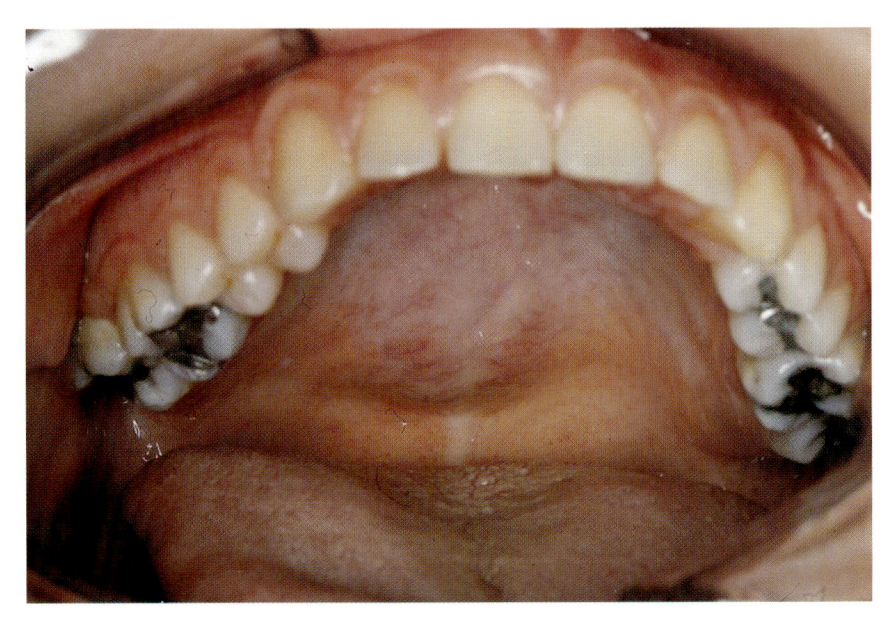

Fig. 3-5a. Slight bony swelling in the midline of the palate in an apparently healthy 14-year-old girl. The biopsy revealed a giant cell granuloma-like lesion. Serologic examination showed the presence of hypercalcemia, hypophosphatemia, and an increased serum alkaline phosphatase activity, leading to the finding of an adenoma in one of the parathyroid glands.

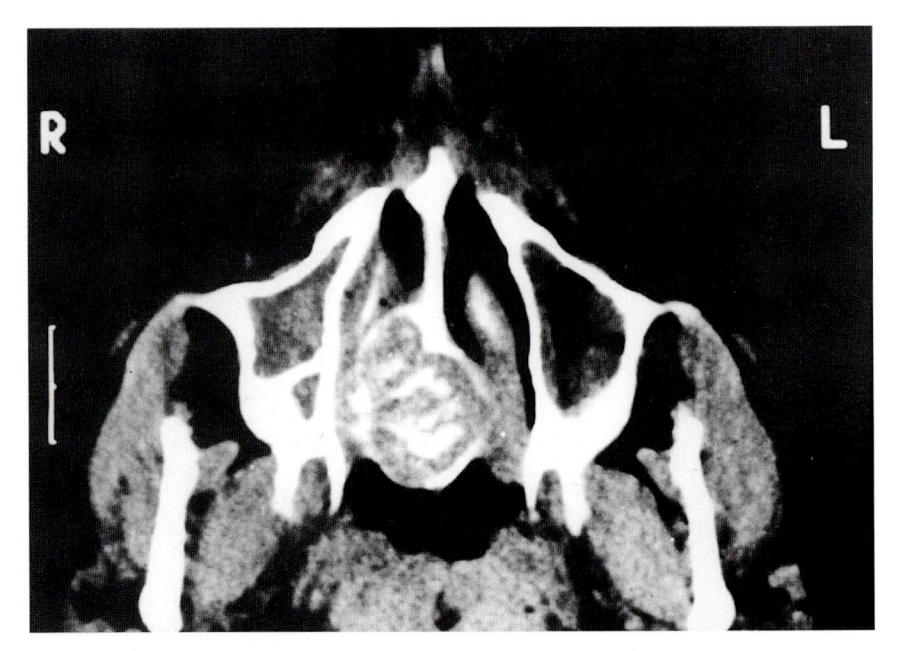

Fig. 3-5b. The CT-scan showed a rather well-circumscribed lesion. There is evidence of secondary bone formation.

Fig. 3-5c.
The skull film revealed a so-called "pepper and salt" appearance.

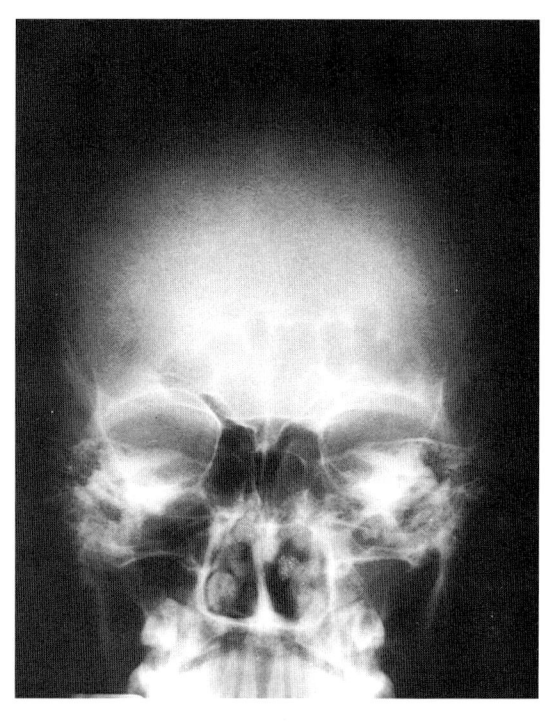

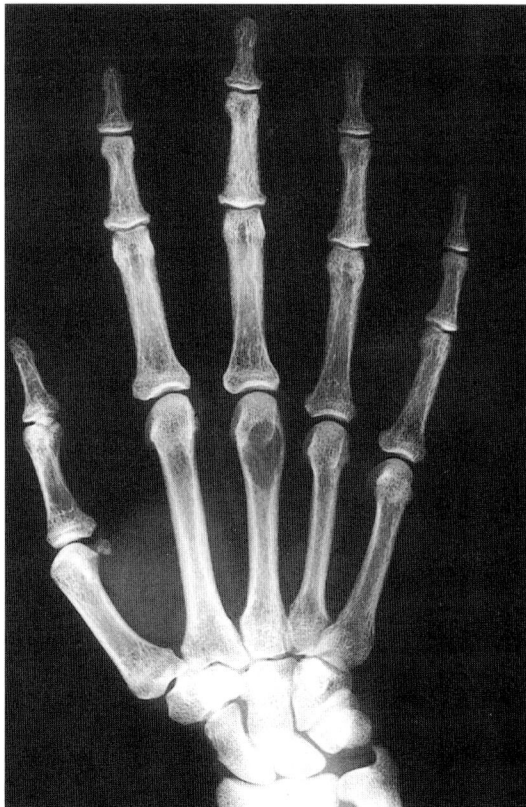

Fig. 3-5d.
Furthermore, cystlike rarefication in a metacarpal bone was detected. Notice also the cortical thinning of the phalanges.
(Courtesy Prof.dr. J. Valk, The Netherlands).

Giant cell tumor

A giant cell tumor is an aggressive tumor characterized by richly vascularized tissue consisting of rather plump, spindle-shaped or ovoid cells and by the presence of numerous giant cells of osteoclast type, which are uniformly distributed throughout the tumor tissue. Relatively little collagen is present[500]. As a synonym, the term osteoclastoma has been used.

In an ultrastructural study nuclear inclusions were observed morphologically that were identical with the 12-15 nn tubules characteristic of the nuclei of osteoclasts in Paget's disease of bone[379].

Giant cell tumors are rare and are more or less limited to the age group of 20-40 years. The sites of involvement are the ends of the long bones[365]. There is much debate about the question of whether this tumor does occur in the jaw bones[382,558], as has also been discussed in the paragraph on histologic aspects of the central giant cell granuloma.

CHAPTER 4

Fibrous dysplasia

Fibrous dysplasia

Definition and terminology

Fibrous dysplasia is a benign condition, presumably developmental in nature, characterized by the presence of fibrous connective tissue with a characteristic whorled pattern and containing trabeculae of immature non-lamellar bone[500]. In some cases heredity plays a role[436].

Lesions of fibrous dysplasia may be monostotic or polyostotic. The use of the term monostotic would actually require a radiographic or scintigraphic survey of the whole body. In view of the rather harmless nature of fibrous dysplasia, and the rarity of the polyostotic type, such a survey is usually omitted. The prefix "monostotic" is also used in case of involvement of multiple craniofacial bones, i.e. maxillary and frontal bone, and also in case of simultaneous occurrence in the mandible and maxilla in the absence of lesions elsewhere in the skeleton. In such instances the term craniofacial fibrous dysplasia may be used. The prefixes "aggressive" or "active" are merely based on clinical behavior and not on histologic criteria.

Monostotic fibrous dysplasia

Epidemiology

The monostotic type of fibrous dysplasia is comparatively rare in the jaws, but is more common than the polyostotic type. The estimated incidence is one per million population per year. Monostotic fibrous dysplasia shows no preference for males or females. The disease occurs particularly in children and young adults.

Clinical aspects

The first symptom of fibrous dysplasia is a non-tender slowly growing swelling of the bone, either in the mandible or the maxilla (Fig. 4-1). In Europeans, aggressive growth in fibrous dysplasia occurs infrequently, in contrast to fibro-osseous lesions in Africans[10].

62 • Fibrous dysplasia

Fig. 4-1a.
Fibrous dysplasia affecting left side of face. No further symptoms present.

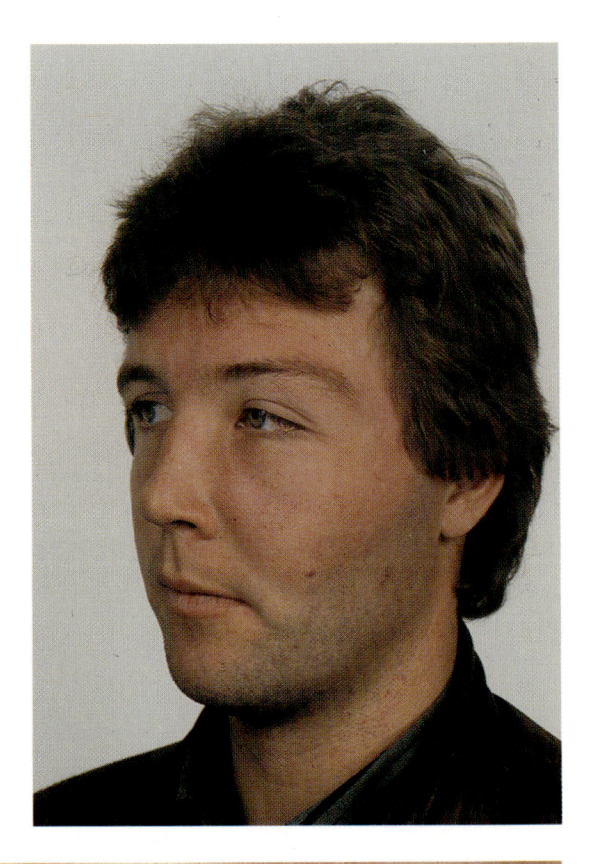

Fig. 4-1b.
There is a bony hard swelling at the buccal aspect of the maxilla.

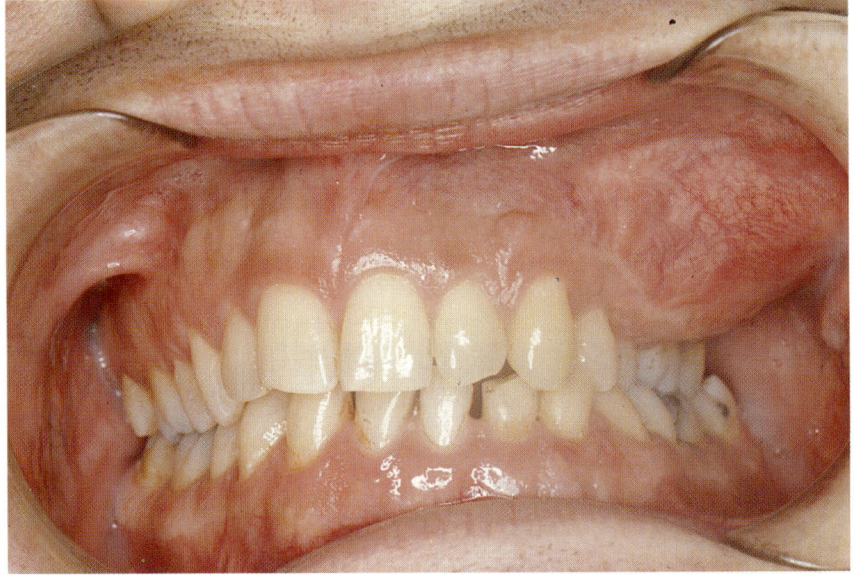

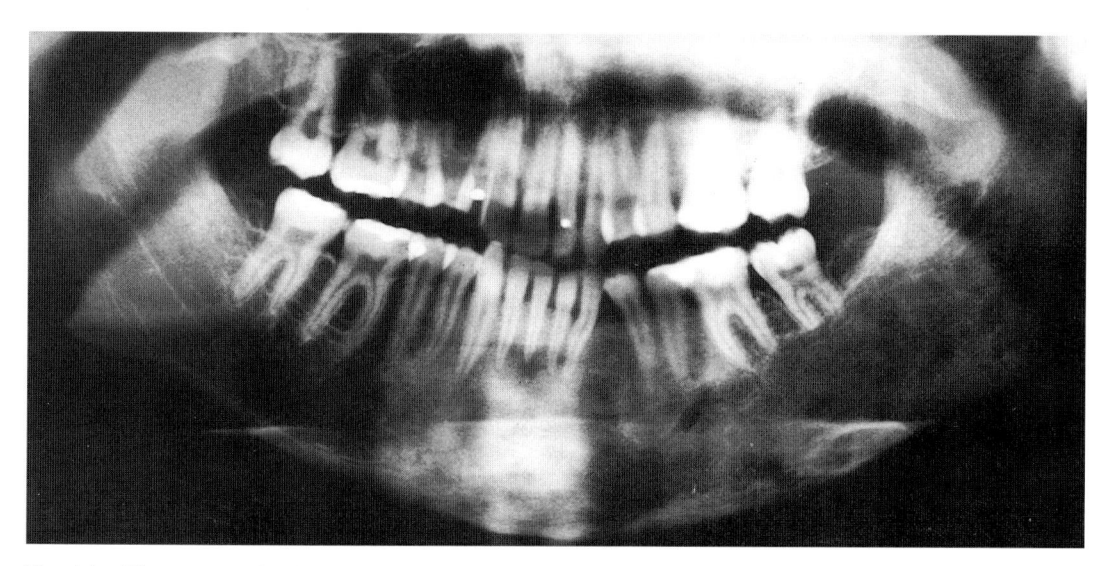

Fig. 4-1c. The panoramic view shows that also the mandible is involved.

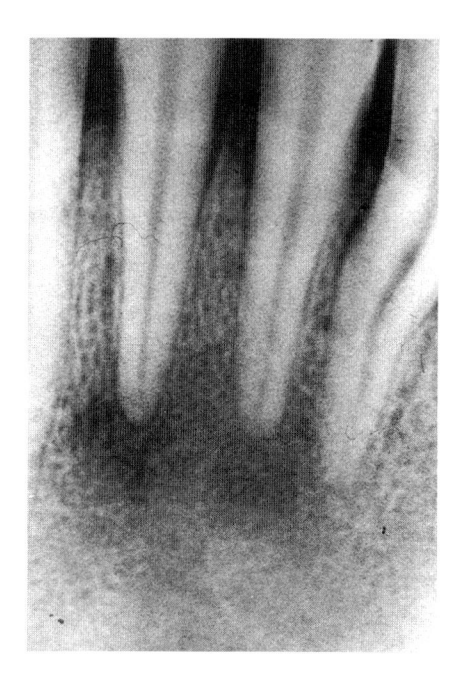

Fig. 4-1d.
The periapical film of the lower anterior teeth shows diffuse radiolucent changes of the apices.

The overlying mucosa remains intact. The consistency of the swelling may vary from firm elastic to bony hard. There is usually no displacement of teeth and the occlusion of the dental arches remains undisturbed. In rare instances chronic osteomyelitis is superimposed.

64 • **Fibrous dysplasia**

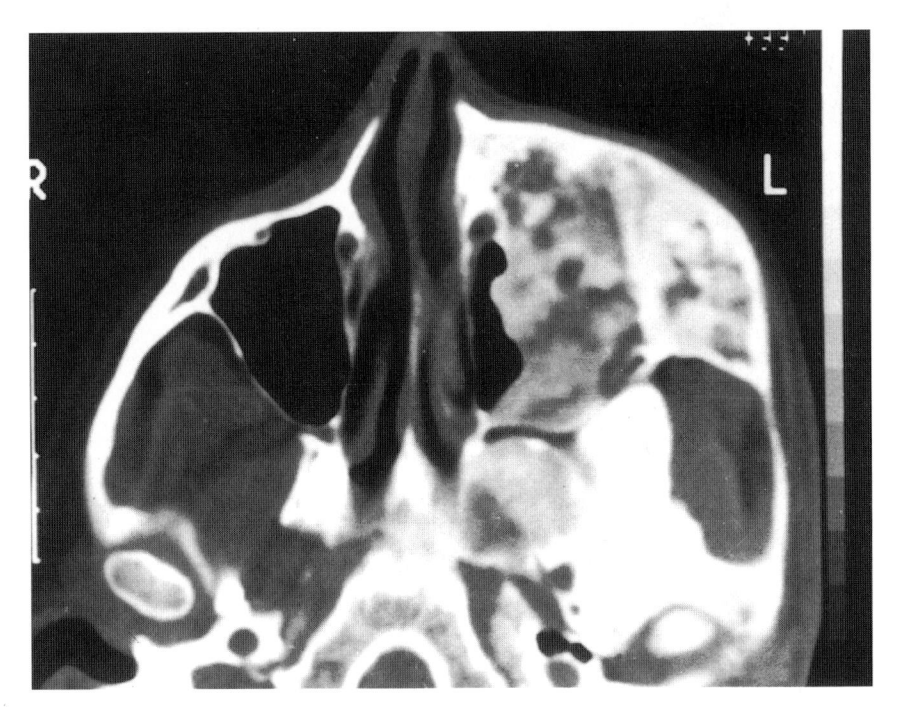

Fig. 4-1e. The extent of the disease is further demonstrated by the CT-scan

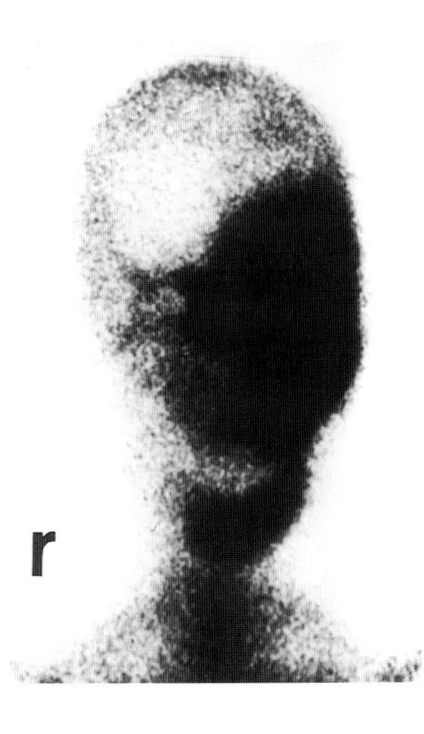

Fig. 4-1f.
and by scintigraphy. (Courtesy
Prof.dr. J. Valk, The Netherlands).

Fig. 4-2.
Ground-glass appearance of fibrous dysplasia of the mandible.

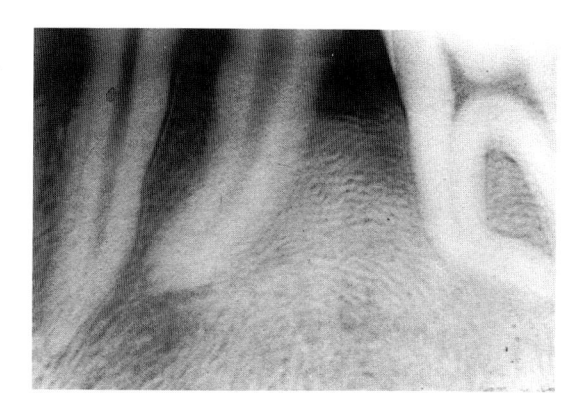

An unusual case of fibrous dysplasia and concomitant dysplastic changes in the dentin has been reported[604].

Laboratory findings

Serum values of calcium, phosphate and alkaline phosphatase remain unchanged.

Radiographic aspects

In the immature stage monostotic fibrous dysplasia may be a multilocular radiolucent lesion with ill-defined borders. In the mature stage a more or less distinct trabecular pattern may be recognized. The lesion may also be opaque with a ground-glass appearance (Fig. 4-2). Resorption of apices is rare. The cortical bone may become extremely thin due to the expansive nature of the lesion. However, true perforation seldom occurs. There is usually no distinct periosteal reaction. The disease may spread from the maxillary bone into the zygomatic bone, the frontal bone and other craniofacial bones, including the base of the skull.

In a group of 25 patients with fibrous dysplasia of the craniofacial bones, six radiologic types were recognized: "Peu d'orange", whorled plaques, diffuse sclerotic, cystlike, Pagetoid, and chalky[409]. The cystlike appearance can be caused by the simultaneous presence of a solitary bone cyst[273].

Scintigraphic aspects

Scintigraphy usually shows an increased accumulation[630]. It is not clear whether or not the findings of bone scintigraphy correlate with the biologic activity of fibrous dysplasia.

Histologic aspects

The microscopic features may vary widely. Classically, a cellular fibrous connective tissue is seen, sometimes showing a whorled pattern. There may be an abundance of connective tissue with little formation of bone. In other cases the formation of bone is more prominent, with little stroma present. The bone trabeculae

66 • Fibrous dysplasia

Fig. 4-3. Cellular fibrous connective tissue and irregularly arranged bone trabeculae in fibrous dysplasia. A few osteoclasts can be observed.

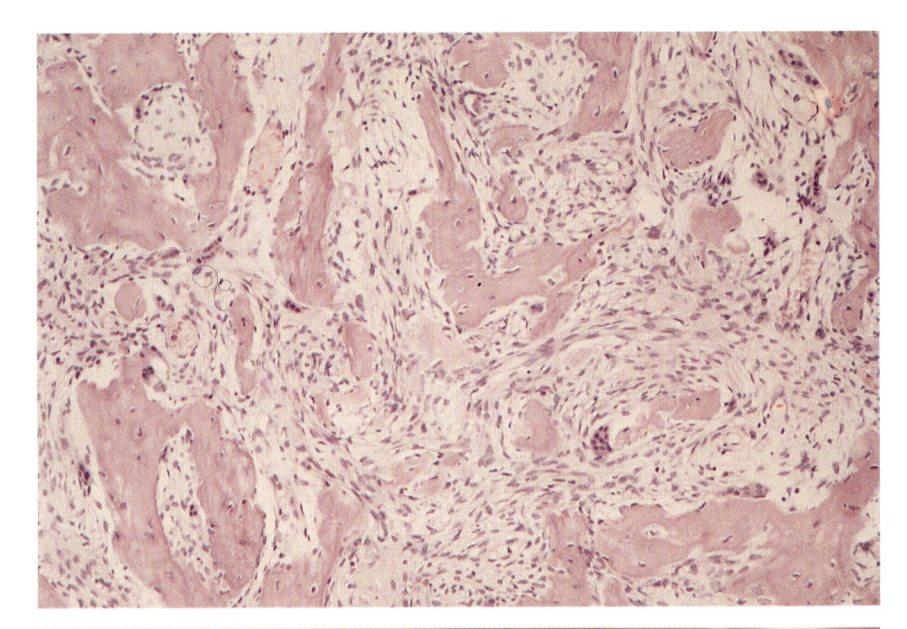

Fig. 4-4a. Bony hard swelling of the maxilla in a 55-year-old woman. The lesion had been present since childhood.

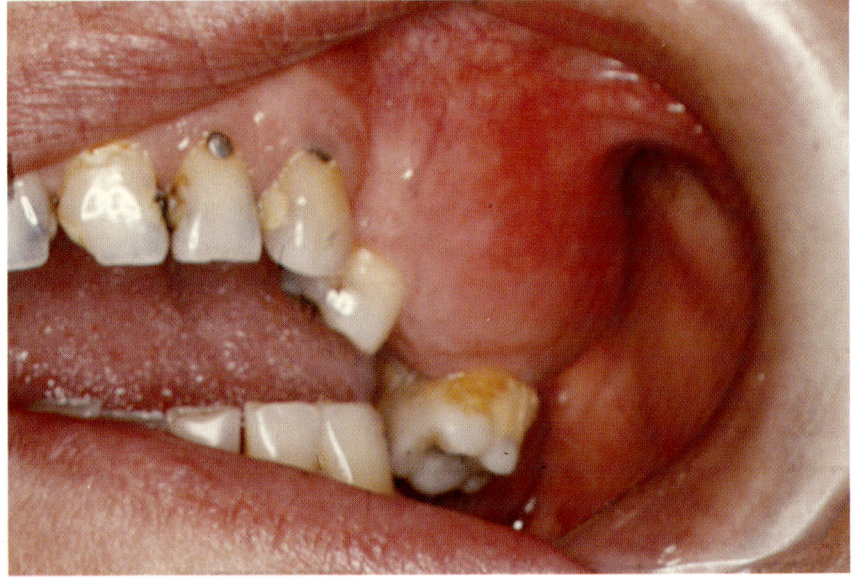

have an irregular outline and have been referred to as "Chinese characters". In addition to signs of bone formation, there are also signs of resorption with sometimes distinct osteoclasts present, even to the extent of resembling a giant cell granuloma (Fig. 4-3). Occasionally, cementum-like structures are observed. The bone trabeculae mainly consist of plexiform (woven) bone, but particu-

Fig. 4-4b.
The radiograph shows a ground glass appearance, suggestive of fibrous dysplasia.

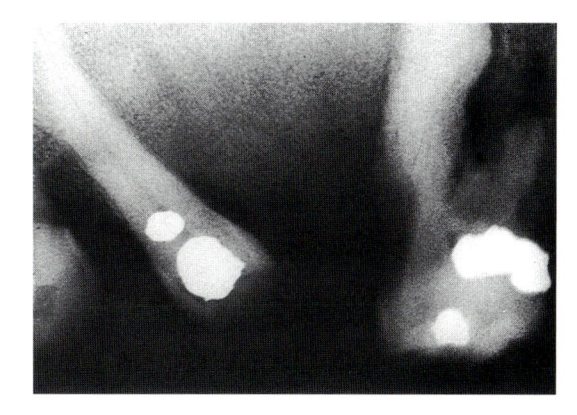

Fig. 4-4c.
The biopsy revealed parallel arrangement of bone trabeculae in a fibrous stroma. Fibrous dysplasia (?).

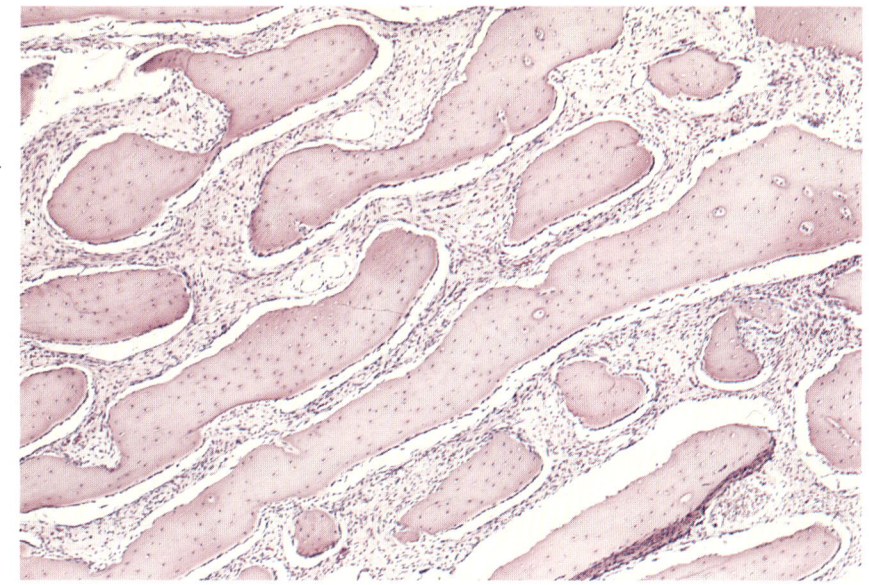

larly in fibrous dysplasia of the jaws one may occasionally observe lamellar bone, sometimes being arranged in a parallel fashion, which actually is not in accordance with the previous definition (Fig. 4-4). In Makek's classification of fibro-osseous cemental diseases of the cranio-facial and jaw bones such a lesion, showing parallelism of the bone trabeculae, is referred to as "osseous keloid"[352].

In contrast to fibrous dysplasia elsewhere in the skeleton, osteoblastic rimming of the trabeculae is generally accepted as part of the histologic features in fibrous dysplasia of the jaws as well.

The microscopic features may mimic those of an ossifying and cementifying fibroma (OCF), if such an entity exists (see p. 225).

68 • Fibrous dysplasia

Fig. 4-5a. Patient suffering from polyostotic fibrous dysplasia. Apart from the craniofacial bones some of the long bones were affected as well.

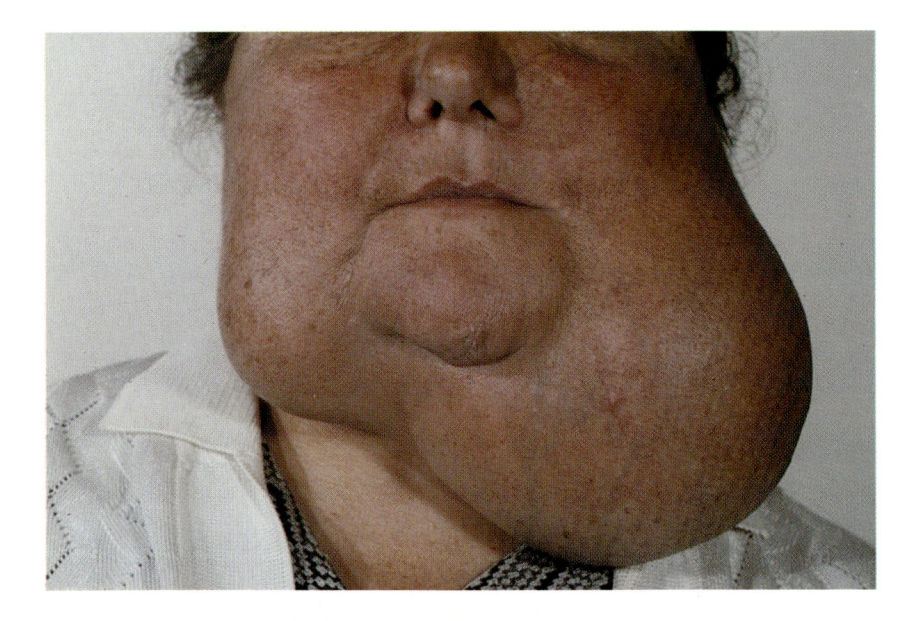

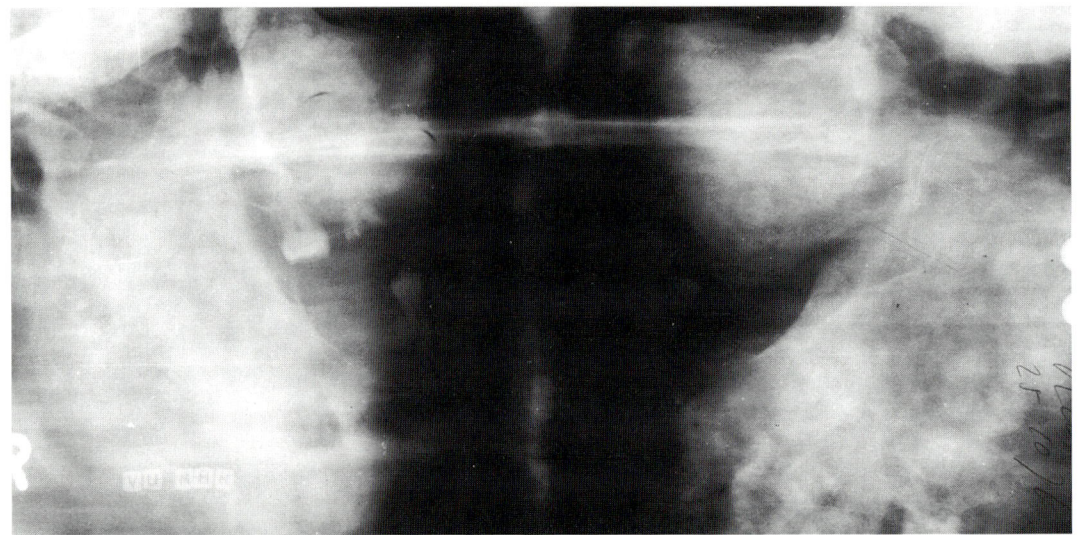

Fig. 4-5b. The panoramic view shows the extent of the mandibular and maxillary involvement.

Some pathologists adhere to the concept that an ossifying and cementifying fibroma should have a distinct capsule. Others claim to be able to distinguish fibrous dysplasia and OCF based on the cellularity of the lesion or on the presence, shape and distribution of cementumlike sphericals.

Occasionally, even with the help of microscopic examination, it is impossible to determine whether one is dealing with fibrous dys-

Fig. 4-5c.
Notice the involvement of the occiput.

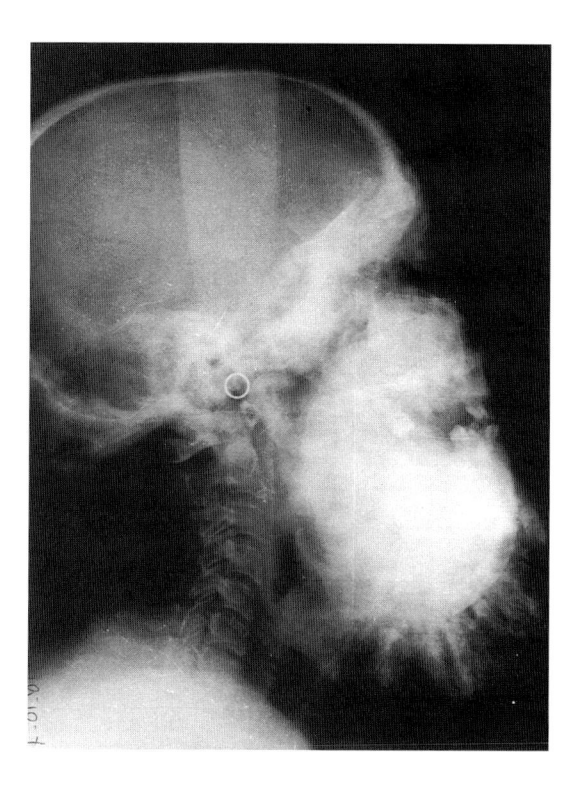

plasia with secondary inflammation or primarily with chronic osteomyelitis. Furthermore, some osteosarcomas may mimic fibrous dysplasia[646].

Due to its tendency to blend into the adjacent normal bone, fibrous dysplasia of the jaws can actually never be removed *in toto*. Fibrous dysplasia usually becomes inactive at age of 20 to 25 years. When a surgical correction is performed during childhood, a recurrence is to be expected within a short period of time, sometimes even in a matter of months. In asymptomatic patients in whom the lesions are slow-growing or have stopped growing, expectant therapy is, indeed, preferred[449].

Irradiation is contraindicated because of the potential risk of inducing malignant changes[384]. Spontaneous malignant transformation has been reported, but is extremely rare in the monostotic type of fibrous dysplasia[446]. In such instances the question arises whether the original diagnosis of fibrous dysplasia had been made correctly.

Polyostotic fibrous dysplasia

The polyostotic type of fibrous dysplasia usually arises at an early age. This type can be subdivided into 1) Jaffe's type, with skin pigmentations called café-au-lait spots, and 2) Albright's syndrome, a more serious type in which skin pigmentations are accompanied by endocrine disturbances of the pituitary gland, the thyroid gland, the parathyroid glands, and the ovaries[245,662].

The affected bones may show expansion and sometimes also deformation. Often the craniofacial bones are involved, especially the occiput and base of the skull (Fig. 4-5)[561]. Pathological fractures are a serious complication.

The radiographic aspects cannot be distinguished from those of the monostotic type. This is also true for the histologic features.

Laboratory examinations demonstrate no characteristic findings in the serum or urine.

Treatment of polyostotic fibrous dysplasia is not possible. If necessary, a modelling correction can be carried out. The chance of malignant transformation is remote, but is more common than in the monostotic type.

CHAPTER 5

Non-odontogenic cysts

In this chapter only cysts will be discussed that are located in or close to the jaw bones and that are not of odontogenic origin. The latter group is discussed in chapter 6. Several of these non-odontogenic cysts do not meet one of the criteria of a cyst, being "lined by epithelium". Instead, the term cyst is often based on the radiographic appearance of a well-circumscribed radiolucency.

Aneurysmal bone cyst

Definition The aneurysmal bone cyst (ABC) is an expanding osteolytic lesion consisting of blood-filled spaces of variable size separated by connective tissue septa containing trabeculae of bone or osteoid tissue and osteoclast giant cells[500].

The etiology and pathogenesis are not well understood[557]. In many instances the ABC is accompanied by another lesion of bone[357], i.e. a solitary bone cyst, fibrous dysplasia and central giant cell granuloma.

Epidemiology ABC's mainly occur in children and adolescents, without sex preference, involving the shafts of the long bones, the vertebral column, the clavicles and the ribs. Only a few cases occur in the jaws. The cyst may occur in the maxilla, but is more common in the mandible, occasionally even bilaterally[488]. Some 70 cases of involvement of the jaws have been reported[578].

Clinical aspects Clinically, the ABC gives rise to a firm, asymptomatic or slightly painful swelling. The duration may vary from a few weeks to several years.

Radiographic aspects The radiograph may show a uni- or multilobular, well-circumscribed lucency, sometimes showing a honeycomb appearance and often an eccentric ballooning (Fig. 5-1). There may be destruction

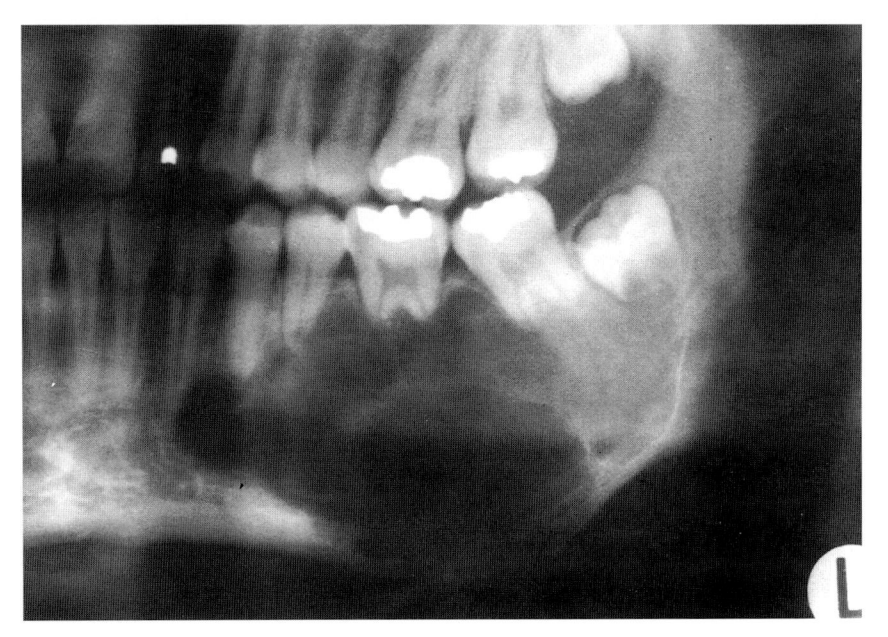

Fig. 5-1. Honeycomb appearance of aneurysmal bone cyst. (Courtesy Dr. E. van Roessel, The Netherlands).

of the cortical bone. Displacement or resorption of the roots of the teeth is not uncommon. Taken together, the radiographic features are not pathognomonic. The differential diagnosis includes such lesions as central giant cell granuloma, ameloblastoma and odontogenic myxoma[46].

Scintigraphic aspects The radionuclide picture is usually "hot". Angiography may show a diffuse filling of the lesion.

Histologic aspects The histologic features consist of connective tissue in which spaces and clefts, filled with erythrocytes, can be seen. Thrombus formation sometimes takes place in these spaces. The presence of multinucleated giant cells is also common. In most cases osteoid formation is observed (Fig. 5-2). In the differential diagnosis the possibility of a central giant cell granuloma should be considered.

Fig. 5-2. Biopsy from aneurysmal bone cyst showing cellular connective tissue with numerous clefts. Note the presence of osteoid and the large number of multinucleated giant cells.

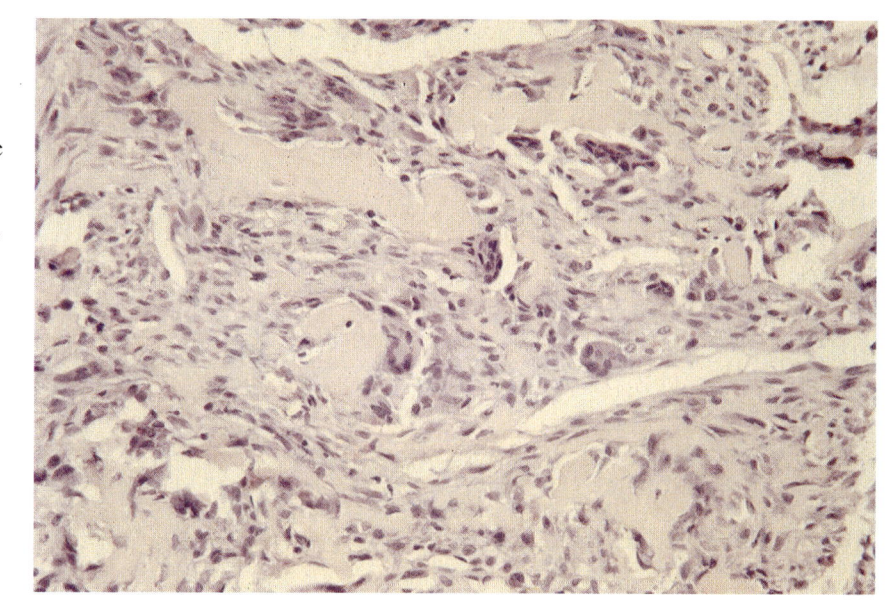

A separate paper has been devoted to the ultrastructural, the enzyme histochemical and immunohistological aspects[591].

Treatment Treatment consists of thorough curettage, which may be accompanied by severe bleeding. Recurrences are not uncommon[344]. In some cases cryosurgery or radiotherapy have been instituted[161].

Dermoid cyst

Dermoid cysts may occur in the oral soft tissues, especially in the floor of the mouth. In rare instances, sebaceous glands and sebaceouslike cells may be present in the wall of dentigerous or odontogenic keratocysts[81]. True dermoid cysts occurring within the jaw bone are extremely rare[114,132].

Fig. 5-3.
Pear-shaped radiolucency between vital 12 and 13, compatible with the clinico-radiologic diagnosis of "globulomaxillary cyst". Histologic examination showed the features of an odontogenic keratocyst.

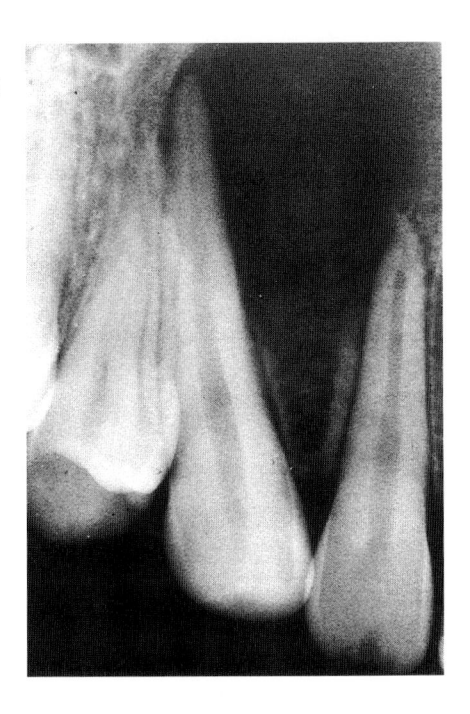

Globulomaxillary cyst

The globulomaxillary cyst has for many years been regarded as a fissural cyst, developing from proliferation of epithelium that has been enclosed during the fusion of the median nasal process and the maxillary processes. According to the "classic" descriptions, the cyst is found between the lateral incisor and the canine in the maxillary bone, presenting as a well-confined lucent anomaly that in some instances displaces the radices of the lateral incisor and the canine (Fig. 5-3).

According to present views, one is in most instances dealing with an odontogenic cyst, such as a radicular cyst (especially of the lateral incisor), a lateral periodontal cyst, a primordial cyst or a keratocyst[637].

Lingual cortical defect of the mandible

Definition and epidemiology

Stafne cyst, latent or static bone cyst, and lingual mandibular salivary gland depression cyst are all used as synonyms for the lingual cortical defect of the mandible (LCDM).

The "defect" represents a concavity of the lingual aspect of the mandibular bone or a cavity within the bone due to the enclosure

Lingual cortical defect of the mandible • 75

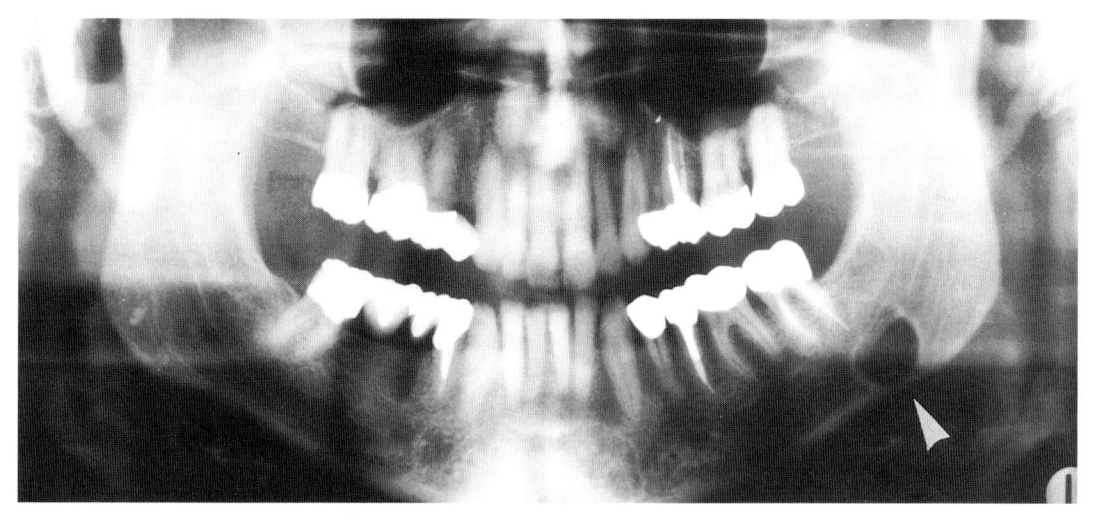

Fig. 5-4. Lingual cortical defect of the mandible at the left side.

of salivary gland tissue during the embryologic stage[623]. However, the phenomenon has also been ascribed to a resorptive process caused by hyperplasia of salivary gland tissue, to an anomaly in the facial artery or to functional adaptation of the bone[491].

The prevalence is estimated at about 0.1-0.4%[128]. The defect is much more common in men than in women. In children it is rare.

Clinical aspects The LCDM is asymptomatic and is almost invariably detected as an incidental finding on the radiograph, especially since the availability of panoramic radiographs.

Radiographic aspects Radiographically, the defect is round to oval and is almost always located near the angle of the mandible, usually inferior to the mandibular canal (Fig. 5-4). Location above the mandibular canal is, indeed, rare[1]. Some lesions have been reported in the anterior region of the mandible (Fig. 5-5)[52,383]. Bilateral occurrence is exceptional, as is a bilocular or multilocular appearance[226,521]. In rare instances the location of the defect may mimic the presence of an odontogenic cyst, e.g. a dentigerous cyst of a wisdom tooth[487].

The LCDM may vary in size from a few millimeters up to several centimeters. The radiolucency is partially or completely surrounded by a dense radiopaque line.

Chen and Ohba have proposed a classification system of these defects based on the position and location of lesions relative to the mandibular canal and the cortical plate of the border of the mandible[108].

Fig. 5-5.
Anterior location of lingual cortical defect of the mandible. (Courtesy Drs. S. Becker and F. Härle, F.R.G.).

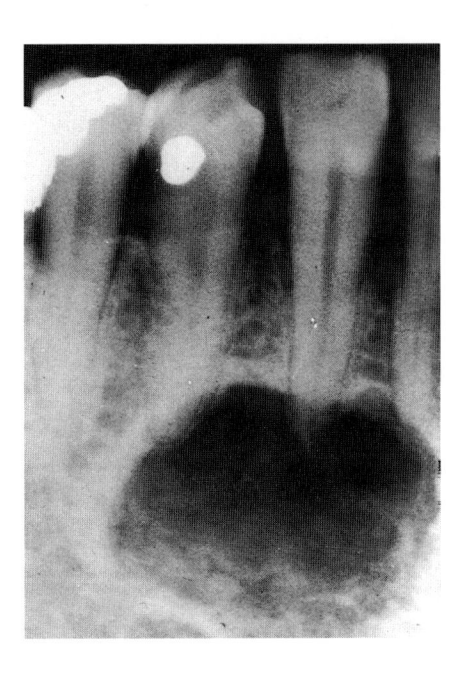

Histologic aspects   In the majority of the surgically explored cases salivary gland tissue was encountered. Also the presence of lymphoid tissue or a lymph node has been reported.

Treatment   The absence of symptoms, the specific site, and the radiographic aspect are usually sufficient for the final diagnosis, making surgical exploration redundant. Surgical exploration is indicated only when the nature of the lesion remains unclear on clinical and radiographic grounds. No follow-up is required.

Median mandibular cyst

In the past, the median mandibular cyst was regarded as a fissural cyst. The present concept, however, is that of an odontogenic origin, based on cysts, such as a lateral periodontal cyst, that happen to be localized in the midline[147,212]. Therefore, the term median mandibular cyst should only be used in a clinico-radiographic sense (Fig. 5-6).

Fig. 5-6.
So-called median mandibular cyst. Histologically, a diagnosis of odontogenic keratocyst was made. (Courtesy Drs. P. Bok, J. Schoen, J.M. Onland and R.M. Berns, The Netherlands).

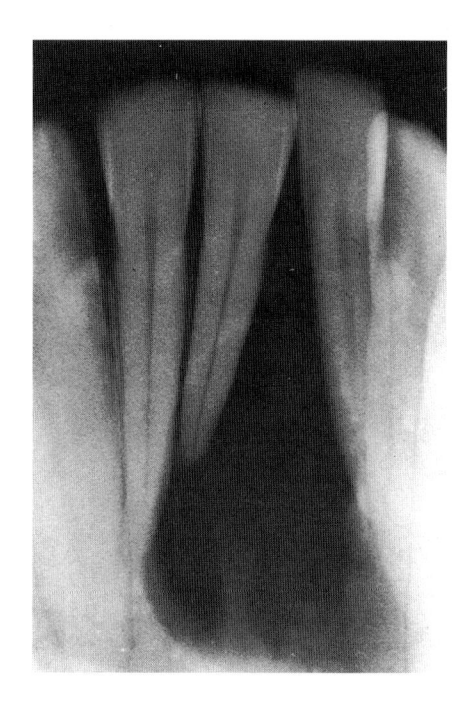

Median palatal cyst

Current views hold that a median palatal cyst is not a separate cyst[660]. It probably is a slightly dorsally located nasopalatine duct cyst. Several textbooks still deal with the cyst as a separate entity. Therefore, the term is mentioned here for sake of completeness.

Nasolabial cyst

The nasolabial cyst is mentioned here for sake of completeness. The cyst primarily develops in the soft tissues and most likely originates from epithelial remnants of the lower part of the nasolacrimal duct[24].

Clinically, the cyst may appear as a swelling of the mucobuccal fold in the upper lateral incisor and canine region, or as a swelling of the nasolabial fold.

In large cysts some erosion of the underlying bone may take place, mimicking a periapical disorder when projected close to the apex of a tooth.

Histologically, pseudostratified cylindric epithelium is the most common finding.

Treatment consists of intraoral enucleation.

Fig. 5-7. Clinical aspect of nasopalatine duct cyst. All teeth are vital.

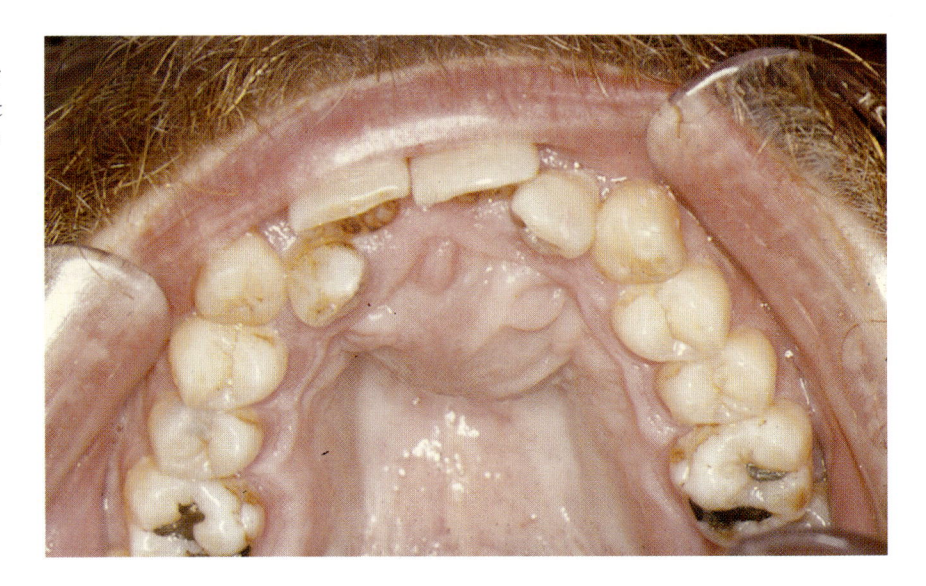

Nasopalatine duct cyst

Definition and epidemiology

The paired nasopalatine ducts arise at the junction of the palatine processes and the premaxilla. In these canals, which are usually closed at both the nasal and oral side, epithelial remnants may be present, occasionally giving rise to the formation of a cyst.

The prevalence is estimated at about 0.1 % or even less. The cyst may occur at all ages, but is usually diagnosed between the ages of 30 and 50 years. There is no sex preference.

Clinical aspects

The cyst may produce a swelling in the midline of the maxilla at the palatal side of the maxillary anterior central incisors or at the palatal aspect of the edentulous maxillary ridge (Fig. 5-7). However, in most cases clinical signs or symptoms are absent.

Radiographic aspects

The nasopalatine duct cyst is often found during routine radiologic examination. It is a round, oval or heart-shaped, usually symmetrical, and well-confined lucent lesion (Fig. 5-8). Sometimes the radices of the central maxillary incisors appear to be somewhat pushed apart. On the basis of the radiograph alone, distinguishing this cyst from a radicular cyst of one of the maxillary incisors is not always possible. In such instances, a vitality test of the related teeth can be decisive. In case of missing teeth, the radiograph may mimic the picture of a residual cyst.

Histologic aspects

The lining of the cyst is composed of stratified squamous epithelium, pseudo-stratified ciliated cylindric epithelium, cubic epithe-

Fig. 5-8.
Occlusal view showing an oval-shaped nasopalatine duct cyst.

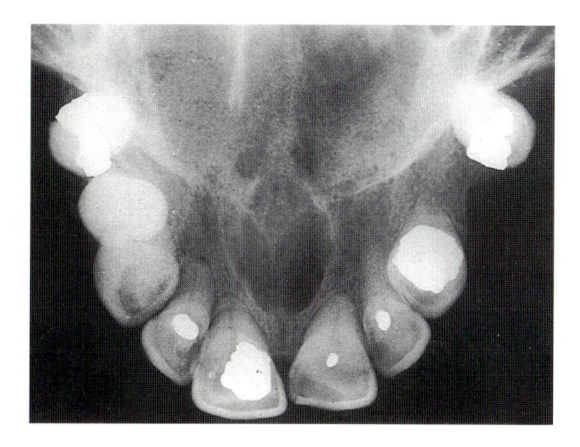

Fig. 5-9.
Wall of nasopalatine cyst. The lining partly consists of stratified squamous epithelium and partly of pseudostratified cylindric epithelium. Note the thickened cyst wall due to inflammatory changes.

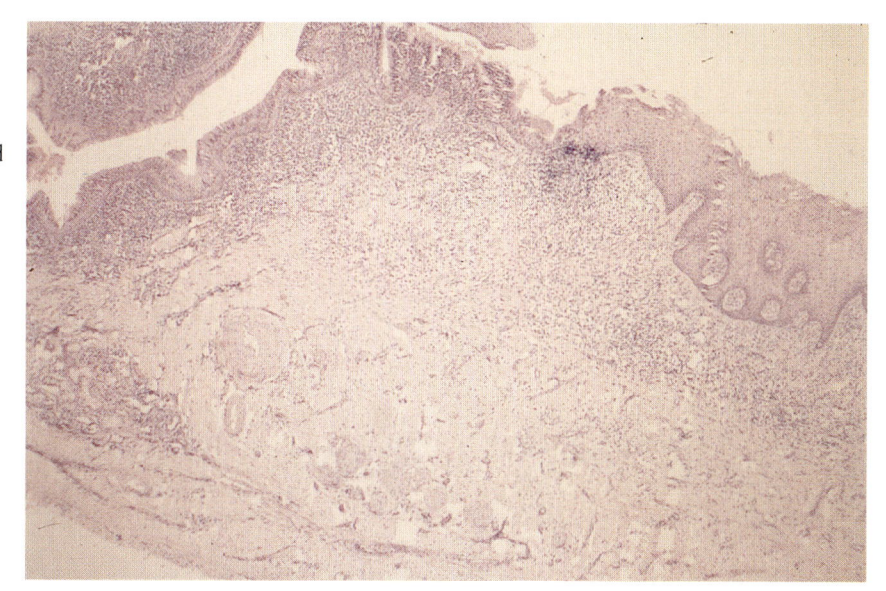

lium, or a combination of these epithelial variants (Fig. 5-9). Large blood vessels and numerous nerve bundles are frequently found in the walls of the cysts, and sometimes also small nests of salivary gland tissue and cartilage. The cartilage commonly occurs in the incisive papilla and is not a distinctive finding in itself. Inflammatory reactions in the cyst wall are rather common[32].

Treatment   The nasopalatine duct cyst is regarded as a harmless lesion. To the best of our knowledge, malignant changes in the epithelial lining have never been reported. Treatment is only required in case of swelling or pain. It is almost always possible to enucleate the cyst in a simple manner, usually via a palatal approach. Recurrences are rare.

Fig. 5-10. Clinical aspect of postoperative maxillary cyst. Notice the scar of the Caldwell-Luc procedure that was performed more than 10 years previously.

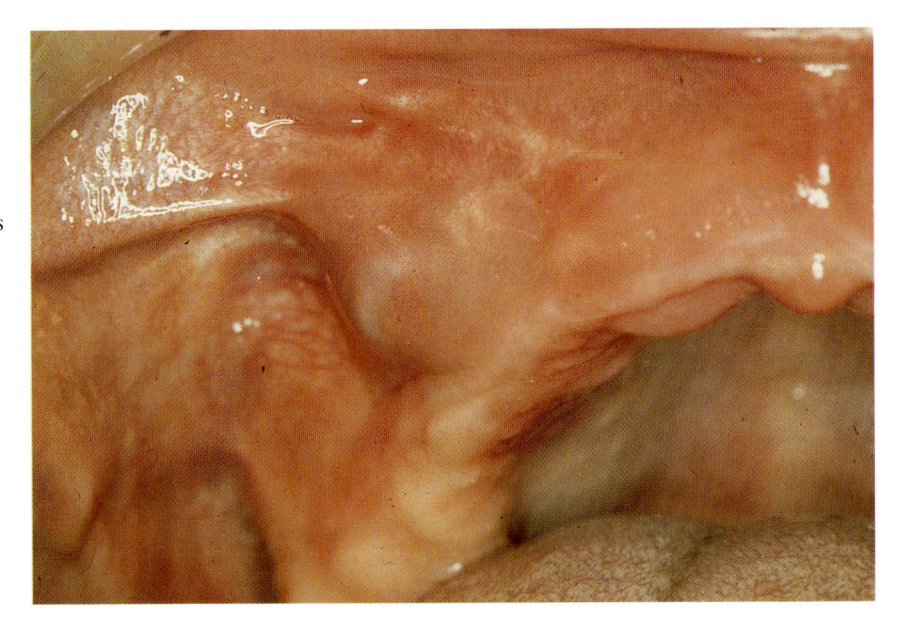

Parasitic cyst

A rare case of mandibular involvement of a hydatid cyst has been reported in a 16-year-old shepherd from India[398]. The mandibular lesion was secondary to a large hydatid cyst that was located in the liver.

Postoperative maxillary cyst

The postoperative maxillary cyst (PMC) develops as a result of entrapment of epithelium from the maxillary sinus into the surgical wound, for instance after a Caldwell-Luc procedure. Initially, the term "surgical ciliated cyst" was applied to this cyst.

Clinically, the common presentation is that of an intraoral or extraoral swelling (Fig. 5-10).

In a series of 60 cases of PMC most cases revealed radiographically a unilocular cystic lesion (Fig. 5-11)[644].

It has been suggested that a characteristic electrophoretic pattern of glycosaminoglycans from fluid aspirates of this cyst facilitates preoperative diagnosis[541].

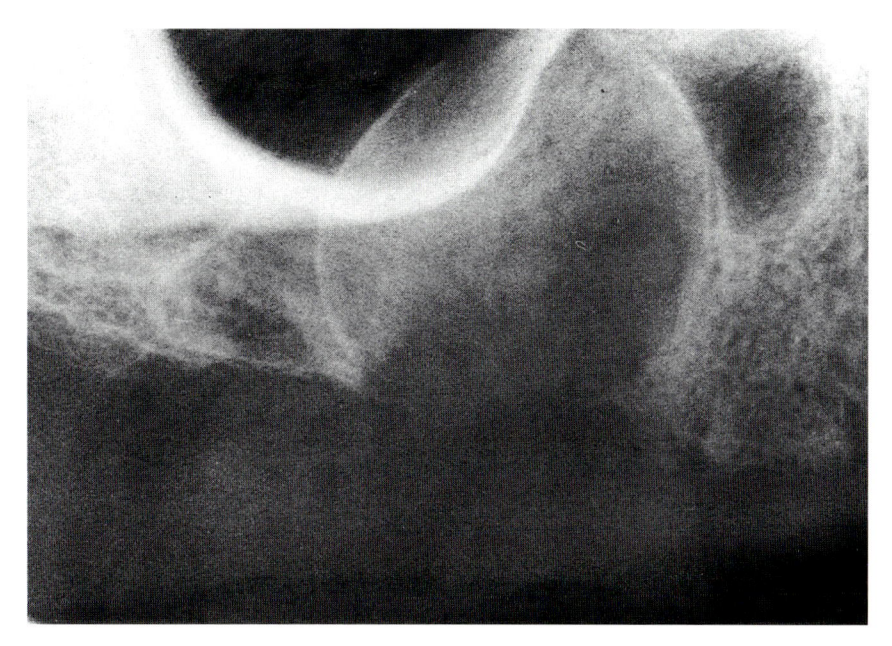

Fig. 5-11. Well-circumscribed lesion produced by a postoperative maxillary cyst.

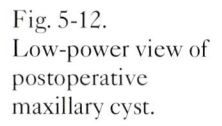

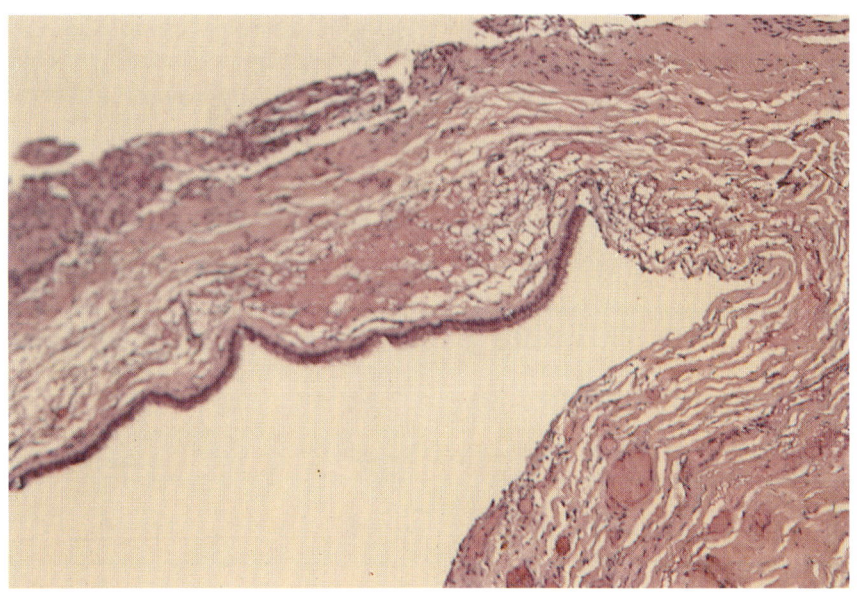

Fig. 5-12. Low-power view of postoperative maxillary cyst.

Histologically, cuboidal, squamous, and mixed epithelial cyst linings have been observed, although the basic lining is the ciliated columnar type (Fig. 5-12)[644].

Treatment consists of enucleation or marsupialization[651].

Solitary bone cyst

Definition and epidemiology

A solitary bone cyst (SBC) is a unicameral cavity filled with clear or sanguineous fluid and lined by a membrane of variable thickness, which consists of loose vascular connective tissue showing scattered osteoclast giant cells and sometimes areas of recent or old hemorrhage or cholesterol clefts[500]. Synonyms that have been used are traumatic, hemorrhagic, simple or idiopathic bone cyst.

Solitary bone cysts occur not only in the jaws but are observed elsewhere in the skeleton as well, especially in the metaphysis at the upper end of the humerus and the femur. The etiology is unknown.

There is no preference for either sex. The cyst is seen particularly in children and adolescents.

Clinical aspects

The SBC is almost always localized as a solitary lesion in the mandible, occasionally bilaterally[60, 305]. Most of these cysts are located in the body or symphysis of the mandible; location in the ramus or even the condyle is rare[323]. Only a few cases of maxillary involvement have been reported[619].

The lesion seldom gives rise to complaints and is usually discovered as an incidental finding on a radiograph. The vitality of the teeth in the involved area remains intact.

Radiographic aspects

The radiograph shows a well-circumscribed lucency, located above the mandibular canal. The outline of the cyst may be lobulated and corticated (Fig. 5-13). The teeth are seldom displaced and the lamina dura remains intact. There is no resorption of the apices. On the occlusal view a slight expansion of the cortical bone may be observed. The cyst may vary in size from a few to several centimeters. In some cases the lesion is associated with an impacted tooth[517] or a root remnant[520].

Laboratory findings

Laboratory values are within normal limits.

Histologic aspects

The only way of establishing the diagnosis of SBC is by surgical exploration. It often appears that the cortical bone has remained intact. After fenestration of the cortical plate, a cavity is encountered which sometimes contains a small amount of straw-yellow liquid. The bony wall usually appears to be lined by an extremely delicate fibrous layer without the presence of an epithelial

Fig. 5-13.
Radiographic aspect of solitary bone cyst. All teeth are vital.

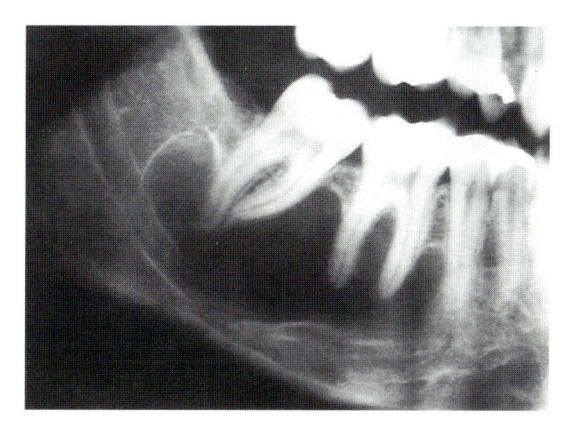

Fig. 5-14.
Lining of the wall of a solitary bone cyst.
No epithelium present. There is some secondary bone formation.

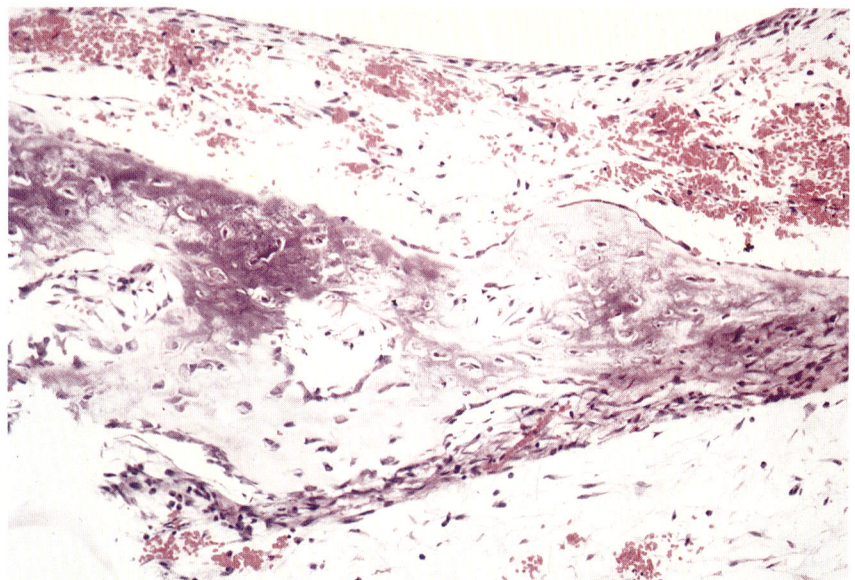

lining (Fig. 5-14)[445]. When the surrounding bone is curetted and examined histologically, fibrous dysplasia-like features are sometimes recognized. It is not clear whether or not there is, in fact, a relationship with fibrous dysplasia, florid fibro-osseous-cemental dysplasia, aneurysmal bone cyst, or central giant cell granuloma, as has been suggested in the literature[305].

Treatment   The exploration required to establish the diagnosis of SBC also implies the treatment. Healing takes place within a year. Some clinicians advocate provoking some bleeding by carefully scraping the surrounding cavity wall. This would enhance the healing of the defect. Others have reported the successful injection of autogenous blood into the cavity[444]. There is little experience with regard to the injection of methylprednisolone acetate. That method has been reported to be successful in SBC's in other sites of the skeleton[499].

Recurrences are rare[187, 196]. The majority of traumatic bone cysts probably heal spontaneously, remaining unnoticed, since the diagnosis is seldom made in patients over 40-50 years of age. Also a case of regression following aspiration has been reported[107].

CHAPTER 6

Odontogenic cysts

Odontogenic cysts are cysts lined by epithelium that is or has been involved in the formation of teeth. In this chapter both the intraosseous and extraosseous odontogenic cysts are dealt with. The calcifying odontogenic cyst will be discussed in the chapter on odontogenic tumors. It is not clear yet whether the botryoid odontogenic cyst is a true entity[304]. The latter cyst will be mentioned in the paragraph on the lateral periodontal cyst.

The odontogenic cysts can be subclassified into developmental cysts and inflammatory cysts (Table 6-1).

Table 6-1. Classification of odontogenic cysts

1. Developmental cysts

    1. Dental lamina cyst of the newborn
    2. Dentigerous cyst
    3. Eruption cyst
    4. Gingival cyst of the adult
    5. Keratocyst
    6. Lateral periodontal cyst (incl. Botryoid odontogenic cyst)
    7. Primordial cyst
    8. Sialo-odontogenic cyst (Glandular odontogenic cyst)

2. Inflammatory cysts

    1. Paradental cyst
    2. Radicular cyst
    3. Residual cyst
    4. Mandibular infected buccal cyst

Developmental cysts

Dental lamina cyst of the newborn

The dental lamina cyst of the newborn is a small extraosseous cyst that develops from epithelial rests of the dental lamina in newborns. Some authors have classified this cyst, together with the gingival cyst of the adult (see p. 95), under the heading of parosteal (peripheral) developmental cysts[277]. Although these (micro)cysts are very common in the fetal stage[388], they are not very often observed at birth.

The diagnosis is primarily based on the clinical appearance and the location (Fig. 6-1). A biopsy should only be carried out in case of doubt.

Histologically, these cysts almost always appear to be filled with keratin. Just on the basis of histopathological features these cysts could be regarded as epidermoid cyst (Fig. 6-2).

Treatment is not required. The cysts will disappear spontaneously, usually within a few weeks or months[429].

Fig. 6-1.
Multiple dental lamina cysts in a newborn on buccal aspect of the lower alveolar ridge.

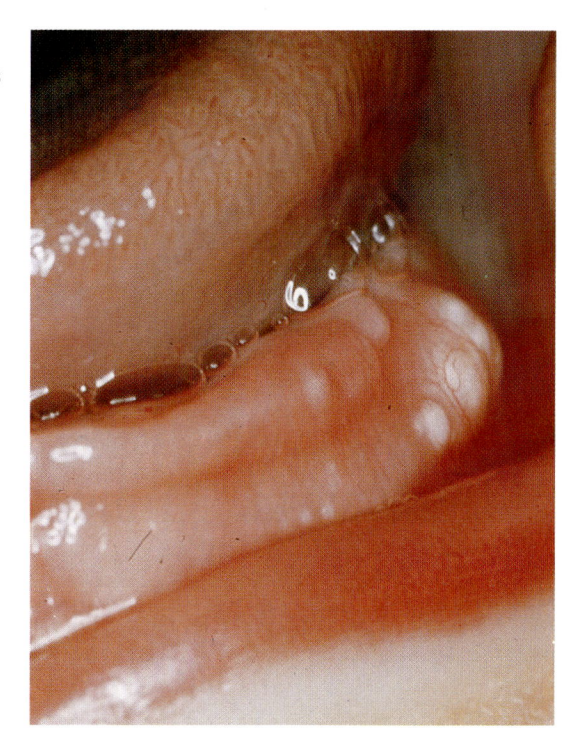

Fig. 6-2.
Low-power view of dental lamina cyst.

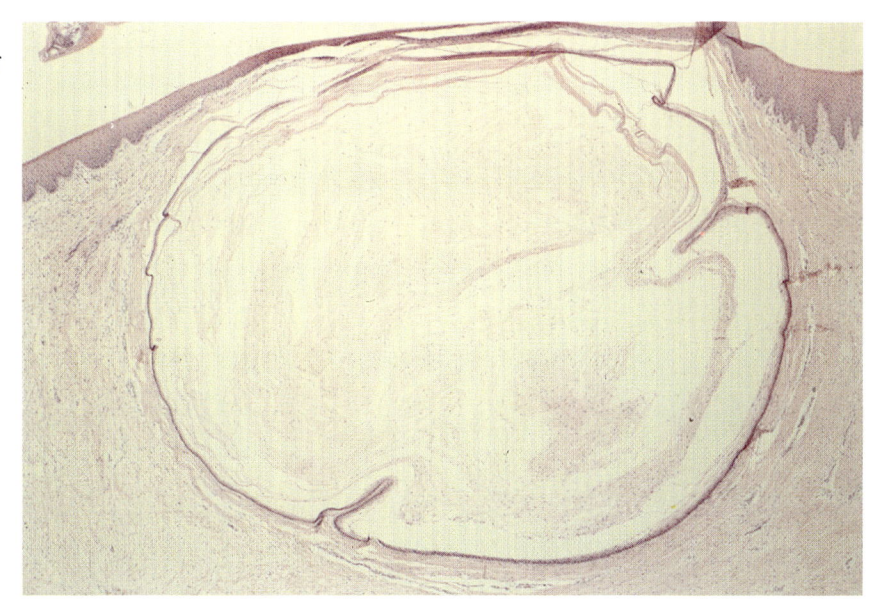

Fig. 6-3a. Cystic swelling in upper right canine area. All teeth were vital.

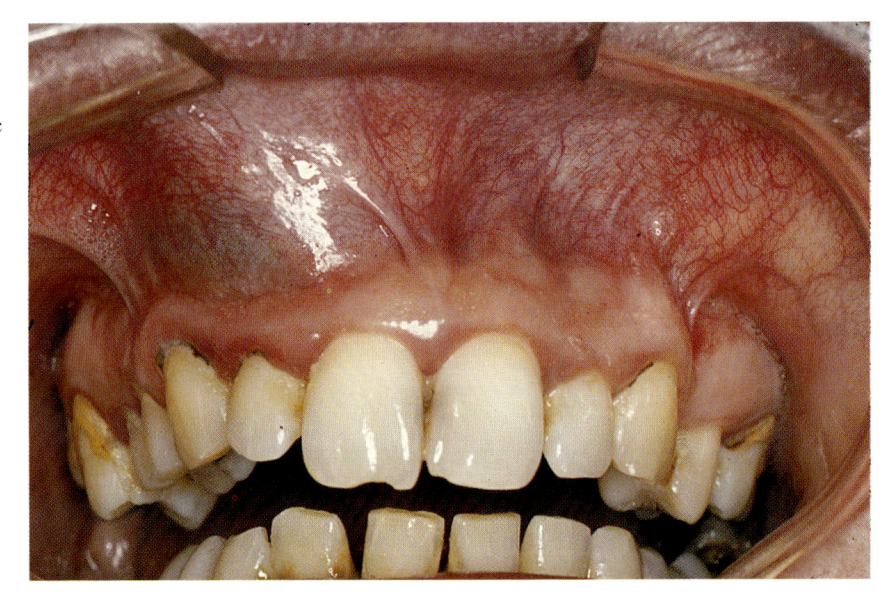

Dentigerous cyst

Definition and epidemiology

The dentigerous cyst, also called follicular cyst, is presumed to develop in the reduced enamel epithelium of a tooth that has not yet erupted. It is a clinical-radiologic diagnosis that requires histologic confirmation.

The dentigerous cyst is a very common cyst that almost exclusively occurs in the permanent dentition, especially in association with impacted third molars in the mandible and impacted canines in the maxilla. There is no sex preference.

Clinical aspects

Clinical features only rarely include enlargement of the maxilla or mandible or displacement of teeth (Fig. 6-3). Indeed, in most cases the cyst is asymptomatic, being detected as an incidental finding on a radiograph. In some instances infection of the cyst induces the formation of an abscess.

Even in very large cysts the inferior alveolar nerve remains undisturbed.

Radiographic aspects

Radiographically, a dentigerous cyst can be described as a unilobular, sometimes multilobular, well-confined, corticated lucency around the crown of an impacted tooth. If the width of the radiolucency around the crown is less than about 2 mm, it is considered to reflect a normal tooth follicle. Dentigerous cysts may become

Fig. 6-3b.
The radiograph is suggestive of a dentigerous cyst of a mesiodens.

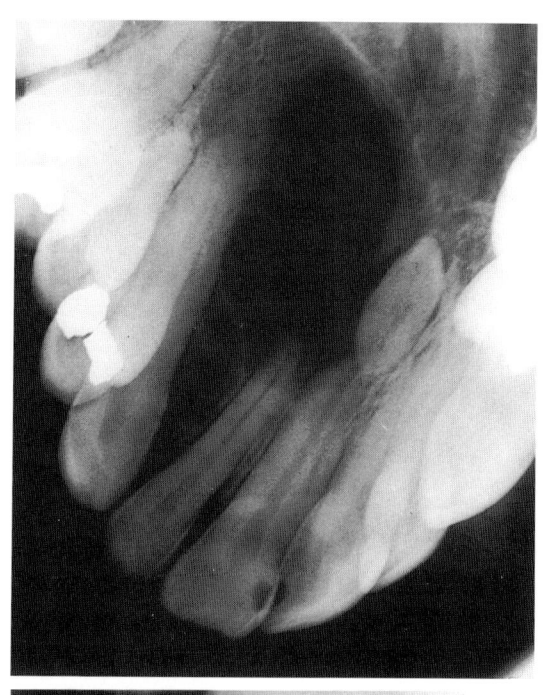

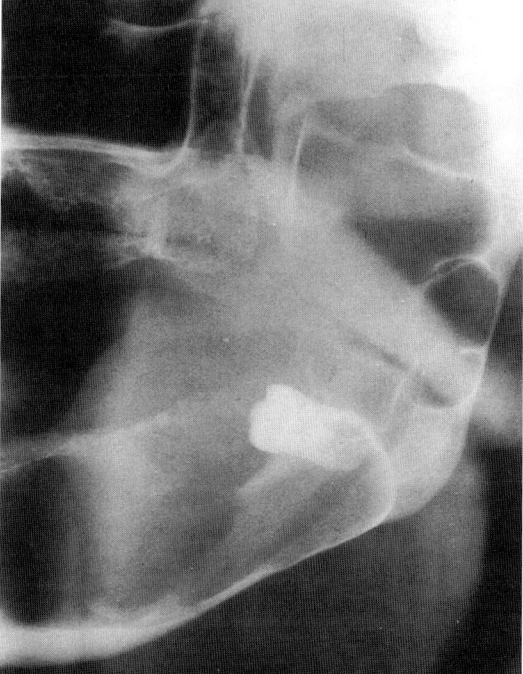

Fig. 6-4.
Multilobular, well-confined radiolucency in association with impacted 38.
The radiologic differential diagnosis includes, apart from dentigerous cyst, an odontogenic keratocyst and an ameloblastoma.

rather large, but rarely cause expansion or perforation of the cortical plates or resorption of adjacent teeth. The mandibular canal sometimes seems to be displaced.

Radiographic differentiation between a dentigerous cyst and an odontogenic keratocyst or an ameloblastoma is barely possible (Fig. 6-4). If patchy calcifications are seen in the lucency, one should consider the possibility of an adenomatoid odontogenic tumor or a calcifying odontogenic cyst.

One should consider taking a biopsy in the presence of unusual radiographic features such as expansion of the bone or resorption of the roots of adjacent teeth.

Histologic aspects

The lining of a dentigerous cyst is composed of stratified squamous epithelium, rarely showing keratinization (Fig. 6-5). Mucous-producing cells are not uncommon. From time to time, the histologic features of a keratocyst are seen in a lesion that was clinically and radiographically diagnosed as a dentigerous cyst. This lesion must then be diagnosed as a keratocyst. Other rather uncommon lesions that may be seen in what look clinically and radiographically like a dentigerous cyst are an ameloblastoma and a squamous cell carcinoma[76]. Therefore, it is advisable to have each dentigerous cyst examined histologically.

Treatment

Treatment of dentigerous cysts consists of enucleation and removal of the associated tooth. Recurrences are rare.

Fig. 6-5a. Cross-section of a dentigerous cyst, showing the crown of an impacted tooth in the cyst lumen.

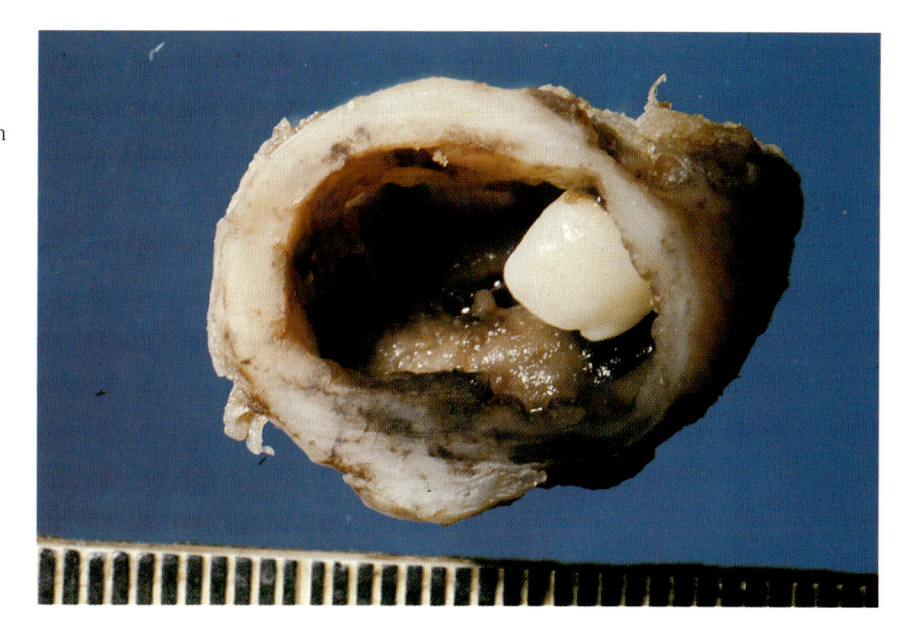

Fig. 6-5b. The lining consists of non-keratinizing stratified squamous epithelium that can not be distinguished from a number of other odontogenic cysts, such as the residual and radicular cyst.

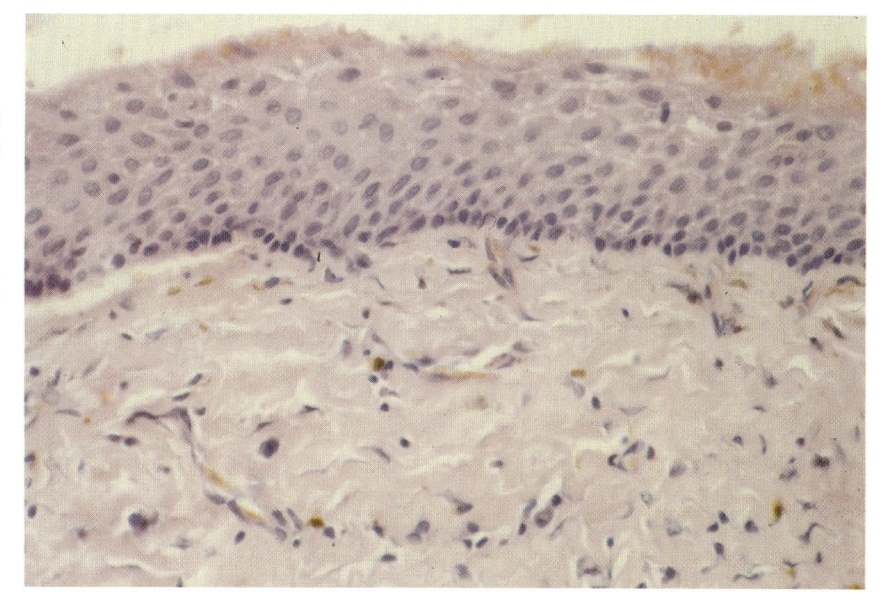

Eruption cyst

An eruption cyst lies superficially to the crown of an unerupted tooth and is regarded by many as a form of dentigerous cyst[437].

The eruption cyst occurs mainly in the primary, but may also occur in the permanent dentition.

Clinically, the cyst is characterized by an asymptomatic blue cystic swelling on the alveolar ridge at the site of eruption of a tooth. In general, the diagnosis can be made with confidence on the basis of the clinical appearance alone. If there is doubt about the diagnosis, a radiograph should be taken and, if necessary, a biopsy as well (Fig. 6-6). The histologic features are similar to those of a dentigerous cyst.

Treatment is not necessary. The involved tooth will, perhaps with some delay, erupt normally[514].

Developmental cysts • 93

Fig. 6-6a.
Clinical aspect of eruption cyst.

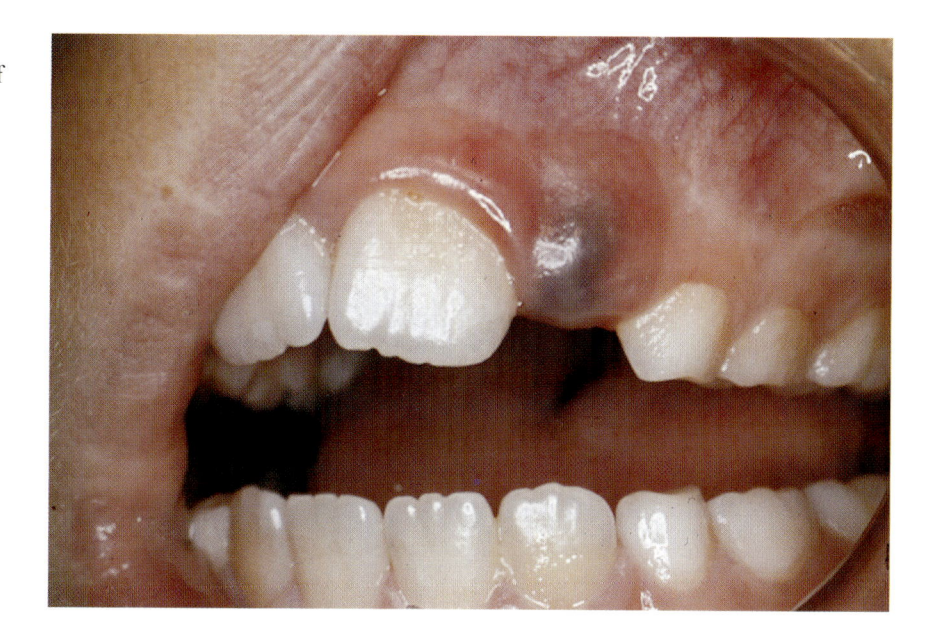

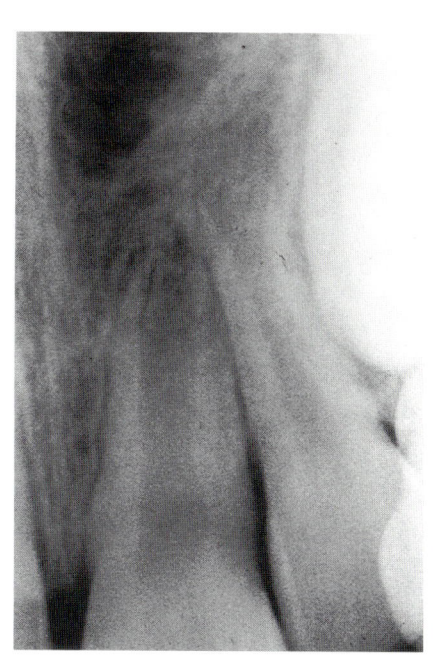

Fig. 6-6b.
A radiograph may be taken in order to exclude a possible underlying disorder in the bone. The 22 is about to erupt.

94 • Odontogenic cysts

Fig. 6-7a.
Gingival cyst between 43 and 44 in an adult.

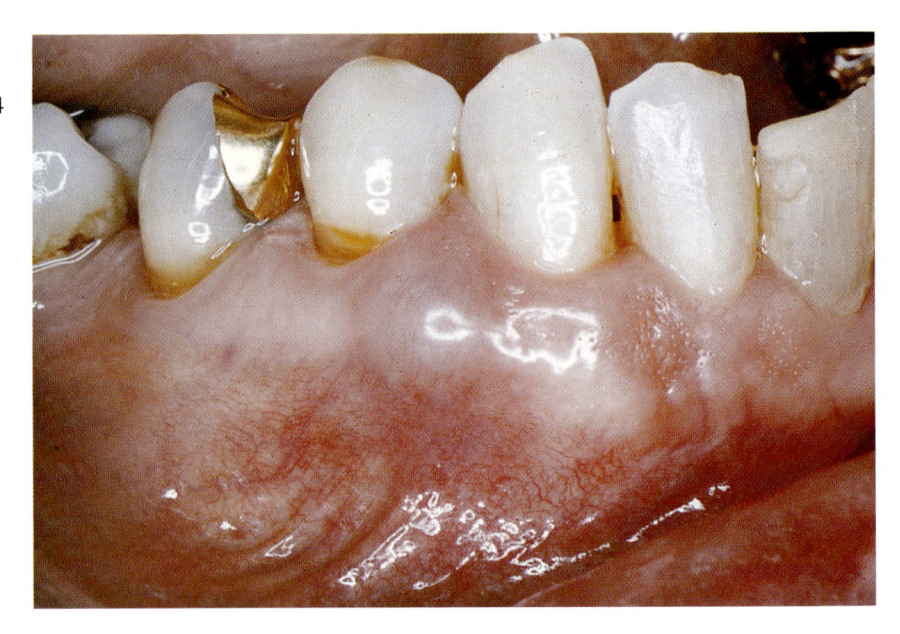

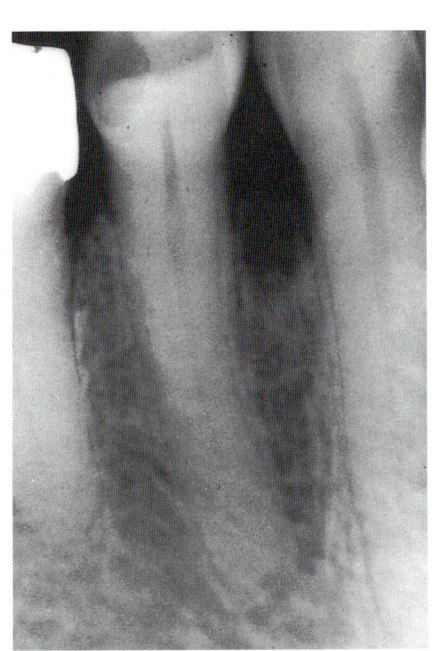

Fig. 6-7b.
The radiograph shows subtle lucent changes at the height of the alveolar bone between 43 and 44.

Fig. 6-7c. The lumen is (secondarily) filled with erythrocytes. Note the delicate epithelial lining with plaque-like thickening as may be seen in a lateral periodontal cyst. (Courtesy Drs. G. Zijlstra and Th.C. Vriezen, The Netherlands).

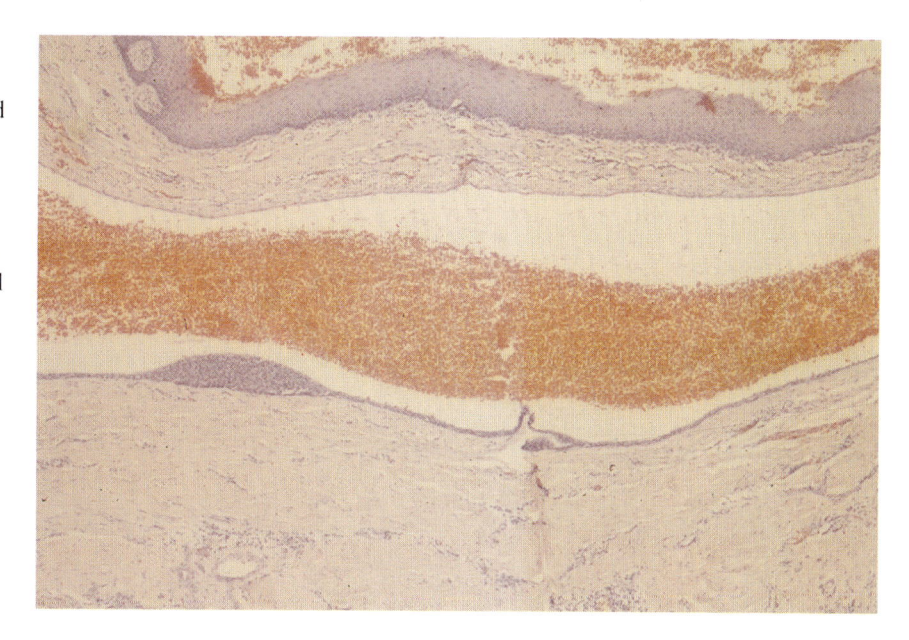

Gingival cyst of the adult

A gingival cyst arises from epithelial cell rests in the gingiva of an adult, and is more or less comparable to the dental lamina cyst of the newborn. Some consider the gingival cyst an extraosseous variant of the lateral periodontal cyst[6,36]. Also the possibility of traumatic implantation of epithelium should be considered in the etiology.

The gingival cyst is nearly always located in the mandible, presenting clinically as a small cystic swelling of the gingiva and producing no, or only subtle, radiographic changes (Fig. 6-7).

Histologically, the epithelial lining may be either very thin - resembling the lining of a lateral periodontal cyst - or may consist of stratified squamous epithelium. The lesion may be multicystic[95].

Treatment consists of surgical removal.

Fig. 6-8a. Basal cell nevi in a patient suffering from basal cell nevus syndrome.

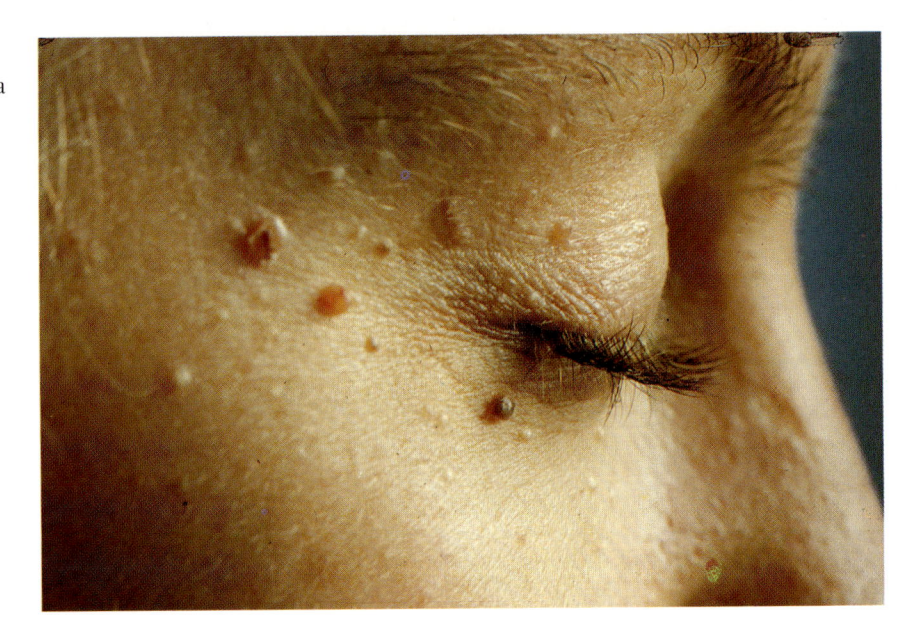

Keratocyst

Definition and epidemiology

The diagnosis of keratocyst, first described by Philipsen in 1956[433], is based on histologic features only, to be described later.

The cyst presumably arises from remnants of the dental lamina or from epithelium of the enamel organ. Some keratocysts possibly develop from the basal cell layer of the oral mucosa. Several authors consider keratocyst and primordial cyst to be synonymous terms. Because of its sometimes aggressive, persistent behavior, some authors have suggested considering this cyst as a benign cystic tumor[13].

Most keratocysts are diagnosed between the ages of 20 and 40. There is no distinct sex preference. In a large series of odontogenic cysts approximately 7% keratocysts were encountered[553].

When multiple keratocysts are found in the jaws, nevoid basal cell carcinoma syndrome appears to be involved in about half of the cases. This syndrome is characterized by multiple keratocysts, basal cell nevi of the skin, and the occurrence of one or more bifid ribs (Figs. 6-8, 6-9)[240]. It should be emphasized that the multiplicity of the jaw cysts refers to the lifetime history of the patient and does not necessarily imply that more than one cyst is present at any one time[626].

Clinical aspects

In 70% of the cases the keratocyst is found in the mandible, usually in the region of the mandibular angle and the ascending

Developmental cysts • 97

Fig. 6-8b. Low-power view of excised basal cell nevus.

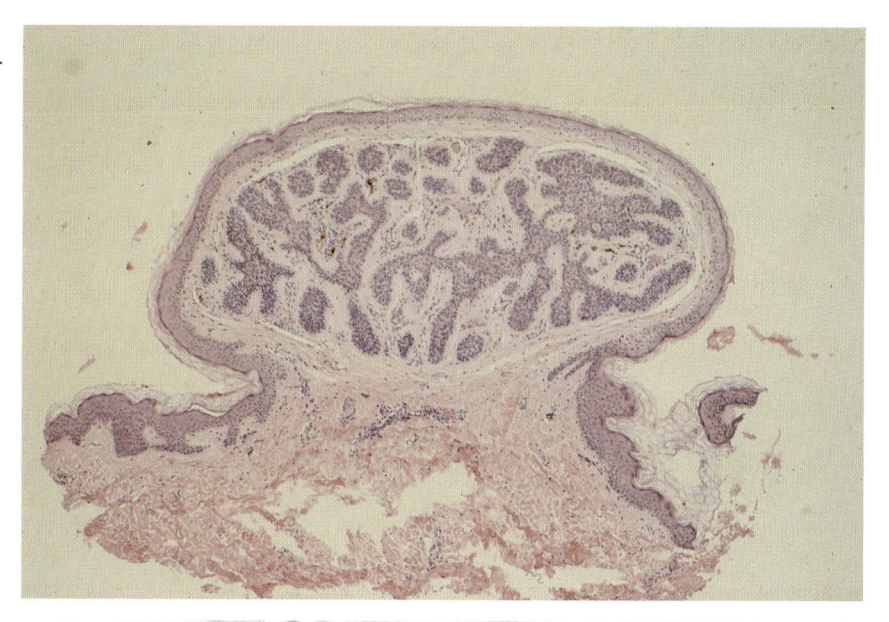

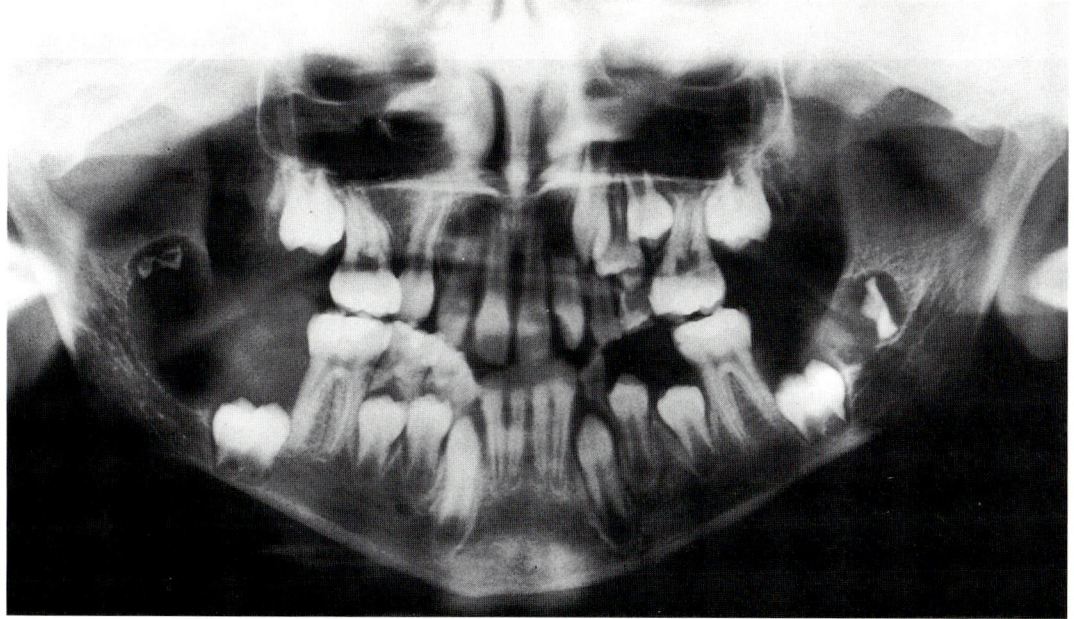

Fig. 6-9a. Odontogenic keratocyst in right and left ascending ramus. In the past, another odontogenic keratocyst has been removed in the upper right bicuspid region. BNS patient.

ramus. In one quarter of the cases a patient with a keratocyst complaints of pain. In a study of 312 patients half had a swelling or an intraoral fistula[80].

98 • Odontogenic cysts

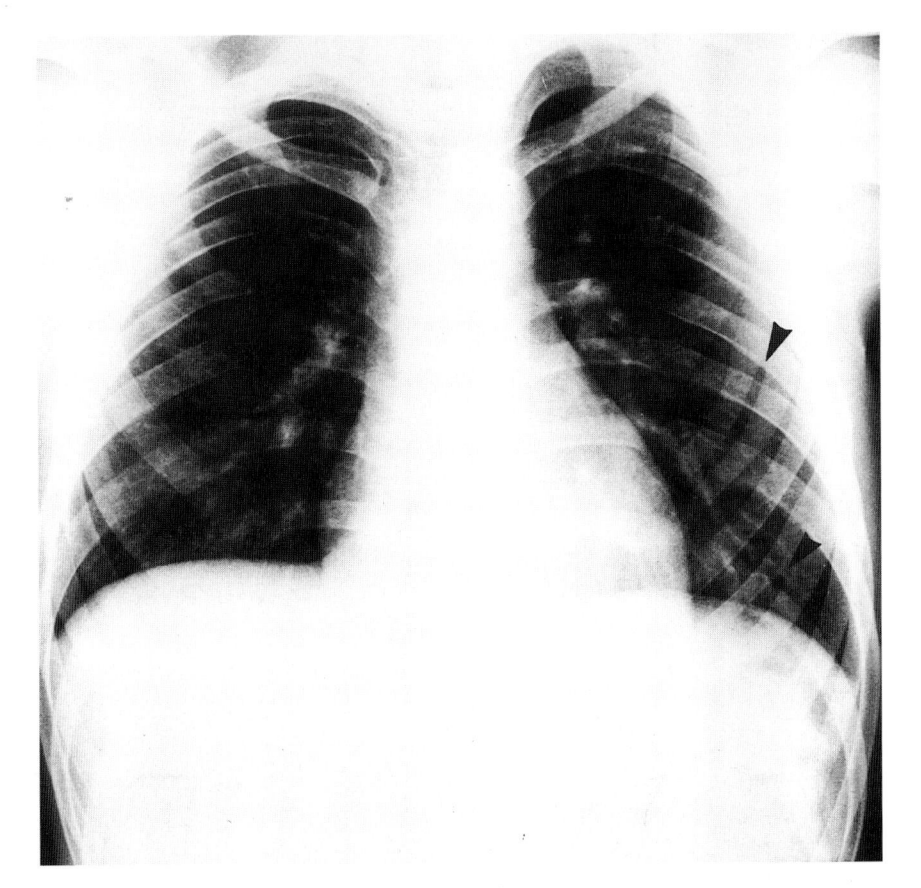

Fig. 6-9b. The chest film shows several bifid ribs.

Radiographic aspects

Radiographically, the keratocyst may present itself in the form of various odontogenic cysts, such as a dentigerous cyst, a lateral periodontal cyst, a primordial cyst, and a residual cyst (Fig. 6-10). Radiographic appearance as a radicular cyst is exceptional[547]. Particularly when the radiograph shows a multilobular cystic lesion, a diagnosis of keratocyst should be considered (Fig. 6-11). A "punching out" and expansion of the cortical bone are indicative of the presence of a keratocyst or an ameloblastoma. In contrast to an ameloblastoma, a keratocyst rarely causes root resorption.

In the radiographic differential diagnosis a central giant cell granuloma and a number of odontogenic tumors, especially the already-mentioned ameloblastoma and an odontogenic myxoma, should be included.

Developmental cysts • 99

Fig. 6-10. Radiographic aspect suggestive of dentigerous cyst of 48. Histologic examination showed the presence of an odontogenic keratocyst.

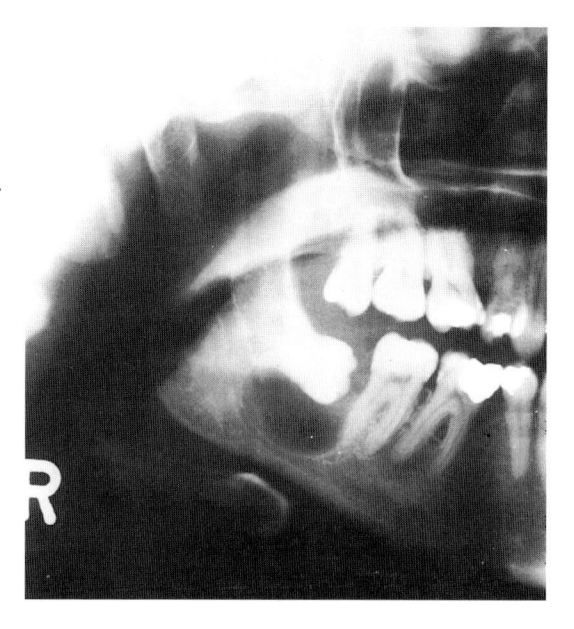

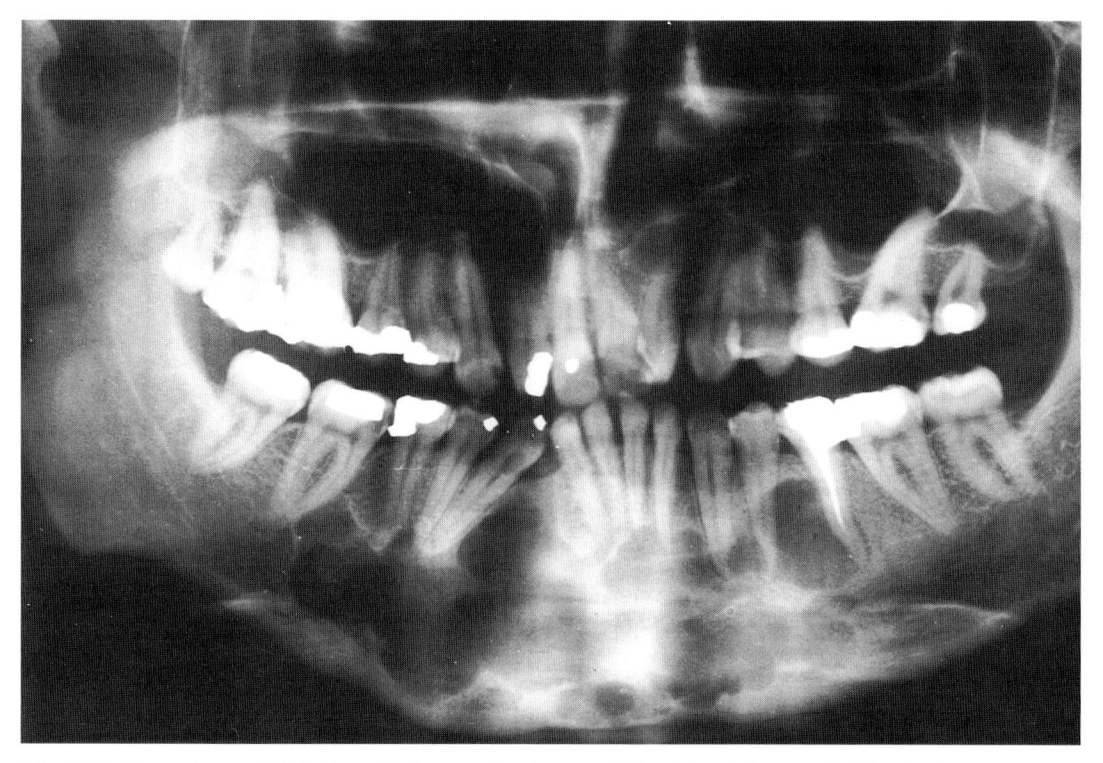

Fig. 6-11. Extensive multilobular radiolucency in the mandible. No missing teeth. Histologic examination showed the presence of an odontogenic keratocyst.

Fig. 6-12a. Low-power view of odontogenic keratocyst. Note the folded appearance of the cyst lumen.

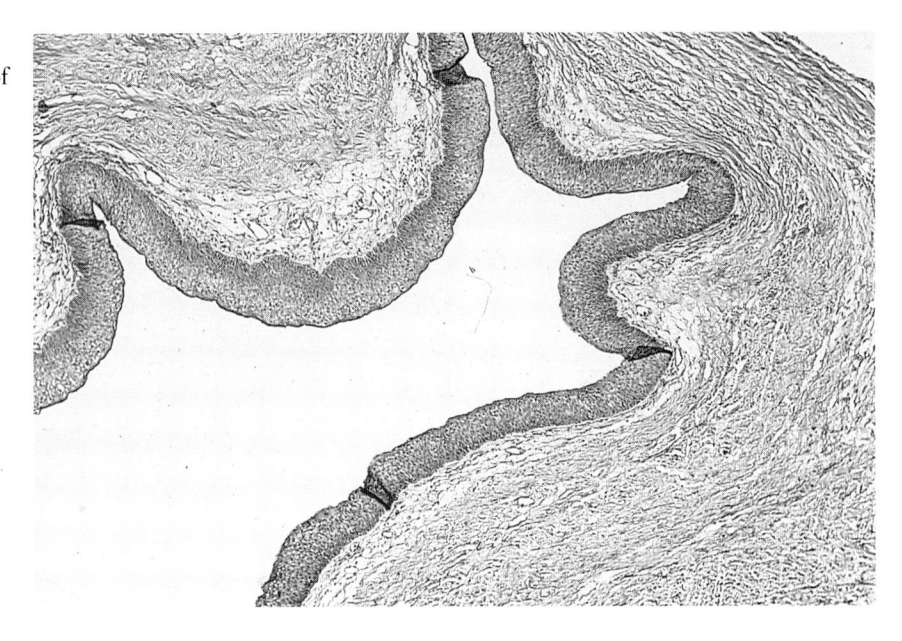

Histologic aspects

The histologic features of a keratocyst are the following (Fig. 6-12):

1. A flat course of the basal cell layer
2. A width of the epithelium of six to eight cell layers
3. Palisading of cells of the basal cell layer
4. A flattening of the cells toward the lumen
5. A corrugated appearance of the epithelium surface
6. Usually parakeratosis, sometimes orthokeratosis of the epithelium
7. Irregular, folded shape of the cyst lumen, that can be filled with keratin
8. Possibly complete absence of inflammatory signs in the cyst wall; sometimes presence of cholesterol crystals, inflammatory cells, and hyaline bodies

In the cyst wall, "daughter cysts" can occur. It is difficult to prove whether these are independent cysts or offshoots from the epithelial lining of the cyst wall. Budding proliferations of the basal cell layer may be indicative of biologically aggressive behavior. Mitoses are not uncommon in the epithelial lining of a keratocyst.

In comparative histologic studies of odontogenic keratocysts in nevoid basal cell carcinoma syndrome and control patients matched for age and site, significant differences between the two groups

Fig. 6-12b. High power view of epithelial lining of odontogenic keratocyst.

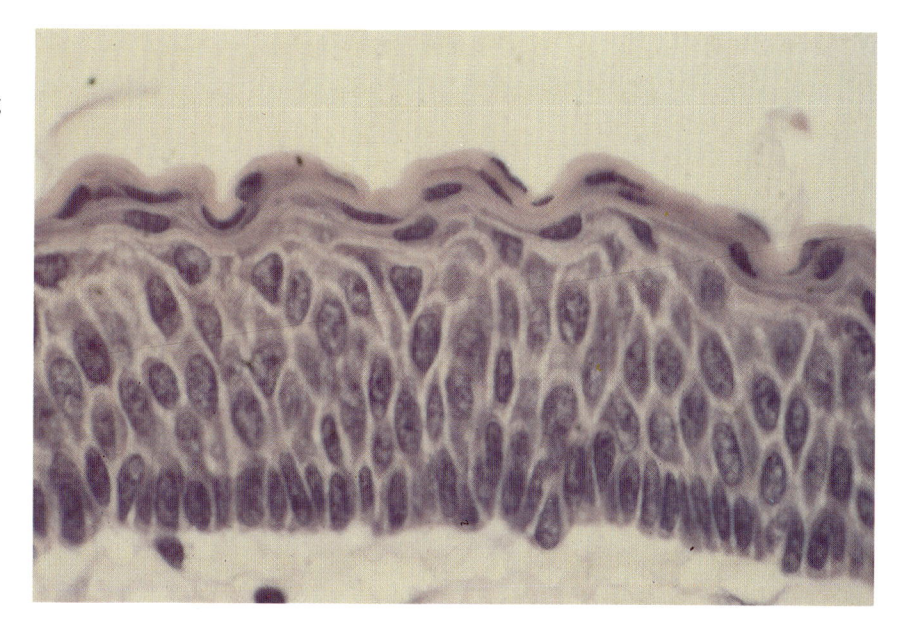

were found in the numbers of satellite cysts, solid islands of epithelial proliferation and odontogenic rests within the capsule, and in the number of mitotic figures in the epithelium lining the main cavity[627, 151]. In a comparative study of the histologic features of recurrent and non-recurrent odontogenic keratocysts no significant histologic differences were observed except for a greater amount of inflammation in the non-recurrent cyst[628].

Ameloblastomatous and malignant changes in the epithelial lining of a keratocyst are unusual[526]. The presence of respiratory epithelium has been reported, as well as of mucous-producing cells, sebaceous glands, and melanin[81].

A distinction should be made between a keratocyst and a keratinizing cyst without the distinctive features of an odontogenic keratocyst. Furthermore, the typical histologic features of a keratocyst may, for the greater part, be lost due to inflammation.

Treatment The keratocyst is distinguished from other odontogenic cysts by a high recurrence rate, which may be more than 50% according to some estimates. Recurrence is probably less frequent in the orthokeratinized variant. Some investigators have shown that the percentage of recurrences does not depend on the type of treatment, e.g. consisting either of enucleation or marsupialization, whereas others show that there is such a correlation (Figs. 6-13, 6-14). In a

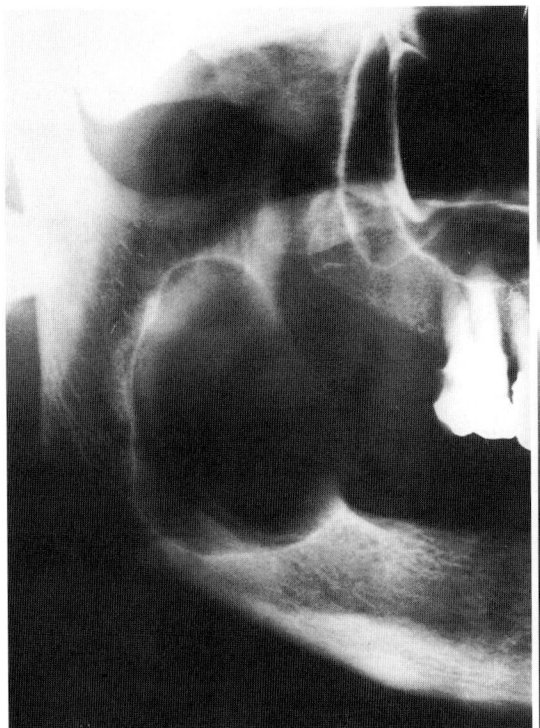

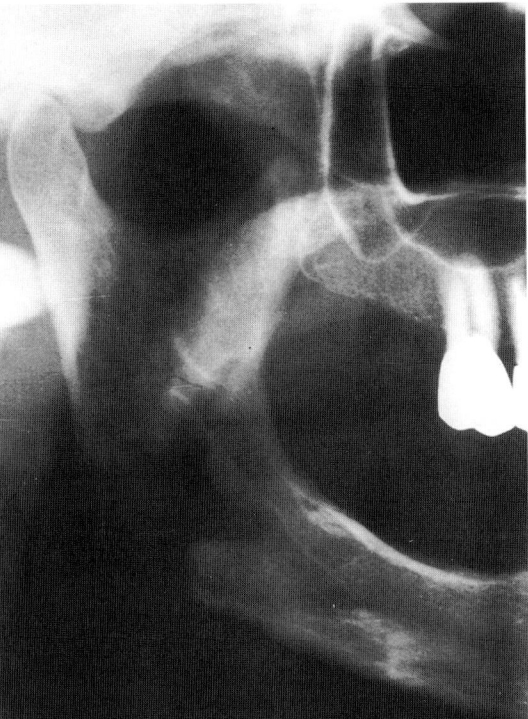

Fig. 6-13a. Odontogenic keratocyst. Treatment consisted of careful enucleation.

Fig. 6-13b. The result one year later.

Swedish study, keratocysts enucleated in one piece recurred significantly less often than cysts enucleated in several pieces; recurrence was also found more frequently in cysts with a multilobular radiographic appearance than in unilobular cysts. On the other hand, the size or the location of the keratocysts did not have an influence on the recurrence rate[197]. In another study the peroperative use of a fixative has been recommended as a measure to prevent local recurrences[593]. Enucleation combined with cryotherapy does not seem to give better results than enucleation alone[295].

It is recommended that patients who have been treated for an odontogenic keratocyst should be followed for at least 10 years at intervals of one to two years.

Developmental cysts • 103

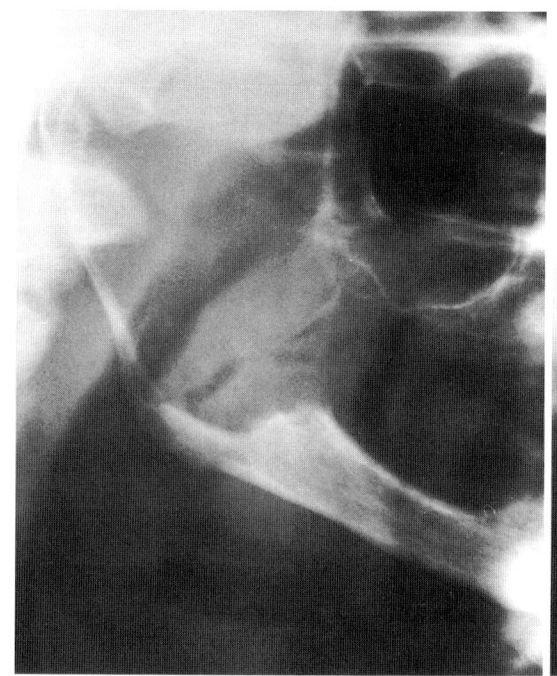

Fig. 6-14a. Odontogenic keratocyst.

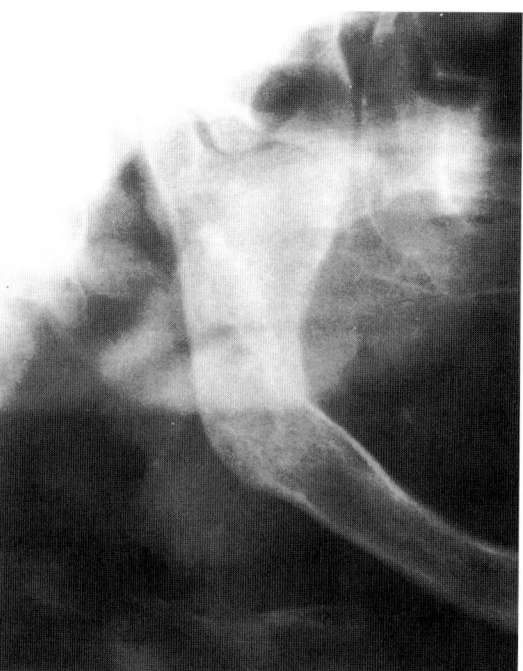

Fig. 6-14c. Treatment consisted of marsupialization. Result one year later.

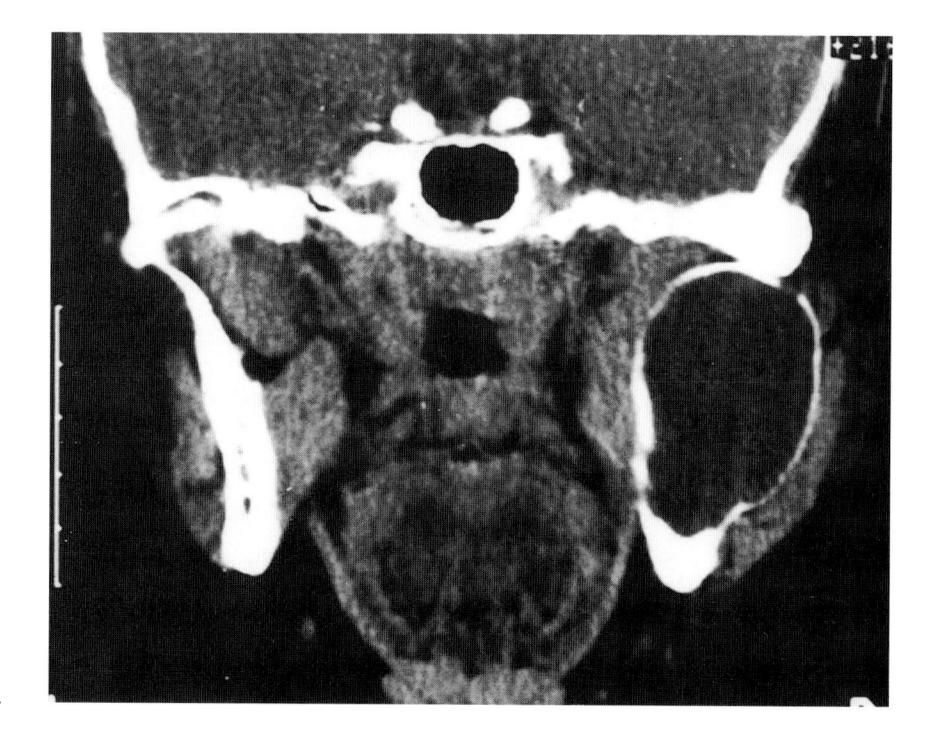

Fig. 6-14b. The CT-scan nicely demonstrates the expansion of the ascending ramus.

Fig. 6-15.
Well-circumscribed radiolucency caused by a lateral periodontal cyst between two vital premolars.
(Courtesy Prof.dr. J.J. Pindborg, Denmark and Prof.dr. M. Shear. U.S.A.).

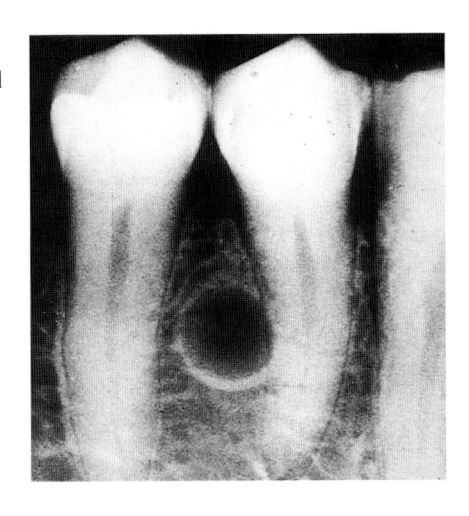

Lateral periodontal cyst (incl. Botryoid odontogenic cyst)

Definition

The lateral periodontal cyst (LPC) is a rather rare developmental cyst that arises in the periodontal ligament of an erupted tooth. The histologic features are rather characteristic.

It is striking that the lateral periodontal cyst occurs almost exclusively in the canine-premolar area of the mandible, an area in which supernumerary teeth are rather common.

There is no sex preference. The diagnosis can be made at all ages.

Clinical aspects

Clinically, LPC rarely if ever gives rise to complaints and is often detected as an incidental finding on the radiograph. The adjacent teeth, remain vital. Otherwise, one is most likely dealing with a laterally located radicular cyst. On probing the gingiva of the adjacent teeth no communication with the cyst should be present. In some cases a slight buccal or lingual expansion may be noticed[165].

Radiographic aspects

Radiographically, the LPC can be described as a well-confined lucency that is seldom larger than 1 cm, situated against the lateral surface of a tooth (Fig. 6-15). The botryoid odontogenic cyst is usually lobulated and reaches beyond the adjacent teeth.

Histologic aspects

Upon microscopic examination, a lining of stratified squamous epithelium can be seen. The epithelial lining is sometimes only one or two cell layers thick. In the typical case, plaquelike thickenings in the epithelial lining are present (Fig. 6-16). In the presence of a multicystic appearance, the term botryoid odontogenic cyst may be appropriate[432].

Fig. 6-16a. Multilobular ("botryoid") lateral periodontal cyst.

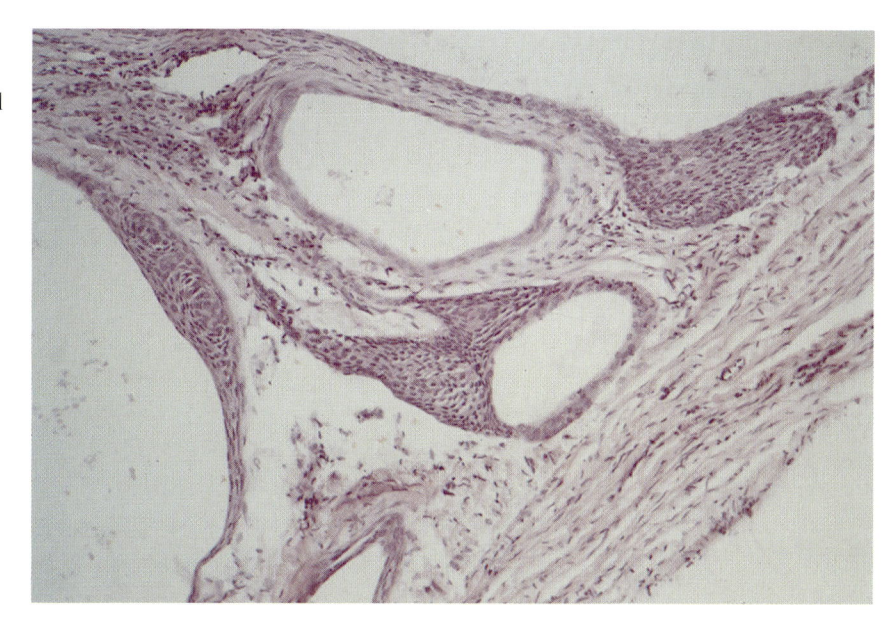

Fig. 6-16b. Notice the plaque-like thickenings of the epithelial lining.

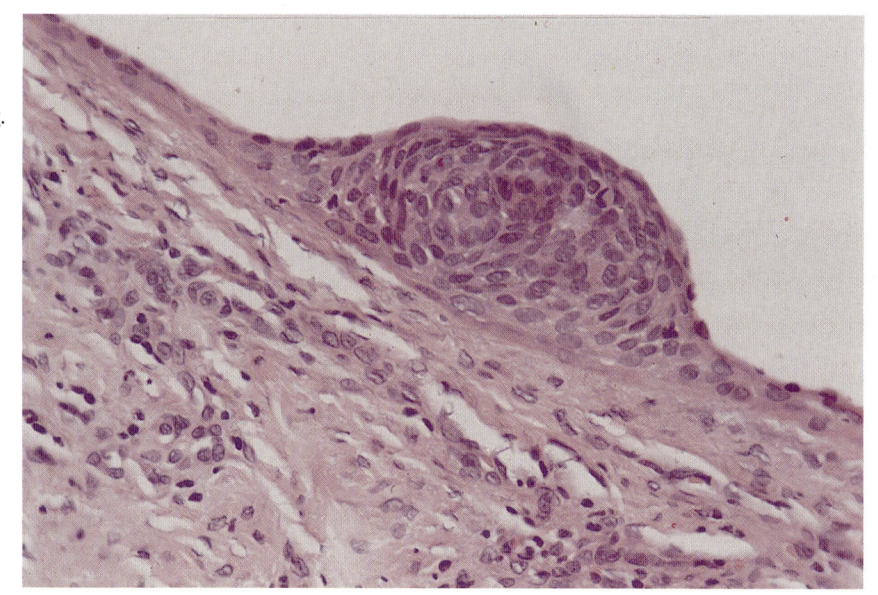

If features of an odontogenic keratocyst are observed[184], a final diagnosis of odontogenic keratocyst should instead be made.

Treatment

Treatment consists of surgical removal. Long-term follow-up is advisable, especially when dealing with the "botryoid" type. Recurrences of the latter type have been reported to occur up to a decade after initial surgery[232].

Primordial cyst

The primordial cyst (PC) is a rather uncommon cyst, located within the bone. The origin of a PC is explained by cystic changes in a developing tooth germ before dentin and enamel matrix have been formed. PC is a clinical-radiologic diagnosis that requires histologic confirmation.

The primordial cyst may cause swelling of the alveolar ridge or displacement of teeth. Radiographically, the primordial cyst may be expressed as a uni- or multilobular circumscribed, lucent lesion. It may be found at a site where a tooth has failed to develop. Otherwise, the cyst may have arisen from a supernumerary tooth germ.

Histologically, the characteristic features of a keratocyst are frequently seen; according to some investigators those features are present in all primordial cysts. Thus, the term keratocyst might be used synonymously or even preferentially. Others prefer to retain the term and entity of primordial cyst[518].

Sialo-odontogenic cyst (Glandular odontogenic cyst)

A few cases have been reported of an intraosseous jaw cyst that shows histologic features, such as the presence of mucin and salivary gland tissue[213, 422]. Furthermore, there is some resemblance to the so-called mucoepidermoid carcinoma. In view of the small number of cases reported so far, it is unsettled yet as to whether the sialo-odontogenic cyst, also referred to as glandular odontogenic cyst, in fact represents a separate entity.

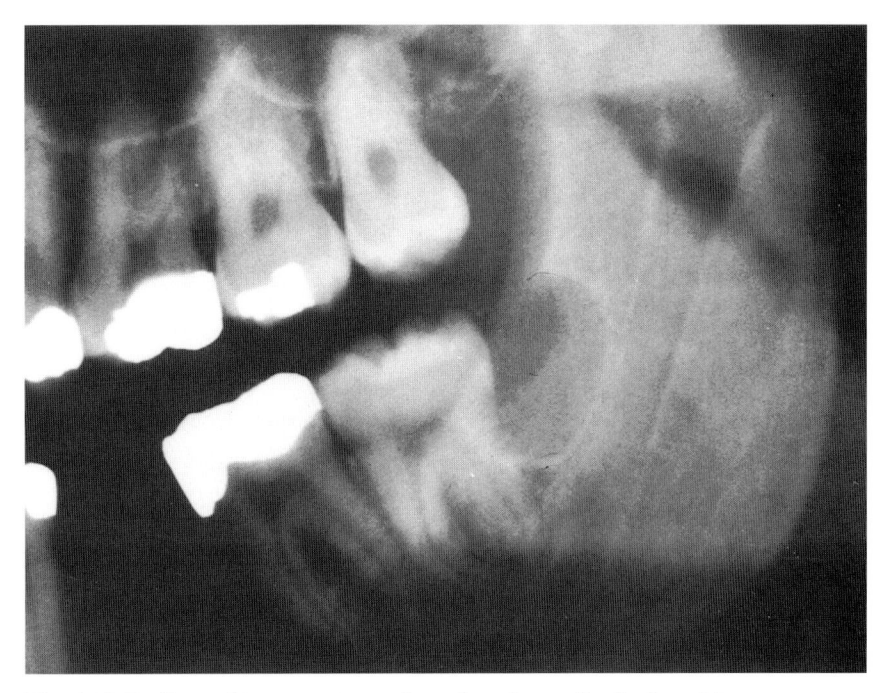

Fig. 6-17. Radiographic appearance of paradental cyst distally from 38.

Inflammatory cysts

Paradental cyst

In 1976, Craig introduced the term paradental cyst[131]. He reported 49 patients with cysts that were almost all situated buccally against the root surface of a partially erupted mandibular third molar, accompanied by pericoronitis (Fig. 6-17). Many of the involved teeth showed an enamel projection buccally at the cemento-enamel junction near the bifurcation.

In a more recent study of 50 cases a marked preponderance in males was noticed[7]. In a series of 27 cases from Denmark no sex difference was observed[586].

The diagnosis of paradental cyst is mainly a clinical one, since many of these cysts are sometimes barely visible on the radiograph. Histologically, a non-keratinized stratified squamous epithelial lining with a dense inflammatory infiltrate in the cyst wall can be observed.

Radicular cyst

Definition and pathogenesis

The radicular cyst is the most common odontogenic cyst. Also the term apical periodontal cyst has been used. The diagnosis of radicular cyst is a clinical-radiologic one that requires histologic confirmation. This radicular cyst develops at the apex of a tooth. It is not clear why in some cases of periapical inflammation cyst formation takes place and in others not. Possibly, in time, each periapical granuloma will develop into a radicular cyst. The rather short time span might be the reason why radicular cysts rarely if ever occur in the deciduous dentition.

The epithelial lining of a radicular cyst probably arises from epithelial rests of Malassez located in the periodontal ligament.

Clinical aspects

Clinically, a radicular cyst may appear as a hard swelling near the apex of the involved tooth. A radicular cyst is often asymptomatic. In some cases, exacerbation of a radicular cyst gives rise to a subperiosteal, submucous, or subcutaneous abscess. In rare instances, transition into intramedullary osteomyelitis may occur[268]. Exacerbation may also enhance the mobility of the tooth. In case of a single-rooted tooth, the vitality test will always be negative. In case of multi-rooted teeth the contents of one root canal might be necrotic - which may induce the development of a radicular cyst - whereas the contents of the other root canal(s) may be vital, as expressed in a positive vitality test.

Radiographic aspects

The radiograph shows a well-circumscribed lucency at the apex (Fig. 6-18). Depending on the position of the apical foramen, the cyst can be located against the lateral surface of a tooth.

If a periapical lucency is present in a tooth that reacts positive to the vitality test, an early stage of a (periapical) fibro-osseous cemental lesion should be considered.

In the lower bicuspids the possibility of projection of the mental foramen to the apex should be taken into account[652].

Histologic aspects

The lining of a radicular cyst consists of non-keratinizing stratified squamous epithelium (Fig. 6-19). In radicular cysts of the maxilla, respiratory epithelium may be found. Radicular cysts rarely display the features of a keratocyst. If they do, the final diagnosis should be changed into "odontogenic keratocyst".

The thickness of the epithelium can vary greatly and appears not to be correlated with the degree of inflammation. Goblet cells may

Inflammatory cysts • 109

Fig. 6-18.
Periapical radiolucency at apex of non-vital 11. The diagnosis "cyst" requires the histologic demonstration of an epithelial lining.

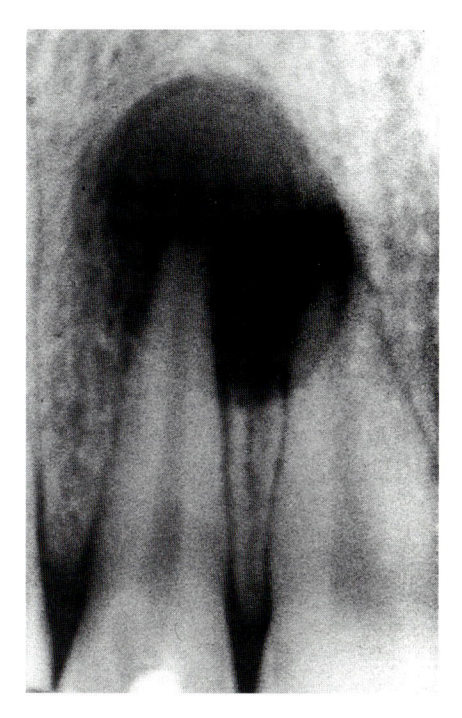

Fig. 6-19.
Low-power view of cross-section through radicular cyst.

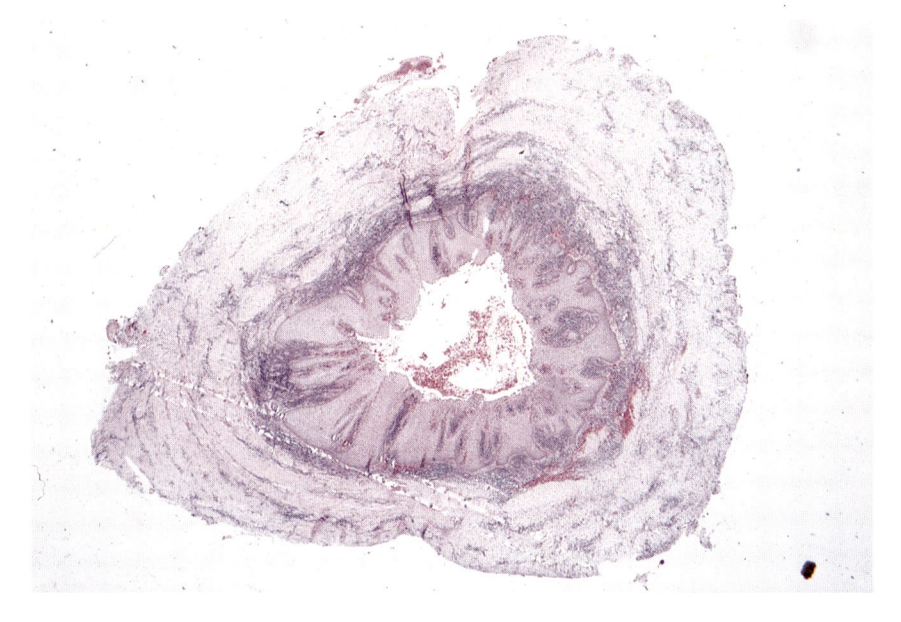

sometimes occur. The cyst wall may contain accumulations of inflammatory cells. Frequently, cholesterol crystals are found, probably as a result of bleeding in the cyst wall. Macrophages with a foamy cytoplasma, called foam cells, are also frequently found. Occasionally, colonies of actinomycetes are found. The development of an ameloblastoma or a squamous cell carcinoma from the epithelium of a radicular cyst is exceptional[595].

Although unfavorable epithelial changes occur less frequently in the radicular cyst than in some of the other odontogenic cysts, it is recommended that each radicular cyst be examined histologically.

Treatment

Root canal treatment alone suffices in case of a small periapical radiolucency of about 1-2 cm, and it does not require surgical elimination of the periapical inflammatory tissue. If radiographic observation after six months does not show a distinct healing of the periapical area, surgical exploration is recommended.

Treatment of a large radicular cyst may consist of extraction of the tooth and enucleation of the cyst, or enucleation of the cyst alone with simultaneously performed apicoectomy and root canal treatment. Some authors have described the successful use of implant material for filling up large cystic defects[573].

Residual cyst

Definition

When a tooth with a radicular cyst is extracted and the cyst is left behind, the cyst may remain unchanged or even increase in size, resulting in a so-called residual cyst. Similarly, after removal of an impacted tooth, parts of a dentigerous cyst or remnants of the follicle may be left behind and develop into a cyst. This, too, could be called a residual cyst. In general, however, the term residual cyst is used to designate a remaining radicular cyst. Some authors, indeed, use the term "residual radicular cyst". It is a clinical-radiologic diagnosis that requires histologic confirmation.

Clinical aspects

Residual cysts mainly occur in the mandibular premolar region. The majority of residual cysts are discovered as an incidental finding on the radiograph. In rare cases swelling is present (Fig. 6-20). Pain is usually absent.

Radiographic aspects

The residual cyst is usually depicted on the radiograph as a solitary, well-circumscribed and corticated lucent lesion. For the radio-

Fig. 6-20a. Swelling caused by a residual cyst.

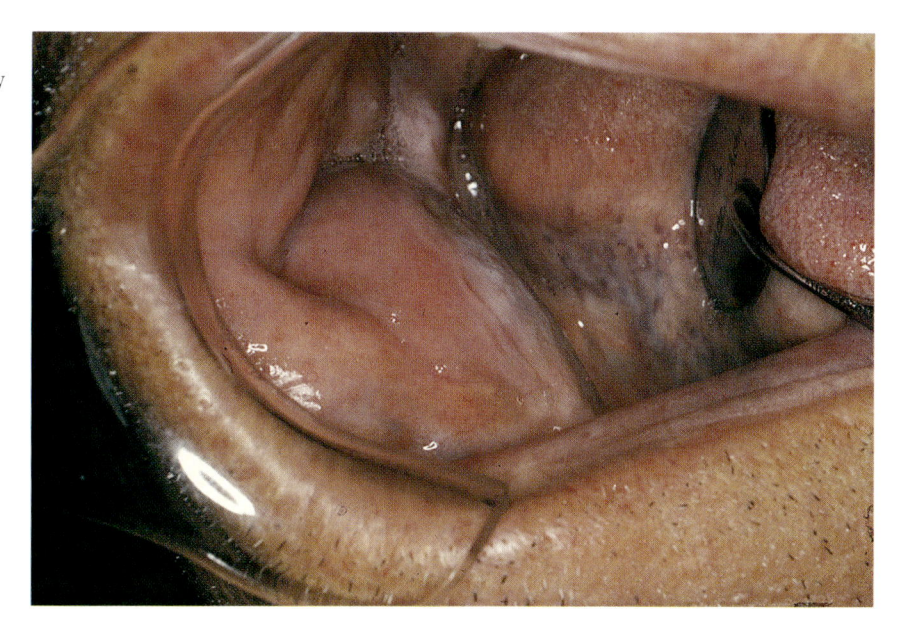

Fig. 6-20b. The radiograph shows a non-characteristic aspect of a residual cyst.

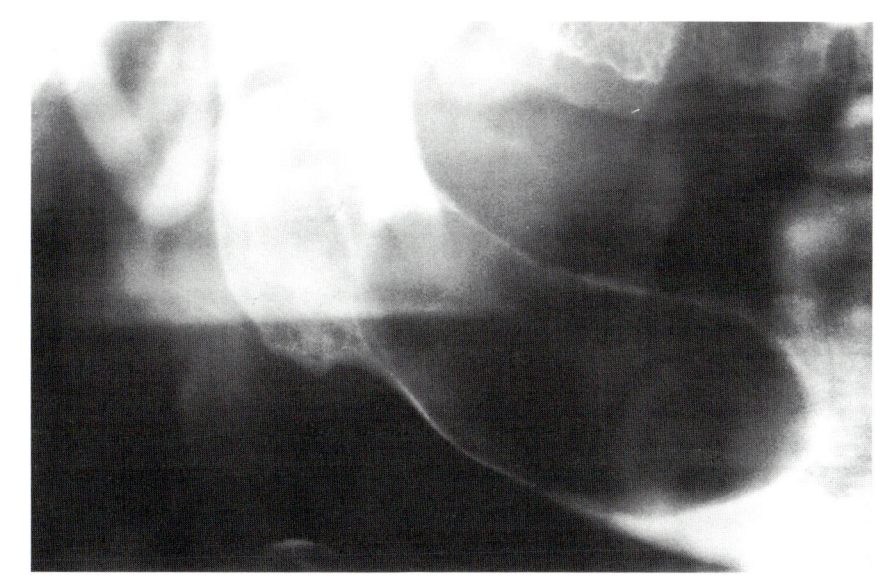

graphic differential diagnosis many possibilities may be considered, such as ameloblastoma, odontogenic myxoma, central giant cell granuloma, primordial cyst, keratocyst, bone cyst, and even a metastatic process.

Fig. 6-21. Hyaline bodies in the epithelial lining of a residual cyst.

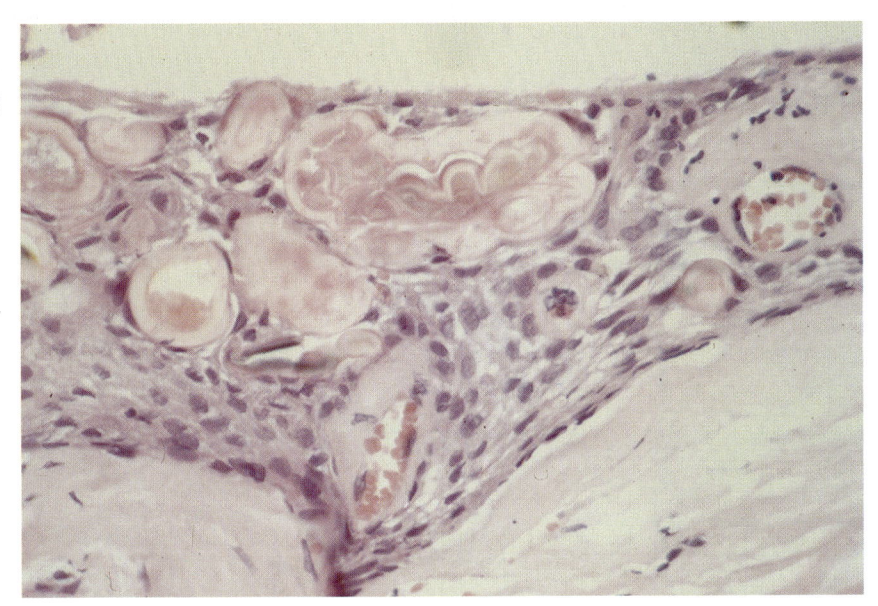

Histologic aspects

Histologically, the residual cyst does not show differences from the radicular cyst. In longstanding cysts dystrophic calcifications may take place[272]. Also hyaline bodies, so-called Rushton bodies, are frequently seen in the epithelium and sometimes also in the cyst wall (Fig. 6-21). Occasionally, the features of a keratocyst or an ameloblastoma may be encountered. Malignant changes are exceptional[595].

Treatment

Treatment of a residual cyst consists of enucleation. In extremely large cysts, in which primary enucleation would enhance the risk of a fracture, marsupialization may be considered.

Mandibular infected buccal cyst

A few cases of so-called mandibular infected buccal cysts occurring in children have been reported[101]. It is questionable at this stage whether this cyst, in fact, represents an entity of its own or merely is a variant of a paradental cyst.

CHAPTER 7

Neoplasms of primary bone origin

In this chapter only neoplasms of primary bone origin will be discussed. Neoplasms of chondroid tissue will be discussed in chapter 8, while neoplasms of other origin will be dealt with in chapters 9 and 10.

Benign neoplasms

Osteoma

Definition and epidemiology

An osteoma is a benign lesion consisting of well-differentiated mature bone tissue, with a predominantly lamellar structure, and showing very slow growth[500].

Osteomas are more or less restricted to the skull and the mandible, and mainly occur in patients between 15 and 30 years of age[501]. An osteoma may also appear as a choristoma in the soft tissues of the oral cavity, in particular in the dorsal surface of the tongue. That entity will not be discussed here any further.

Clinical aspects

True osteomas of the jaws are exceedingly rare and occur almost exclusively in the mandible[470]. They are often asymptomatic and may spontaneously stop growing. The lesion is bony hard.

Multiple osteomas of the jaws are a characteristic feature of Gardner's syndrome, which consists of multiple polyps in the colon and rectum, multiple cutaneous and subcutaneous tumors, osteomas of the long bones, the skull, and the jaws, and multiple impacted, supernumerary teeth (Fig. 7-1)[37, 656]. The disorder is of an autosomal dominant trait. A few cases have been reported in which no hereditary pattern could be recognized[150]. It has been observed that familial polyposis coli is often accompanied by gastric polyps and occult osteomatous changes of the mandible. Therefore, it has

114 • Neoplasms of primary bone origin

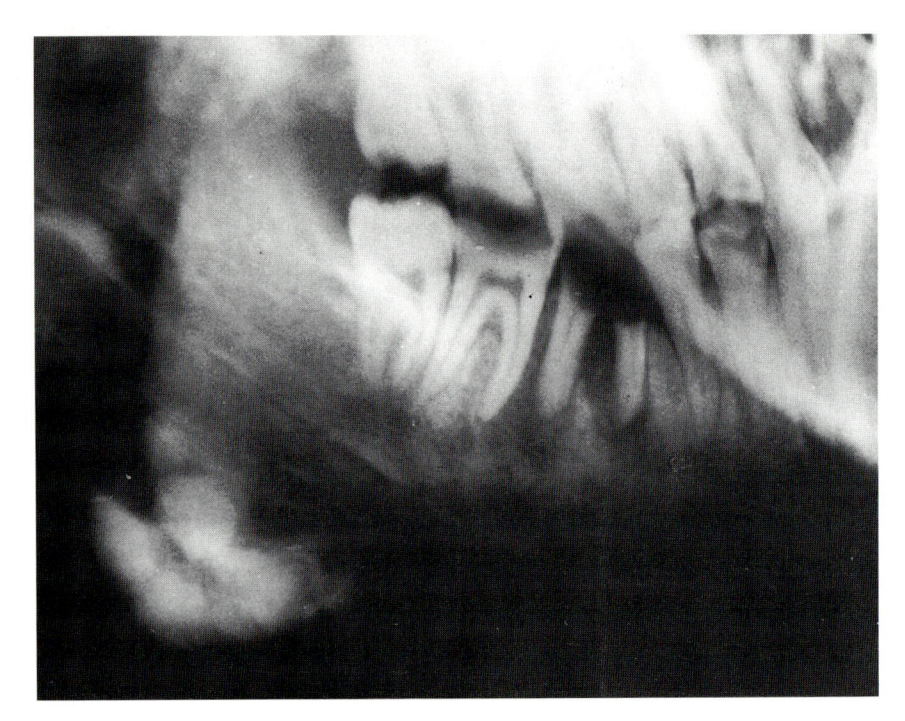

Fig. 7-1a. Osteoma at the angle of the mandible in a 17-year-old boy.

Fig. 7-1b. A surgical correction was performed and a histologic diagnosis of osteoma was made.

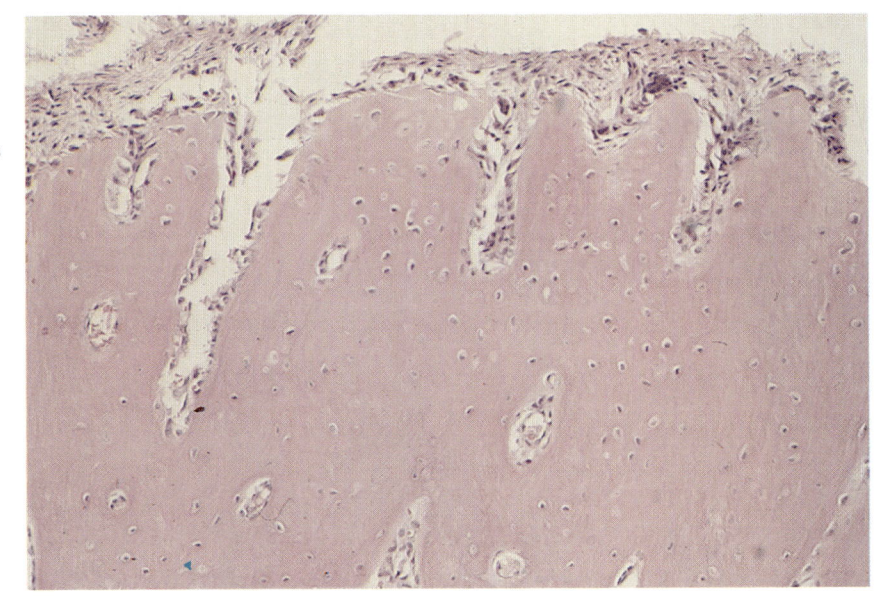

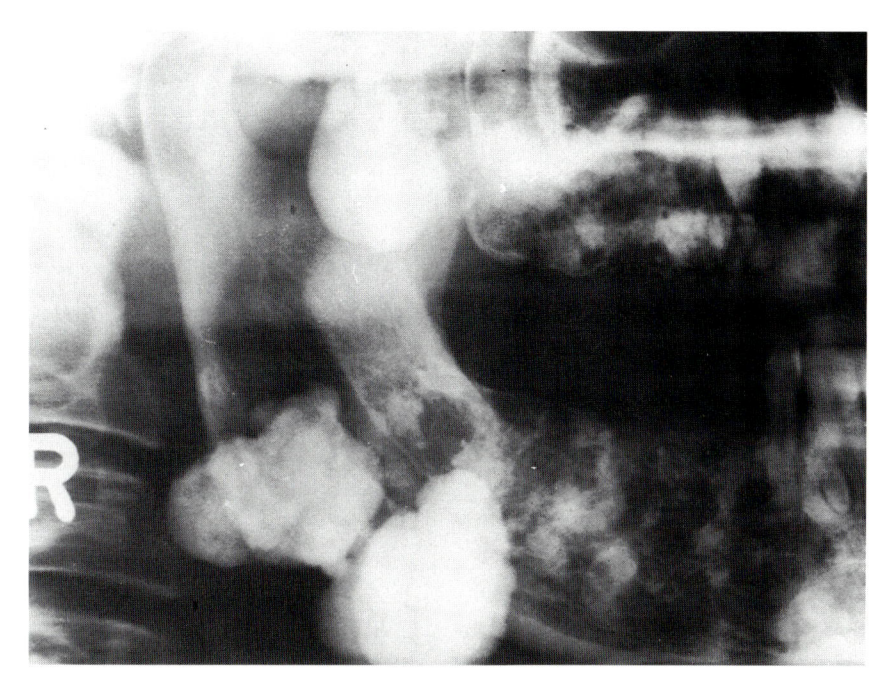

Fig. 7-1c. The patient was seen again after 20 years.

Fig. 7-1d. Only at that time was a diagnosis of Gardner's syndrome made. The patient died two years later from colon cancer.

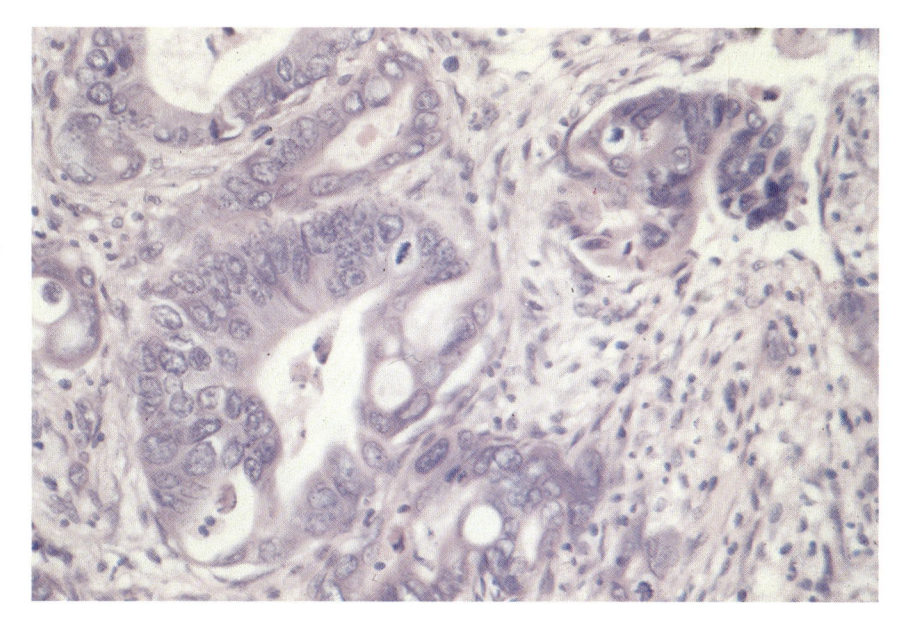

been considered that familial polyposis coli and Gardner's syndrome are substantially the same entity[318].

A single osteoma of the mandible can be the first manifestation of Gardner's syndrome. In a study of 50 patients with familial adenomatosis coli osteomatous jaw changes were seen in 82% as compared with 10% in matched controls; supernumerary teeth, compound odontomas and/or impacted teeth were observed in 30% of the patients compared with 4% of the controls[622]. In a somewhat similar study osteomatous lesions were present in 62% of the patients with adenomatosis coli[303].

By age 40 malignant changes often occur in the intestinal polyps. Because of the inherent risk of malignant change, prophylactic colectomy may be considered as soon as the diagnosis is substantiated.

Radiographic aspects

The radiograph of an osteoma of the jaws shows a rather circumscribed, opaque structure.

Histologic aspects

Microscopic examination shows well-differentiated mature bone tissue, with a predominantly lamellar structure, without the presence of a true capsule. The bony tissue may be exceedingly compact. Apparently, there are no histologic differences between isolated osteomas and osteomas in patients suffering from Gardner's syndrome. Occasionally, foci of cartilage or myxomatous tissue are encountered in an otherwise cellular stroma, in which case the term osteochondroma may be applied[78].

Treatment

Treatment consists of surgical removal. Recurrences are uncommon[74]. Malignant transformation has never been reported.

Osteoblastoma (incl. Osteoid osteoma)

Definition

In the WHO-classification the *osteoid osteoma* is defined as "A benign osteoblastic lesion characterized by its small size (usually less than 1 cm), its clearly demarcated outline, and by the usual presence of a surrounding zone of reactive bone formation. Histologically, it consists of cellular, highly-vascularized tissue made up of immature bone and osteoid bone"[500].

The *osteoblastoma* is defined as "A benign lesion with a histological structure similar to that of osteoid osteoma, but characterized by its larger size (usually more than 1 cm) and by the usual absence of any surrounding zone of reactive bone formation"[500].

Many investigators question whether the osteoid osteoma can be distinguished from the benign osteoblastoma and use the term osteoid osteoma for lesions smaller than 2 cm and the term osteoblastoma for larger ones.

Epidemiology

An osteoid osteoma or an osteoblastoma located in the skeleton is quite rare, usually appears under the age of 20 years, and is more often seen in men than in women.

The literature contains hardly any report of lesions called osteoid osteoma of the jaws. Approximately 80 cases have been reported using the term osteoblastoma[172, 490].

Clinical aspects

In the reported osteoblastomas, the main clinical feature consisted of an expansile, bony hard lesion (Fig. 7-2). In a number of cases other symptoms such as pain or discomfort have been mentioned.

Radiographic aspects

On the radiograph a quite well-circumscribed, radiolucent lesion may be observed. Sometimes a mixed radiolucent-radiopaque aspect is present. In a study in which the findings in osteoblastomas of the jaws were compared with those located elsewhere in the skeleton the radiologic and histologic features in the gnathic and extragnathic sites were shown to be similar[543].

Histologic aspects

Microscopic examination reveals vascular connective tissue with giant cells and proliferation of osteoblasts producing anastomosing trabeculae of osteoid, immature and cementumlike bone. A few mitoses may be present. There is no true encapsulation. The distinction between an osteoblastoma and a low-grade osteosarcoma can at times be difficult from a histopathologic point of view[124].

The division of osteoblastoma into benign and aggressive sub-

118 • Neoplasms of primary bone origin

Fig. 7-2a. Bony hard, palatal expansion caused by an osteoblastoma.

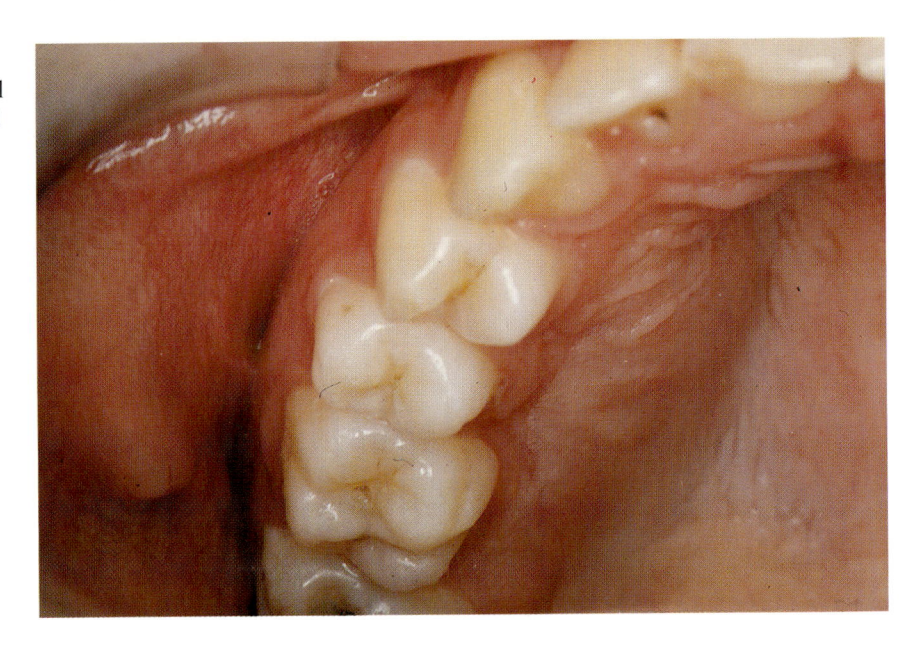

Fig. 7-2b. The periapical film showed mixed radiolucent-radiopaque changes around the apex of 15.

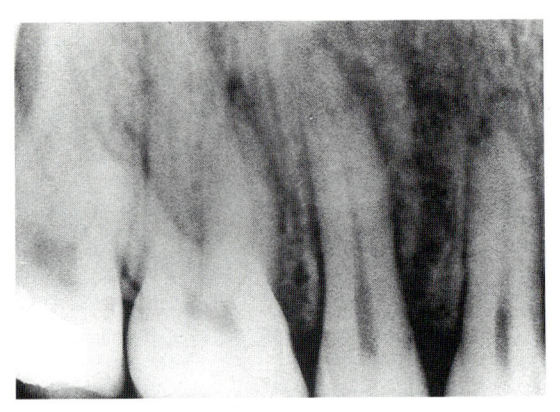

groups, based on histologic criteria only, seems to represent a somewhat artificial classification[412].

Treatment   Treatment consists of curettage or local excision. Some authors advocate performing preoperative embolization[420]. A rare case of spontaneous regression after the taking of a biopsy has been reported[162].

Fig. 7-2c. The biopsy revealed the rather characteristic features of an osteoblastoma.

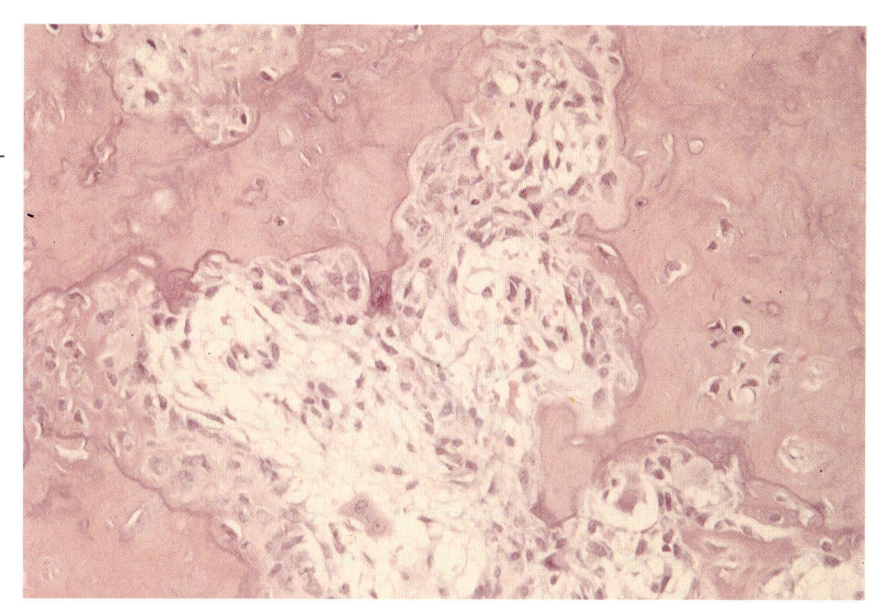

Malignant neoplasms

Osteosarcoma

Definition and epidemiology

An osteosarcoma is a malignant tumor, characterized by the direct formation of bone or osteoid tissue by the tumor cells[500].

The osteosarcoma is seen particularly in patients between 10 and 25 years of age. The lesion appears more often in men than in women, and has a preference for the long bones, particularly the femur and the tibia.

Approximately 6% of all osteosarcomas are located in the jaws, the incidence in the USA being somewhat less than 1 per million population per year. Osteosarcomas occur more often in the mandible than in the maxilla.

Etiology

An osteosarcoma sometimes seems to develop after trauma. However, no definite evidence exists that trauma is actually a causative factor. Occasionally, an osteosarcoma develops in a patient affected by Paget's disease or in a patient who has been irradiated either for a benign bone lesion or for adjacent soft tissue disease[269, 663]. The latent time period may vary widely.

Clinical aspects

Most osteosarcomas of the jaws are centrally located in the bone.

120 • Neoplasms of primary bone origin

Fig. 7-3a. Firm elastic swelling of mandibular mucobuccal fold based on osteosarcoma.

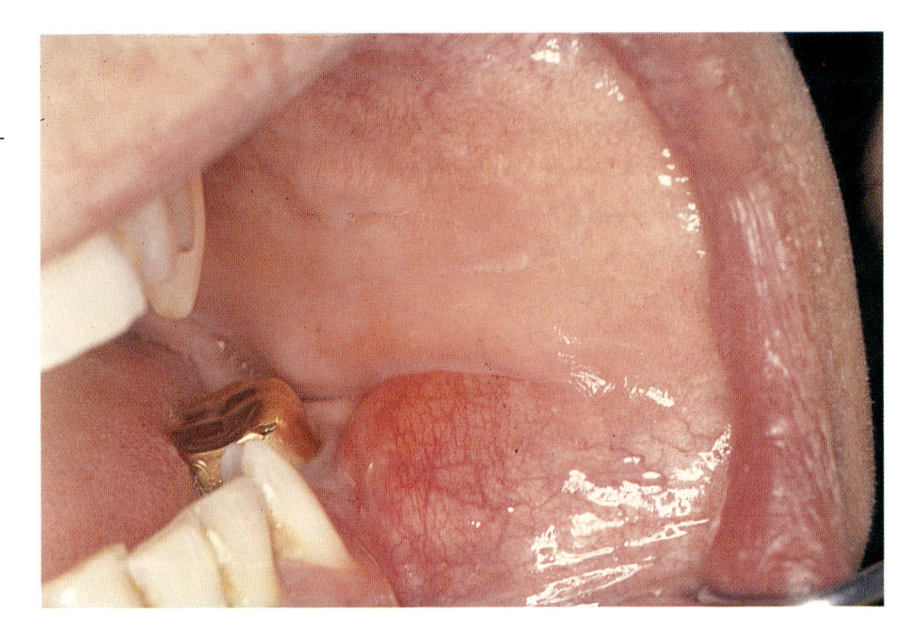

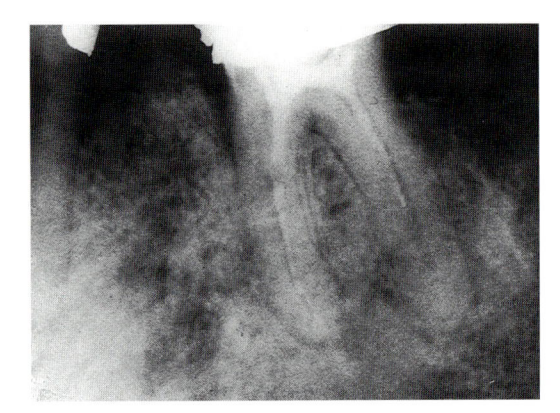

Fig. 7-3b. In view of the poor root canal treatment in 36 a diagnosis of sclerosing osteomyelitis could be suggested.

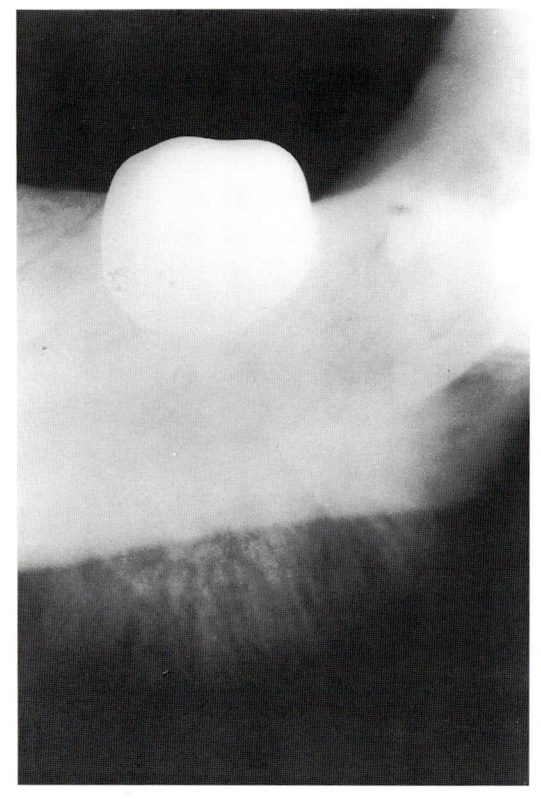

Fig. 7-3c. The occlusal view, however, shows the suspicious "sunray" aspect of an osteosarcoma.

Fig. 7-4a. Palatal swelling caused by osteosarcoma. Some deciduous teeth had been extracted three days previously.

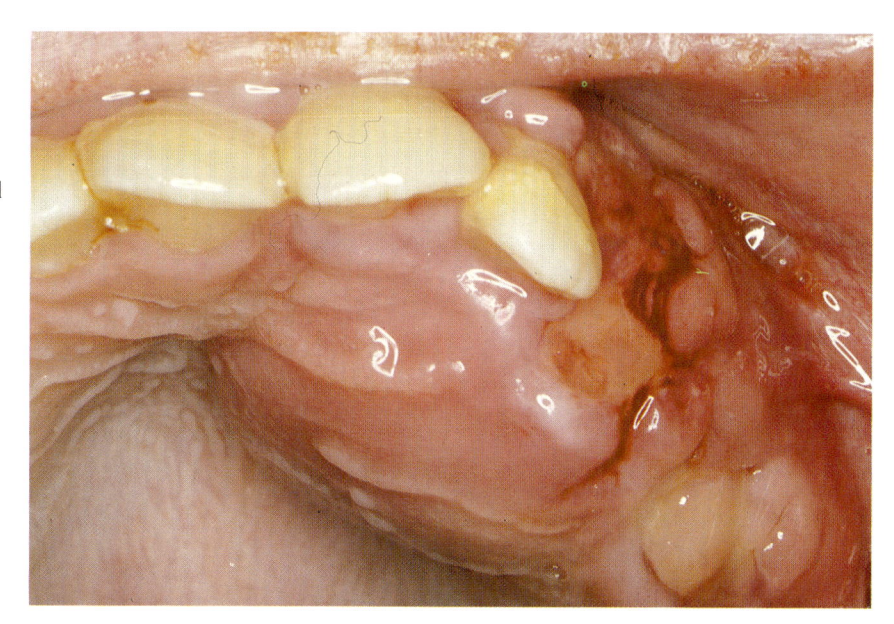

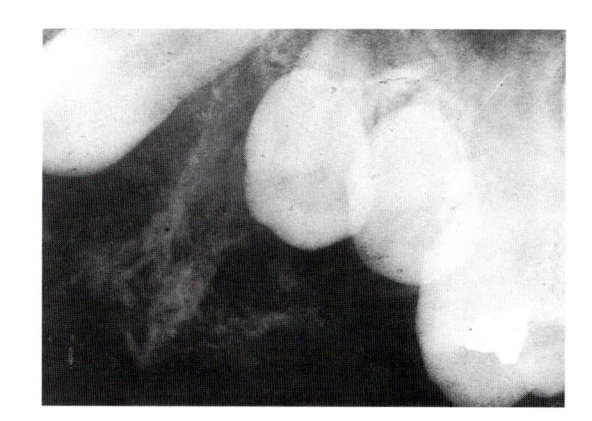

Fig. 7-4b. Effacement of outline of tooth follicles of 23, 24 and 25.

Juxtacortical or parosteal location, which means a location directly to the outer surface of the cortical bone, is somewhat exceptional[82, 667].

The symptoms consist of swelling, mobile teeth, anesthesia or paresthesia, toothache, and nasal obstruction (Figs. 7-3 to 7-6). In many cases there is an apparently unavoidable patient's and doctor's delay.

It is exceptional to come across a metastatic or possible multicentric osteosarcoma[556]. Furthermore, a rare case of simultaneous occurrence in the mandible and maxilla[199], and of an osteosarcoma of the mandible and lung cancer have been reported[414].

122 • Neoplasms of primary bone origin

Fig. 7-5a. Swelling of the maxilla caused by osteosarcoma.

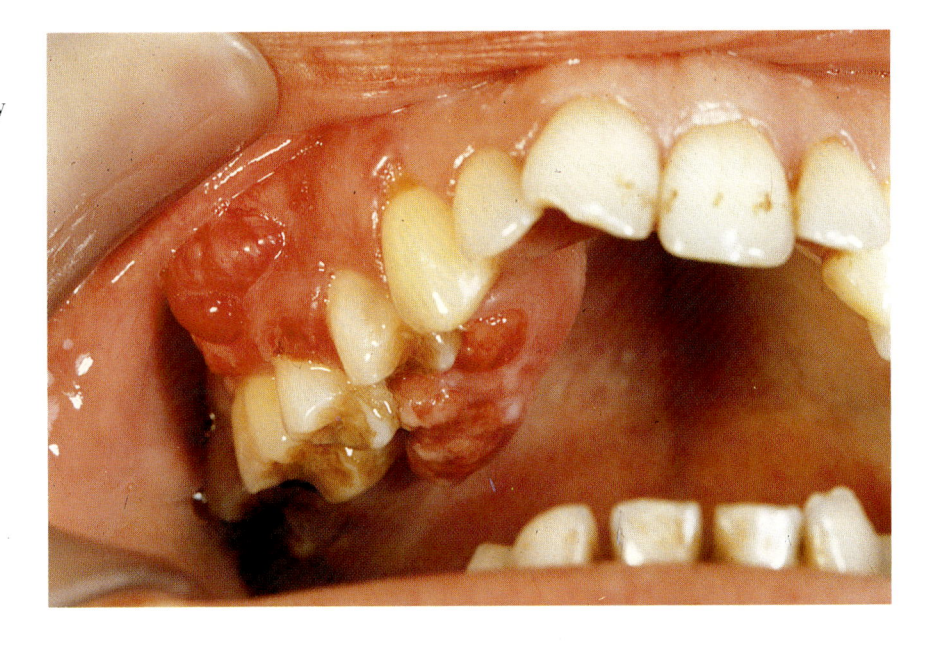

Fig. 7-5b. Notice the more or less symmetrical widening of the periodontal ligament, especially around 14 and 15. (Courtesy Dr. H. Seydell, The Netherlands).

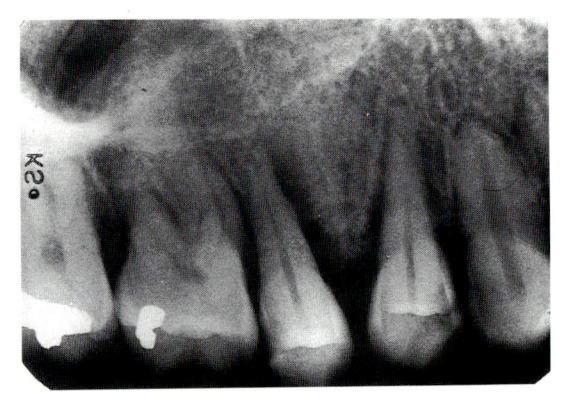

Malignant neoplasms • 123

Fig. 7-6a.
Clinical aspect of osteosarcoma of the maxilla.

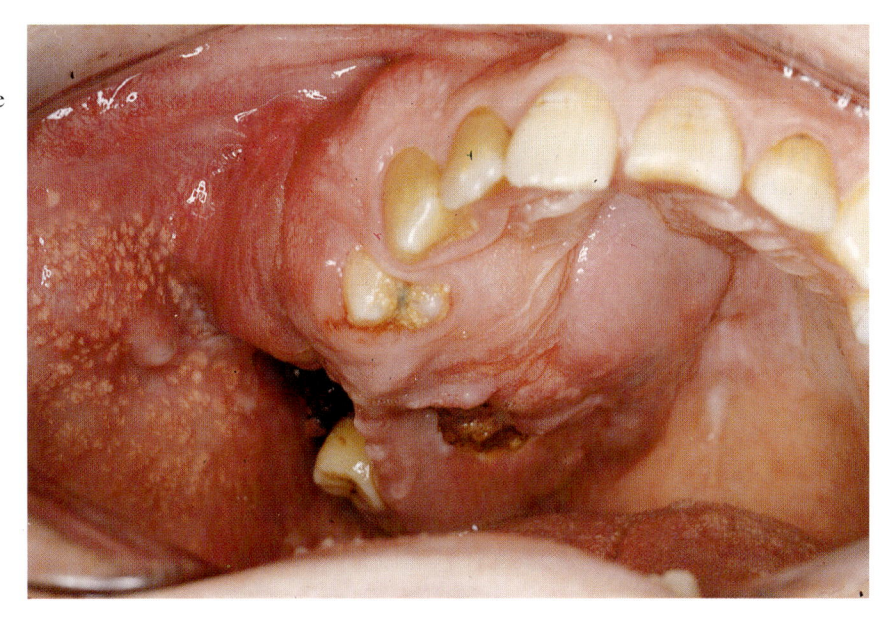

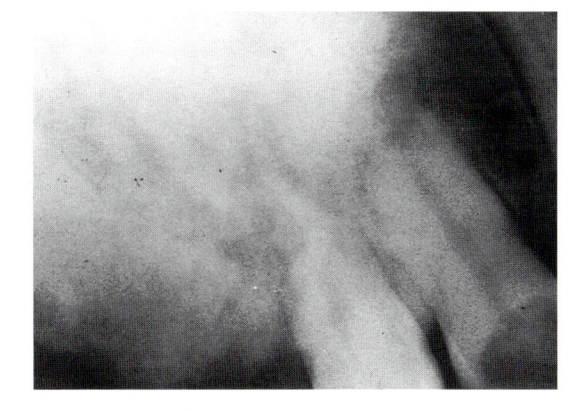

Fig. 7-6b.
Notice the resorption of the apices.

Radiographic aspects In the osteoblastic type the radiograph may show an opaque lesion, with bony trabeculae directed perpendicularly to the outer surface. In this way a "sunray" aspect may be formed. Over time there are expansion and perforation of the cortical bone. The osteolytic type is far less characteristic. It is usually an ill-defined lucency that causes expansion and destruction of the cortical bone. In the presence of teeth a more or less symmetrical widening of the periodontal ligament may be observed even before changes can be noticed elsewhere in the bone[214]. Also effacement of follicular cortices of unerupted teeth is a sign that is highly suggestive of malignancy. Widening of the mandibular canal is another ominous sign[334,535,640].

124 • Neoplasms of primary bone origin

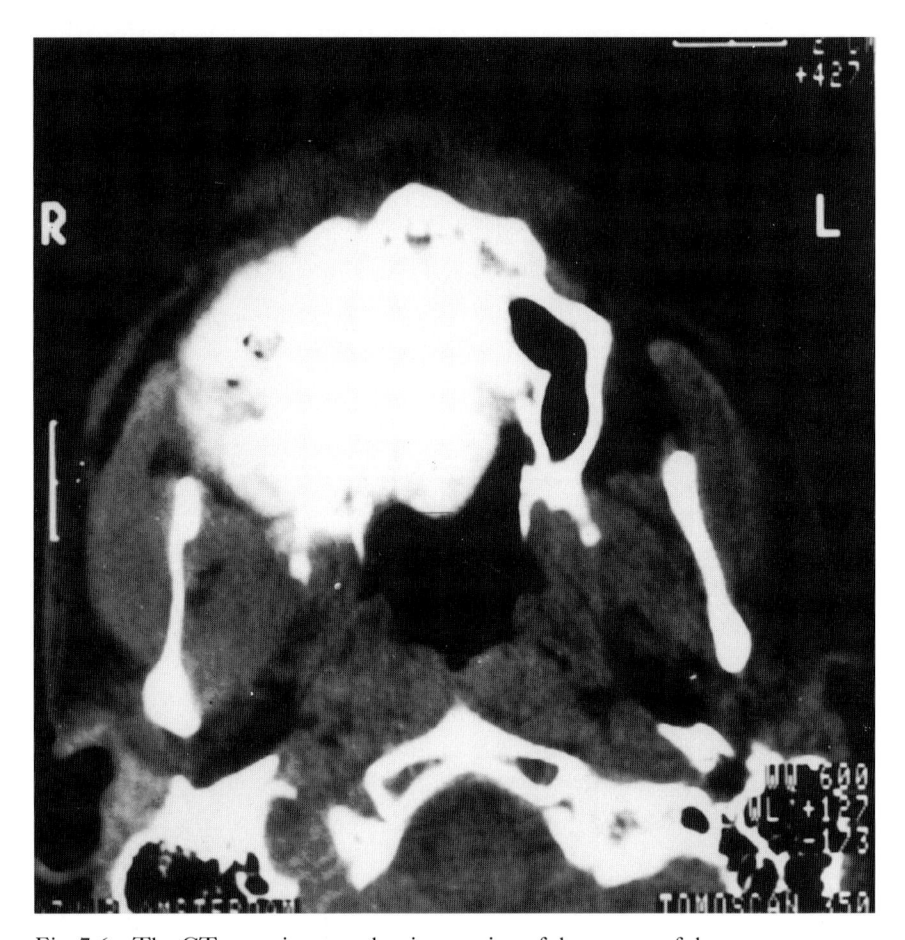

Fig. 7-6c. The CT-scan gives another impression of the extent of the tumor.

Scintigraphic aspects   A scintigram of radiostrontium will show a positive picture. In itself, such finding is not characteristic of osteosarcoma.

Histologic aspects   Microscopic examination shows a proliferation of atypical osteoblasts. Osteoid and bone formation takes place in an irregular pattern. Sometimes a proliferation of anaplastic fibroblasts appears. Vascular clefts may be encountered, resulting in terms like teleangiectatic osteogenic sarcoma[106]. Multinucleated giant cells may be scarce or abundant (Fig. 7-7).

Osteosarcomas of the jaws are, in general, better differentiated than similar tumors in the long bones. Even if the tumor largely consists of malignant-looking cartilage, it is still considered an osteosarcoma whenever osteoid and bone are being formed directly in the stroma. The alkaline-phosphatase positivity of the tumor cells

Fig. 7-7a. Various histologic aspects of osteosarcoma: Osteosarcomatous tissue causing resorption of the preexisting lamellar (normal) bone.

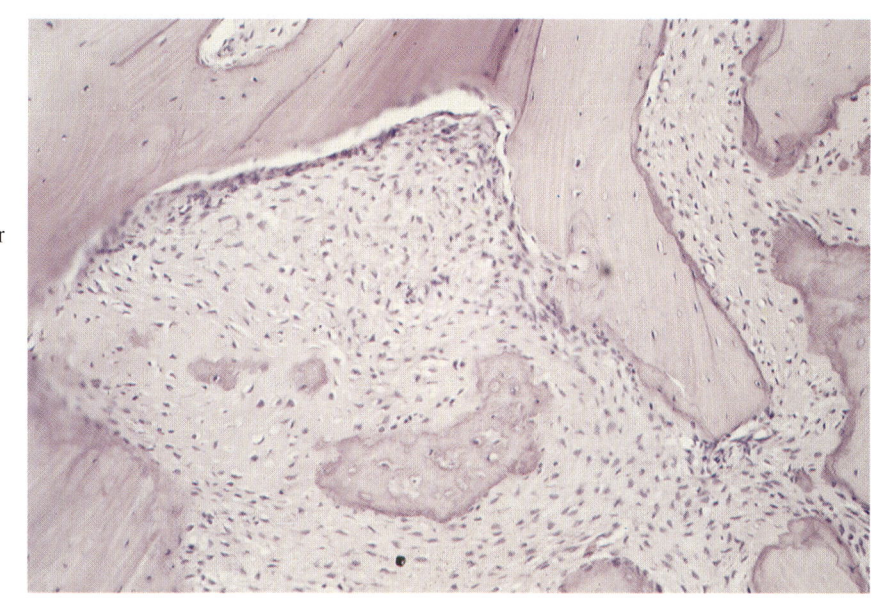

Fig. 7-7b. Fingerlike projections of osteoid at the periphery of an ostosarcoma, explaining the "sunray" aspect as shown in Fig. 7-3c.

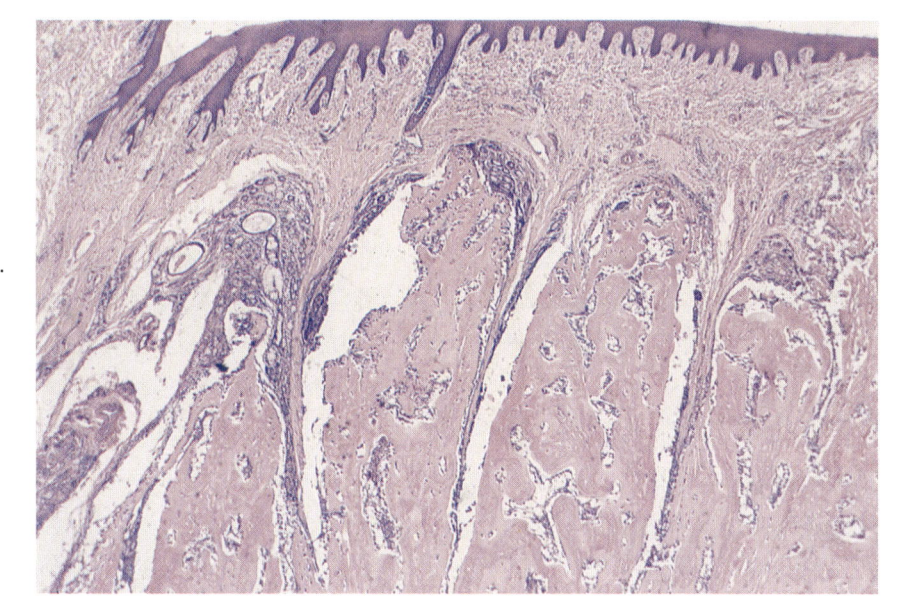

Fig. 7-7c. Area of chondroid tissue in osteosarcoma (chondroblastic type).

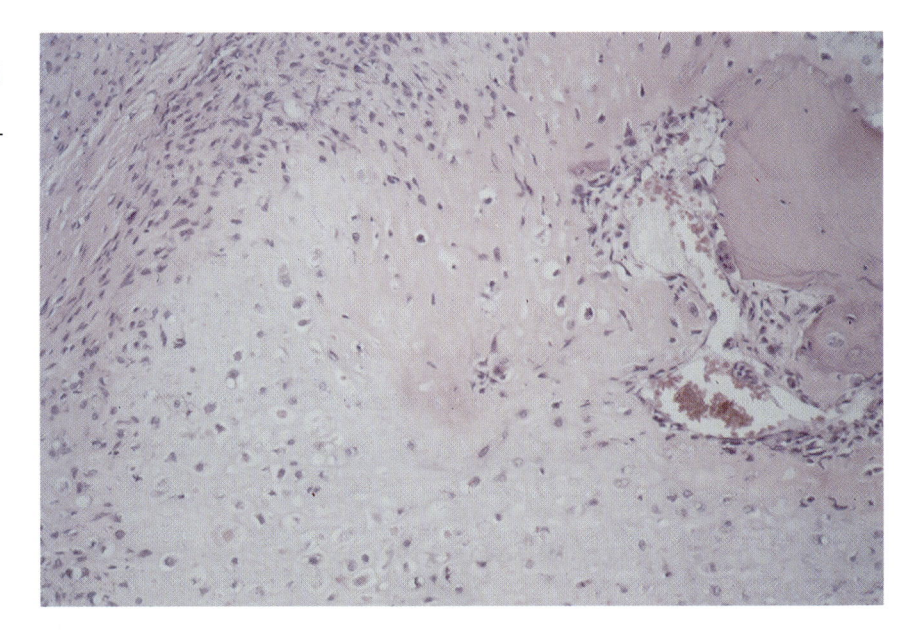

Fig. 7-7d. Sclerotic cementumlike area in osteosarcoma of the jaw.

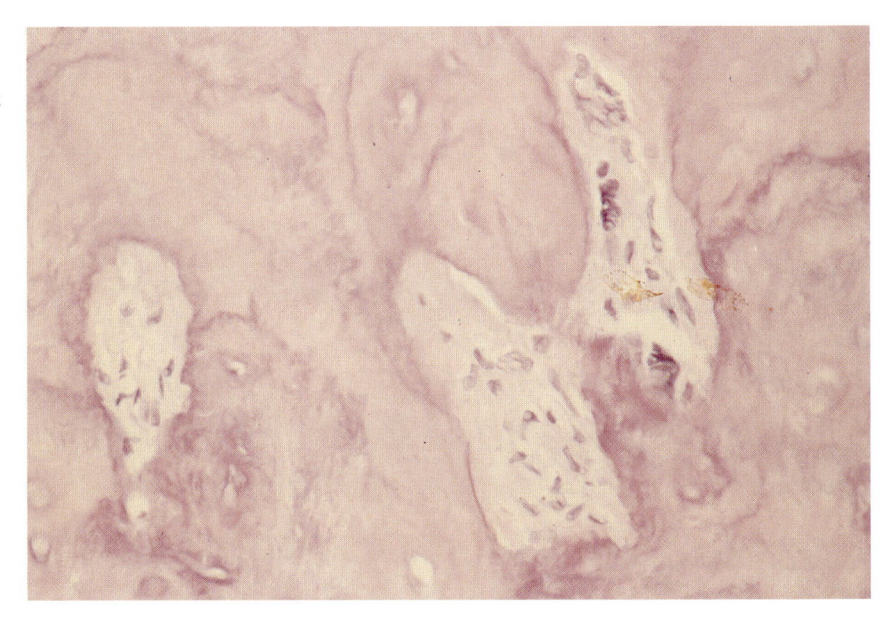

Fig. 7-7e. Proliferation of atypical osteoblasts and osteoid formation. Notice multinucleated giant cells, which may lead to an erroneous diagnosis of giant cell granuloma.

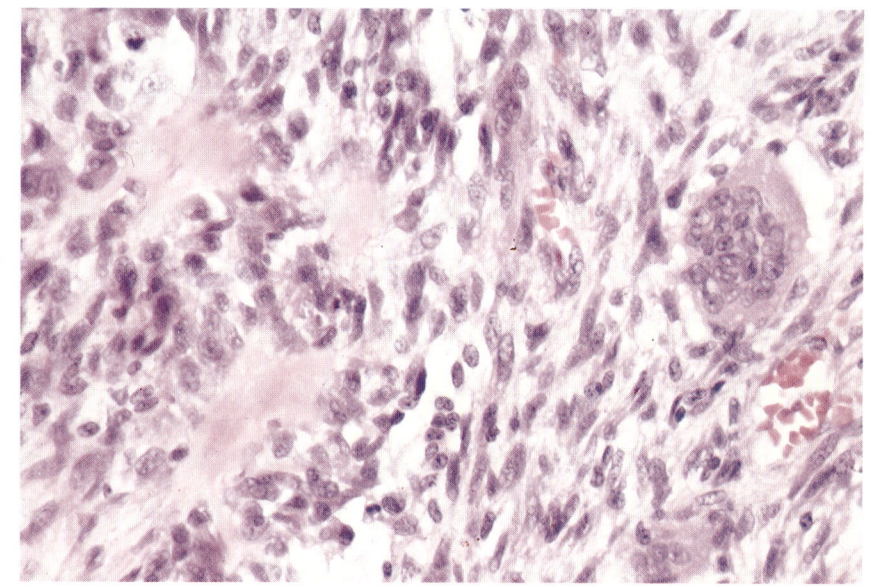

Fig. 7-7f. Irregular bone trabeculae of osteosarcoma that could be mistaken for fibrous dysplasia.

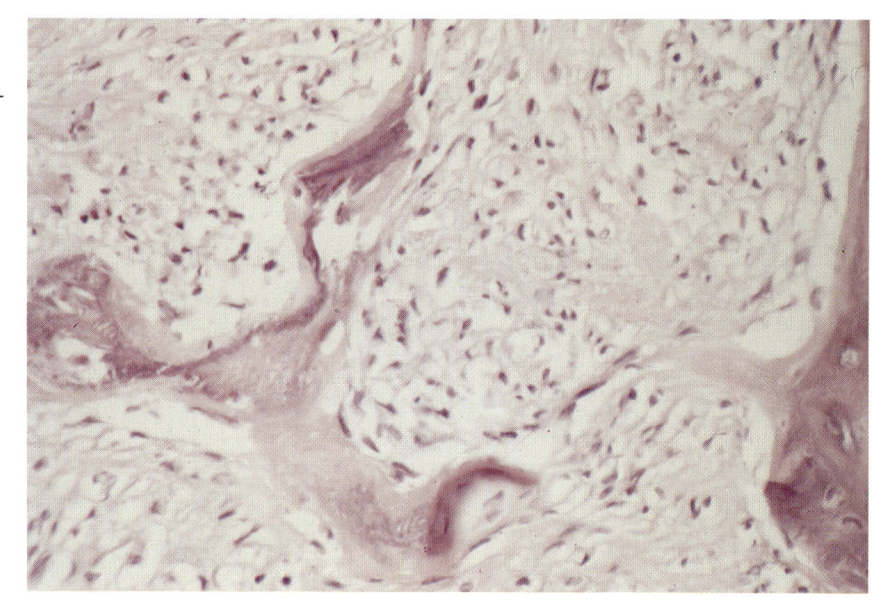

in osteosarcoma is another criterion in the distinction between osteosarcoma and chondrosarcoma[492].

Ultrastructural studies have shown that apart from osteoblasts a number of other cells can be identified in an osteosarcoma. They are, among others, the chondroblast, the osteocyte, undifferentiated cells, and myofibroblasts[461, 504]. The immunoprofile of jaw osteosarcomas and chondrosarcomas seems to be of limited value, with a possible exception for osteonectin[464].

DNA analysis by cytophotometry may be of help in cases presenting histopathological difficulties[49].

Treatment

Treatment consists primarily of aggressive local surgery. Some authors have suggested the use of additional chemotherapy[483]. In about half the cases of osteosarcoma of the jaws there is metastatic spread, usually to the lungs. The prognosis of osteosarcomas of the jaws seems somewhat better than that of osteosarcomas elsewhere in the skeleton, although a reliable comparison is almost impossible due to the small numbers of well-documented jaw sarcomas. The suggested better prognosis may be due to a lower mitotic activity in osteosarcomas in the jaws than in sarcomas elsewhere in the body. Besides, mandibular osteosarcomas seem to have a better prognosis than maxillary ones. Chondroblastic osteosarcomas appear to have a more favorable prognosis[119].

Metastasis is usually via the bloodstream and often occurs within one to two years. Of the patients who die from osteosarcoma, most do so with uncontrolled local disease.

Ewing's sarcoma

Definition

Ewing's sarcoma is a malignant neoplasm for which the cell of origin is somewhat unclear. The tumor is presumably derived from the mesenchyme of the bone marrow. Perhaps the neoplasm arises in a multicentric fashion.

At present two variants are to be distinguished, the typical Ewing's sarcoma and an atypical variant[337]. The typical Ewing's sarcoma consists of immature, blastemic tissue, whereas the atypical variant has a more histiocytic appearance.

Epidemiology

Ewing's sarcoma is more common in men than in women. The age of preference is between 10 and 25 years. The common sites are the shafts and metaphyses of long bones.

The jaws are rarely affected. In Dahlin's series of 299 lesions just three were located in the jaws[138]. In a series of 24 cases of primary tumors and tumor-like conditions of the jaws in children younger than 15 years, two cases of Ewing's sarcoma were encountered[310]. Most of the cases are located in the mandible[41, 56]. Ewing's sarcoma can also be metastatic to the mandible.

Clinical aspects

The neoplasm is characterized by pain and an often rapidly increasing swelling of the soft tissue, somewhat mimicking the features of an inflammatory process (Fig. 7-8). Also loosening and displacement of teeth have been reported. The duration of the signs and symptoms may range from just a few days to several months.

Ewing's sarcoma metastasizes early to the lungs, liver, other bones and also to regional lymph nodes. Bone scans are recommended at presentation and periodically during follow-up[224].

Laboratory findings

Albuminuria and secondary anemia have been reported systemic findings[138].

Radiographic aspects

On radiographic examination the mottled osteolytic, destructive changes may not be very impressive in appearance, since the disease takes place mainly in the cancellous part of the bone. Cortical expansion may occur. It is notable that Ewing's sarcoma penetrates the cortical bone rather rapidly. There may be signs of reactive periosteal bone formation, which may result in an "onion skin" appearance. The radiographic differential diagnosis of Ewing's sarcoma in the jaws includes osteosarcoma, small round cell tumors,

Fig. 7-8a. Intraoral presentation of Ewing's sarcoma.

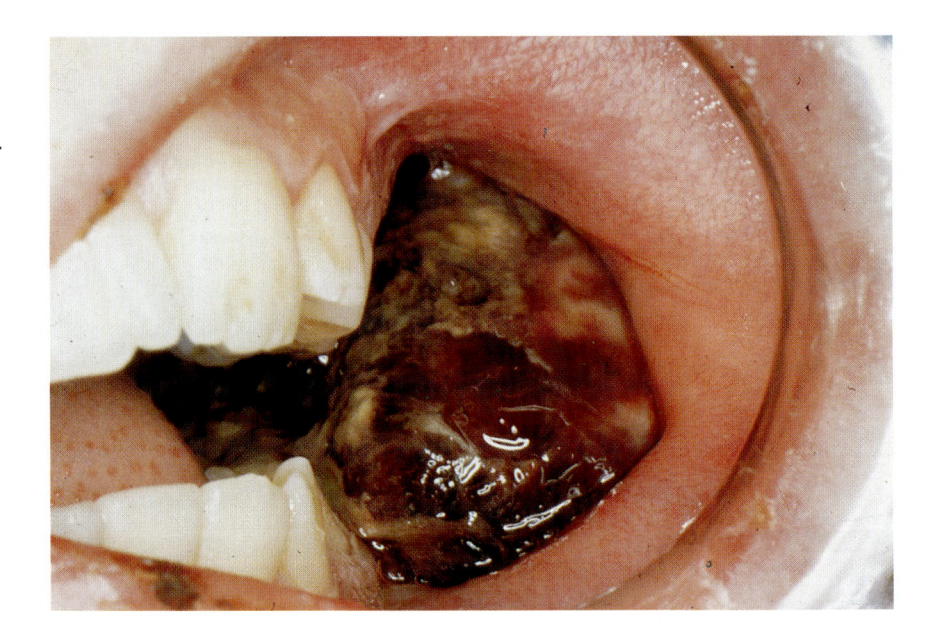

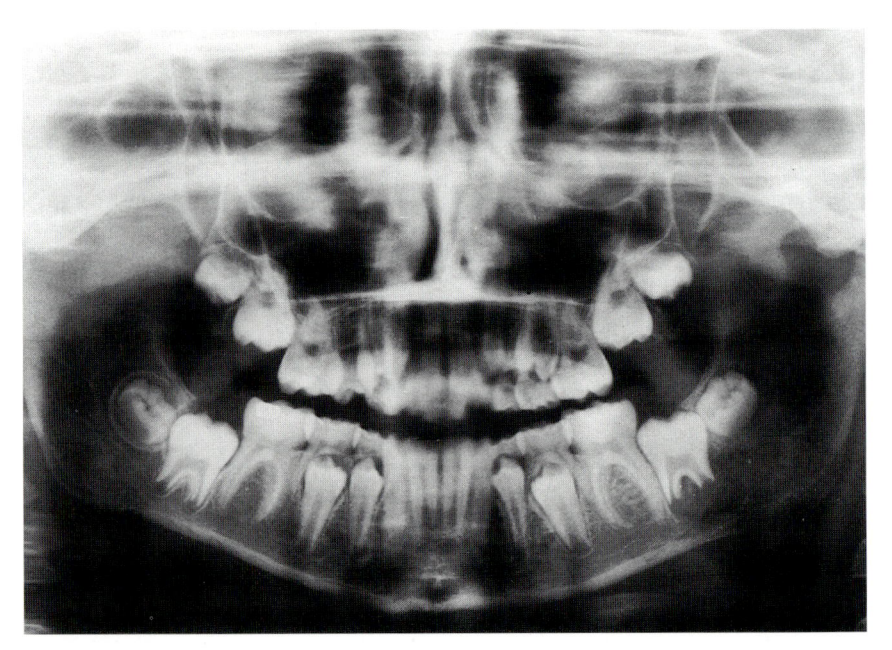

Fig. 7-8b. There is loss of cortication around the developing crown of 38 (compare with 48 at the right side).

Malignant neoplasms • 131

Fig. 7-8c.
Note the osteolytic changes in the ascending ramus and the destruction of the cortical bone at the angle of the mandible.

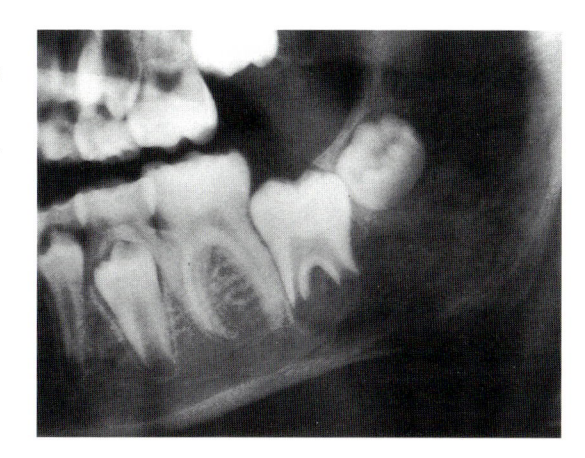

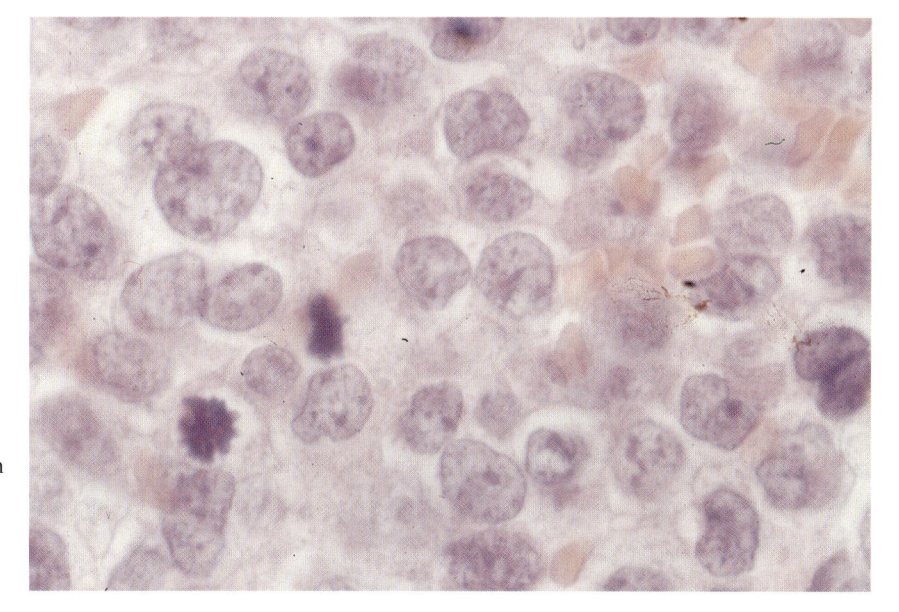

Fig. 7-8d. Densely packed small round cells in Ewing's sarcoma. No distinct cytoplasmic outline visible.

Langerhans' cell granulomatosis (histiocytosis X), metastatic and locally invasive carcinoma, and inflammatory processes[494].

Histologic aspects

On histological examination densely packed small cells are seen without distinct cytoplasmic outlines[500]. The nuclei are usually round to oval. The chromatin pattern is often of a fine granulated nature. There may be more than one nucleolus present. Mitotic figures may be numerous. Sometimes the tumor cells are grouped as pseudo-rosettes around blood vessels, which may suggest a diagnosis of neuroblastoma. Other possibilities in the histologic differential diagnosis include rhabdomyosarcoma and a metastatic neuroblastoma.

In a correlative cytological and histological study of 14 cases it was shown that Ewing's sarcoma has a characteristic appearance in smears and that fine needle aspiration cytology can be used in its primary diagnosis[137].

Treatment   At present, treatment usually consists of a combination of surgery, radiotherapy, and multiple-drug chemotherapy. The prognosis is still rather unfavorable, mainly due to uncontrolled metastatic spread.

Based upon the follow-up of 29 patients with Ewing's sarcoma of the head and neck, the statement has been made that the prognosis of head-and-neck Ewing's is significantly better than Ewing's sarcoma overall[527].

CHAPTER 8

Neoplasms derived from cartilage

Cartilage-forming tumors comprise both benign and malignant types. In this chapter only the chondroma, the benign chondroblastoma and the (mesenchymal) chondrosarcoma will be discussed. Chondromyxoid fibroma is dealt with in chapter 9, while the synovial chondromatosis is discussed in the chapter on disorders of the temporomandibular joint (chapter 13).

Benign neoplasms

Chondroma

Definition and epidemiology

A chondroma is a benign tumor characterized by the formation of mature cartilage, but lacking the histological characteristics of chondrosarcoma, such as high cellularity, pleomorphism and presence of large cells with double nuclei or mitosis[500].

The neoplasm may occur anywhere in the skeleton, but is extremely rare in the jaws[90, 580]. In fact, chondromas seldom appear in bones that have been formed in an endesmal or membranous way, as is the case with almost the entire maxilla and mandible. Many investigators dispute the existence of benign chondroid tumors in the jaws and believe that the reported cases are actually examples of either a chondrosarcoma or a chondroblastic osteosarcoma.

The chondroma may be seen at any age and shows no preference for either sex.

Clinical aspects

If the neoplasm does occur in the oral cavity, it is usually the palate or anterior part of the maxilla that is involved. Occasionally the presence of a chondroma is observed in the soft tissues of the oral cavity, such as in the tongue. Such a lesion should be considered a developmental lesion rather than a neoplasm. In rare instances the formation of cartilage can be seen in chronically inflamed, hyperplastic mucosa along the borders of a denture.

Radiographic aspects   Radiographic examination of a chondroma shows a somewhat ill-defined lucent or spotty opaque lesion.

Histologic aspects   On microscopic examination hyaline cartilage with or without foci of calcification or necrosis can be seen. The chondroid cells are small and contain only one nucleus. The transition from a chondroma into a chondrosarcoma may be extremely smooth.

Treatment   Treatment of a chondroma consists of surgical removal.

Benign chondroblastoma

A chondroblastoma is characterized by highly cellular and relatively undifferentiated tissue made up of rounded or polygonal chondroblast-like cells with distinct outlines, together with multinucleated giant cells of osteoclast type arranged either singly or in groups. On the whole, little intercellular material is seen, but the presence of small amounts of cartilagenous intercellular matrix with areas of focal calcification is typical[500]. Synonyms for benign chondroblastoma are epiphyseal chondromatous giant cell tumor and Codman's tumor.

The tumor is most common at the ends of the long bones, usually occurs in patients under 20 years of age, and is seen twice as often in men as in women. Only a few cases of involvement of the jaws, particularly in the condyles and the palate, have been reported[62]. In the latter location most tumors seem to have originated from the nasal septum or its surrounding tissues.

Fig. 8-1. Swelling of the palate caused by chondrosarcoma.

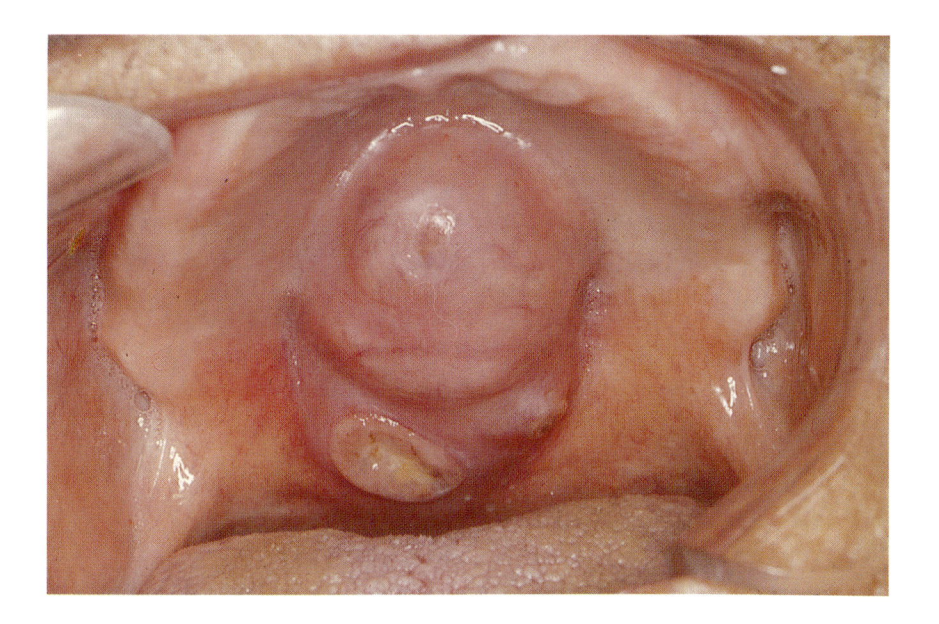

Malignant neoplasms

Chondrosarcoma

Definition and epidemiology

A chondrosarcoma is defined as a malignant tumor characterized by the formation of cartilage, but not of bone, by the tumor cells. It is distinguished from chrondroma by the presence of more cellular and pleomorphic tumor tissue, and by appreciable numbers of plump cells with large or double nuclei. Mitotic cells are infrequent[500]. Sometimes the term secondary chrondrosarcoma is used, indicating malignant transformation in a preexisting benign chondroid neoplasm.

The neoplasm may arise at any age. There is no sex preference.

Chondrosarcomas are found mainly in the pelvis, ribs, shoulder girdle, femur and humerus. An excellent review has been presented of chondrosarcoma in the general skeleton, in the head and neck area, and in extraskeletal soft tissues[216, 217]. Several other reviews of jaw involvement have been published[15, 192, 469].

Clinical aspects

Chondrosarcomas in the maxilla have a predilection for the anterior area and, in the mandible, for the premolar and molar region, the symphysis and the condylar and coronoid processes.

The symptoms of a chondrosarcoma in the oral cavity ususally consist of a painless swelling (Fig. 8-1). Regional lymph node metastasis is unusual. In the later stages of the disease lung metastases are common.

Radiographic aspects

The radiographic picture is not characteristic. Occasionally, radiopaque structures due to calcifications may be seen. Expansion and destruction of the cortex may be observed (Fig. 8-2). Resorption of the roots of the teeth is not uncommon. Widening of the periodontal membrane space is another common observation[217].

Histologic aspects

The microscopic aspects may strongly resemble a chondroma. The cartilage cells are, however, more polymorphous and often have double nuclei. The number of mitoses may be limited (Fig. 8-3).

In the presence of cartilage in lesions of the bones, the possibility of a chondrosarcoma or a chondroblastic osteogenic sarcoma must be considered. It has been stated that the tumor cells of a chondrosarcoma are negative for alkaline phosphatase and positive for an osteosarcoma[492]. In some instances the presence of clear-cells has been reported[531].

Treatment

Treatment of a chondrosarcoma consists of surgical removal. Irradiation seems to be of little use. Adjuvant chemotherapy may be of some value[385]. In general, the five-year survival rate is rather unfavorable, especially with regard to maxillary tumors.

Fig. 8-2.
Expansion of mandible caused by chondrosarcoma.

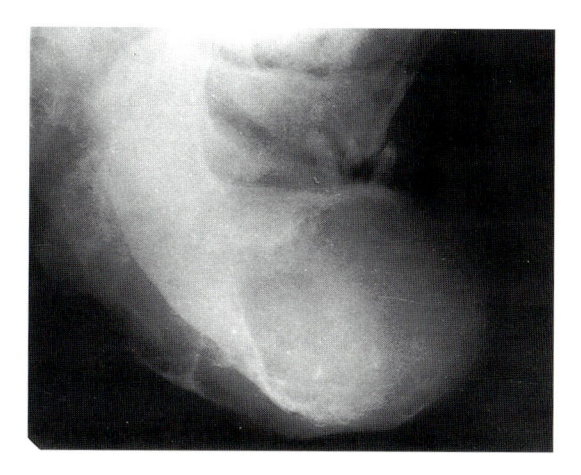

Fig. 8-3.
Histologic section of chondrosarcoma showing moderate cellular and nuclear pleomorphism.

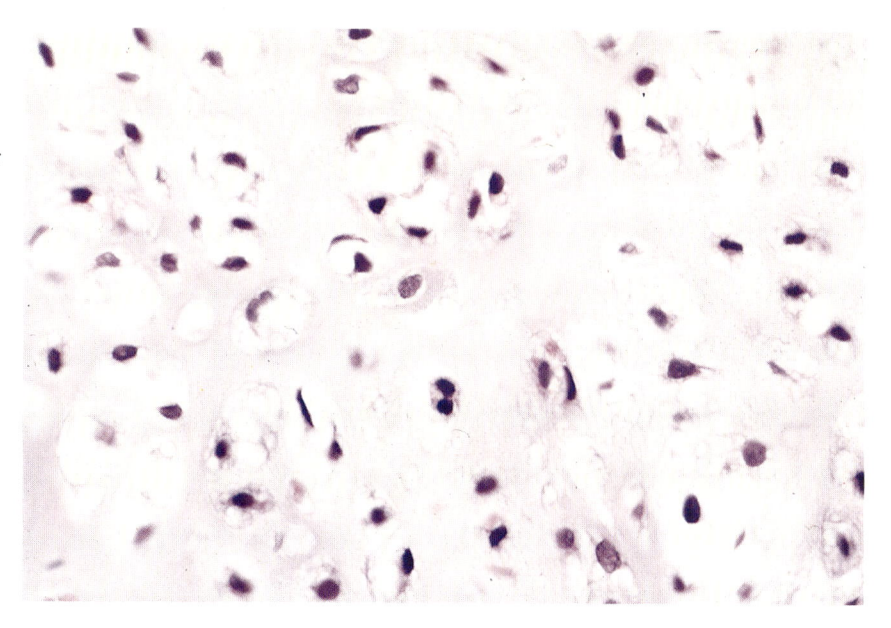

Mesenchymal chondrosarcoma

Definition — The mesenchymal chondrosarcoma should be regarded as a separate variant and is defined as a malignant tumor, characterized by the presence of scattered areas of more or less differentiated cartilage together with highly vascular spindle-celled or round-celled "mesenchymal" tissue[500].

Epidemiology — Occurrence in the jaws is rather exceptional[136]. A 1982 review of the literature described only 23 cases of jaw involvement[113]. The average age was 22 years. There was no preference for either men or women. The neoplasm was observed as often in the mandible as in the maxilla. Following the aforementioned review, a few other cases have been reported[278, 489, 615].

Clinical aspects — A painless mass is frequently the presenting complaint. There may be extension into the soft tissue. When occurring in the mandible, paresthesia may be present.

Radiographic aspects — The radiographs show in most cases a non-characteristic well or poorly demarcated osteolytic lesion.

Histologic aspects — Histologically, the tumor appears often to be rather circumscribed. The neoplasm consists partly of fields of oval to round undifferentiated cells and partly of cartilagelike tissue that is often rather sharply delineated with respect to the undifferentiated cells. The undifferentiated cells are occasionally arranged along capillaries, thereby mimicking the features of a hemangiopericytoma.

Treatment — Treatment is similar to that for "regular" chondrosarcoma.

CHAPTER 9

Non-osseous, non-chondroid neoplasms
(excl. odontogenic tumors)

In this chapter neoplasms of non-osseous and non-chondroid origin will be discussed, with the exception of odontogenic tumors. The latter group will be dealt with in chapter 10.

Chemodectoma

To the best of our knowledge just one case of a chemodectoma, a neuroendocrine tumor involving the mandible, has been reported[94].

Chondromyxoid fibroma

A chondromyxoid fibroma is a benign tumor. Chondromyxoid fibromas form less than 1% of all bone tumors, mainly occur in young adults and do not show preference for either sex.

The most common locations are the proximal metaphyseal regions of the femur and tibia. Only a few cases of chondromyxoid fibroma occurring in the jaws, most often in the mandible, have been described in recent years[206,252,349]. With regard to the occurrence in this particular site a possible role is attributed to remnants of Meckel's cartilage.

Clinical aspects The chondromyxoid fibroma is a slow growing, often painful tumor.

Radiographic aspects The radiologic features are not pathognomonic and consist of a well-circumscribed multilocular lucency of round or oval shape, resembling the features of giant cell granuloma, aneurysmal bone cyst or odontogenic myxoma (Fig. 9-1).

Histologic aspects

A chondromyxoid fibroma is characterized by lobulated areas of spindle-shaped or stellate cells with abundant myxoid or chondroid intercellular material, separated by zones of more cellular tissue rich in spindle-shaped or rounded cells with a varying number of multinucleated giant cells of different sizes. Large pleomorphic cells may be present and can result in confusion with chondrosarcoma[500]. However, chondrosarcomas lack the rather abrupt boundary and admixture of fibrous elements found in chondromyxoid fibromas[48].

In an ultrastructural comparison between chondromyxoid fibroma of the mandible and a typical chondromyxoid fibroma of the femur no basic differences were observed[251].

Treatment

The reported treatment varies from curettage to local resection. Incomplete curettage does not always lead to recurrence. In general, conservative resection is recommended. Radiotherapy should be discouraged because of possible induction of malignant transformation. Spontaneous malignant transformation is exceptional.

Fig. 9-1a.
Rather well-circumscribed radiolucency displacing 23. No characteristic features.

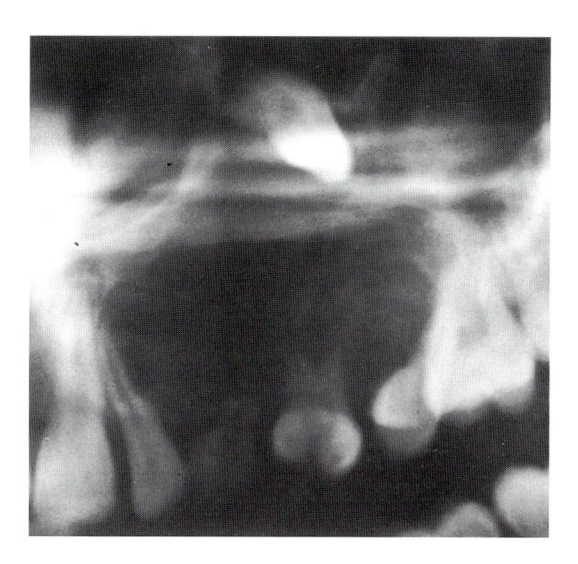

Fig. 9-1b. Histopathologic diagnosis: chondromyxoid fibroma. (Courtesy Dr. J.L.E.M. Starmans, The Netherlands).

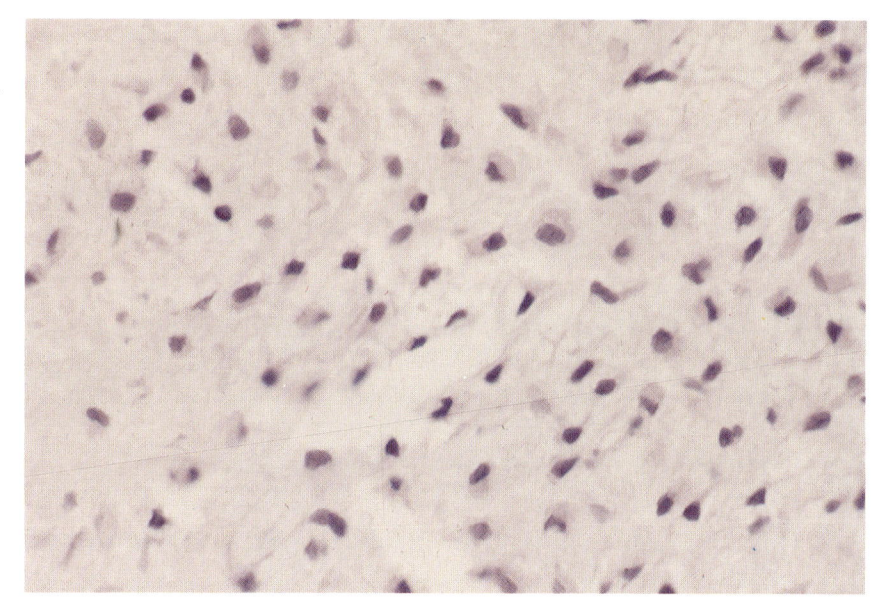

Desmoplastic fibroma

Definition and epidemiology

A desmoplastic fibroma is a benign tumor, characterized by the formation of abundant collagen[500]. It has been stated that desmoplastic fibroma of bone represents the intraosseous counterpart of the soft tissue fibromatoses[585].

The tumor mainly occurs in young adults of either sex and may affect all skeletal sites. More than one-third of all desmoplastic fibromas of the body are located in the jaws. By 1978 some 26 cases had been described in the literature[204]. Since then, several other cases have been added to the literature[324, 585]. In the majority of cases the tumor is located in the mandible. A rare case of maxillary involvement has been reported[218].

Clinical aspects

A desmoplastic fibroma is a slowly growing tumor that sometimes causes discomfort and loosening or displacement of teeth[61, 59, 270].

Radiographic aspects

Radiographically, the neoplasm appears as a lucent, often multilobular and somewhat circumscribed lesion (Fig. 9-2). The cortical bone may be expanded and finally destroyed. The radiographic differential diagnosis includes many lesions such as ameloblastoma, central giant cell granuloma and eosinophilic granuloma.

Histologic aspects

Histologically, the tumor is characterized by the formation of abundant collagen fibers by the tumor cells. A capsule is lacking. The tissue is poorly cellular, and nuclei are ovoid or elongated. The cellularity, pleomorphism, and mitotic activity that are features of fibrosarcoma are lacking[500].

It is sometimes difficult to make the diagnosis with certainty, in particular in respect to a non-ossifying fibroma, a central odontogenic fibroma, an odontogenic myxoma, and a low-grade fibrosarcoma[97, 534].

Treatment

The treatment is often confined to thorough curettage. Recurrences are not uncommon[61].

Fig. 9-2a.
Part of panoramic view of multilobular desmoplastic fibroma of the mandible.

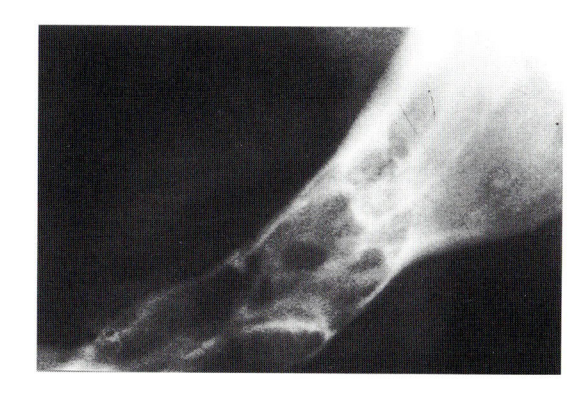

Fig. 9-2b.
Poorly cellular fibrous tissue. Abundant collagen fibers. Desmoplastic fibroma. (Courtesy Dr. J.I.J.F. Vermeeren, The Netherlands).

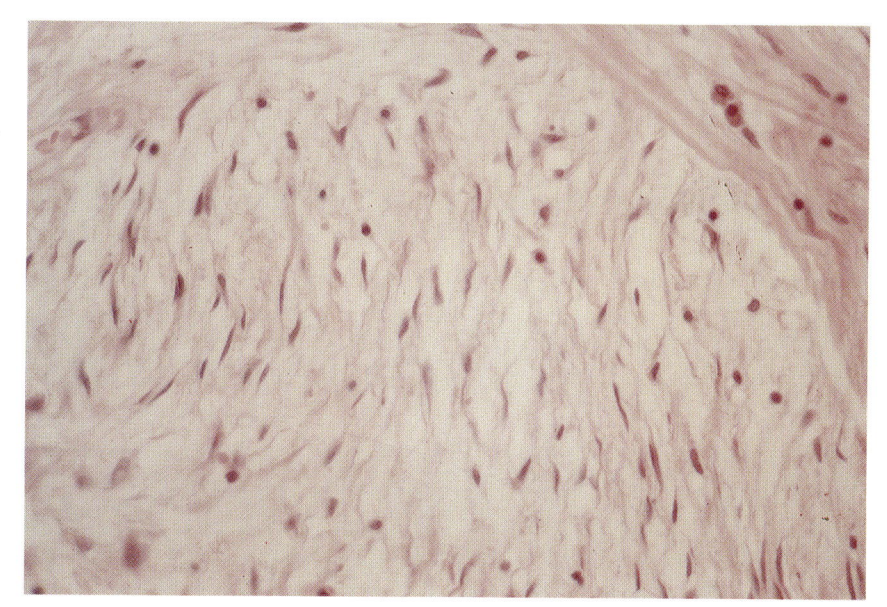

Non-ossifying fibroma
(Non-osteogenic fibroma, Xanthoma, Xanthofibroma, Xanthogranuloma)

Definition and terminology

In 1964 a case was reported of a benign, solitary, so-called xanthogranuloma of the mandible[480]. In a more recent paper a distinction has been made between xanthogranuloma and xanthoma[390]. The xanthogranuloma in that paper was considered to be an inflammatory granulomatous reaction with a "somewhat neoplastic" behavior. The xanthoma was regarded as a degenerative stage in a pre-existing process, i.e. giant cell tumors, fibrous dysplasia, simple bone cyst or aneurysmal bone cyst, without a tendency toward aggressive behavior. Others have confirmed that view, recognizing, however, that the pathologist is not always able to identify the associated lesion[63].

In yet another paper the terms xanthofibroma and fibrous histiocytoma have been proposed for what actually seems to be a lesion similar to the aforementioned xanthoma and xanthogranuloma[610]. Also the term non-osteogenic fibroma has been used[22]. The term non-ossifying fibroma is perhaps as appropriate to designate this lesion, although the objection has been made that the non-ossifying fibroma is classically described as a lesion with a distinct radiographic appearance, located in the metaphysis of a long bone and occurring mainly in children[610]. Nevertheless, a few cases of non-ossifying fibroma of the mandible have been reported[173, 351, 353]. More recently it has been stated that these lesions are histiocytic in nature and range from small, innocuous lesions, which are regarded as the osseous counterpart of non-X histiocytosis, to larger, more destructive lesions diagnosed as benign fibrous histiocytoma of bone[255].

Epidemiology

The small number of cases reported and the inconsistency in terminology do not permit conclusions as to race, age and sex preferences.

Clinical aspects

The lesions may produce an asymptomatic expansion or may be incidentally detected on a radiograph during routine examination.

Radiographic aspects

Radiographic changes may consist of a unilobular or multilobular, rather well-circumscribed radiolucent defect or of a diffuse, lytic process (Fig. 9-3). In some instances a ground-glass appearance may be observed.

Fig. 9-3a.
Rather well-circumscribed radiolucency.

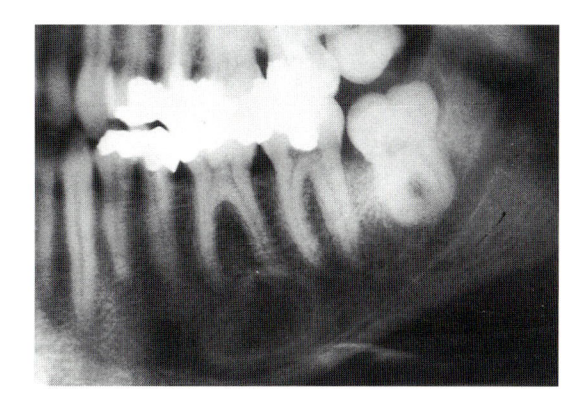

Fig. 9-3b.
On exploration, no relation with 36 was observed. Numerous "foam cells" with remnants of preexisting bone. Histopathologic diagnosis: non-ossifying fibroma ("xanthoma").

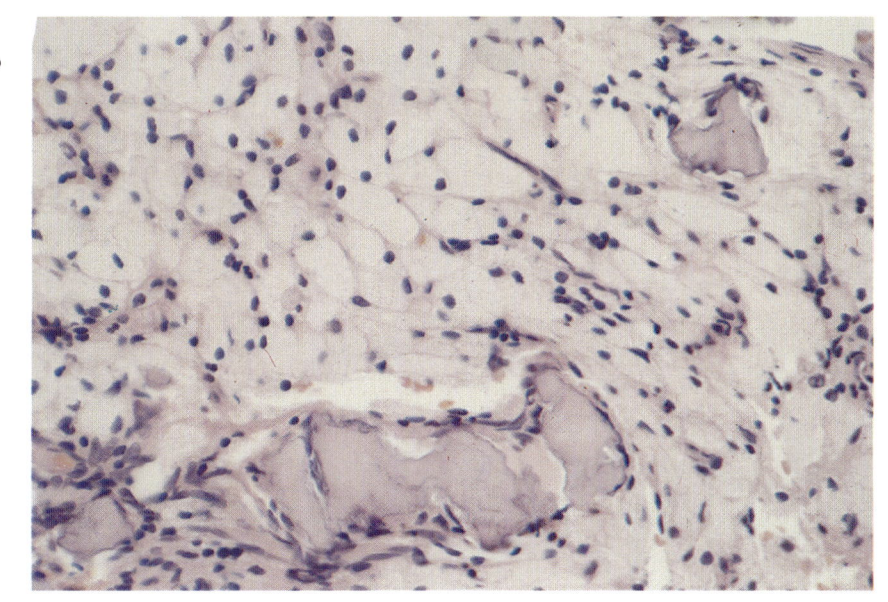

Histologic aspects   Histologically, the lesion consists of large and small nests of lipid-containing foam cells. In such areas the stromal tissue is composed of rather collageneous spindle-shaped connective tissue cells in winding, thick strands or whorled bundles. Irregularly dispersed among the stromal cells are small, often multinucleated giant cells about areas of recent capillary hemorrhage where many of them contain granules of hemosiderin in their cytoplasm. The lipid content is mainly in the form of cholesterol clefts. The absence of bone formation within the lesion's stromal tissue is consistent and striking.

Treatment   In view of the limited number of cases reported, no general statements can be made with regard to treatment.

Fig. 9-4a.
Firm elastic swelling at the lingual aspect of the mandible in fibromatosis.

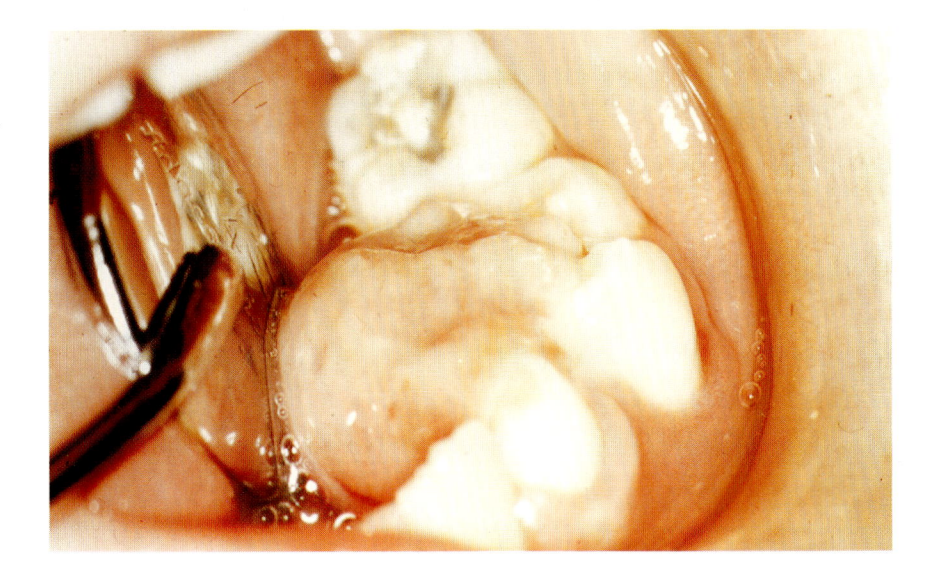

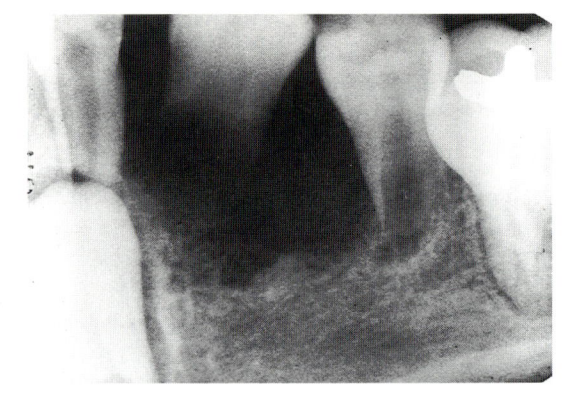

Fig. 9-4b.
The radiograph showed an osteolytic lesion.
(Courtesy Dr. A. Larsson, Sweden).

Fibromatosis

Definition and epidemiology

The fibromatoses form a spectrum of proliferative fibrous lesions, ranging from parvicellular, benign-looking, to very cellular lesions that can barely be distinguished from fibrosarcomas[47]. The prefix "juvenile" is commonly used in lesions in patients up to 15 years of age. The prefix "aggressive" is based purely on the clinical behavior. Some authors use the term "aggressive fibromatosis" and "infantile fibrosarcoma" synonymously. Nodular fasciitis is regarded as a subgroup of fibromatosis[142, 645]. Perhaps, desmoplastic fibroma of bone represents the intraosseous counterpart of the soft tissue fibromatoses[585].

The etiology is unknown, although trauma may play a role.

Fibromatosis occurs particularly in the soft tissues of the

Fig. 9-5. Cellular fibroblastic tissue in fibromatosis. Notice the presence of some multinucleated giant cells.

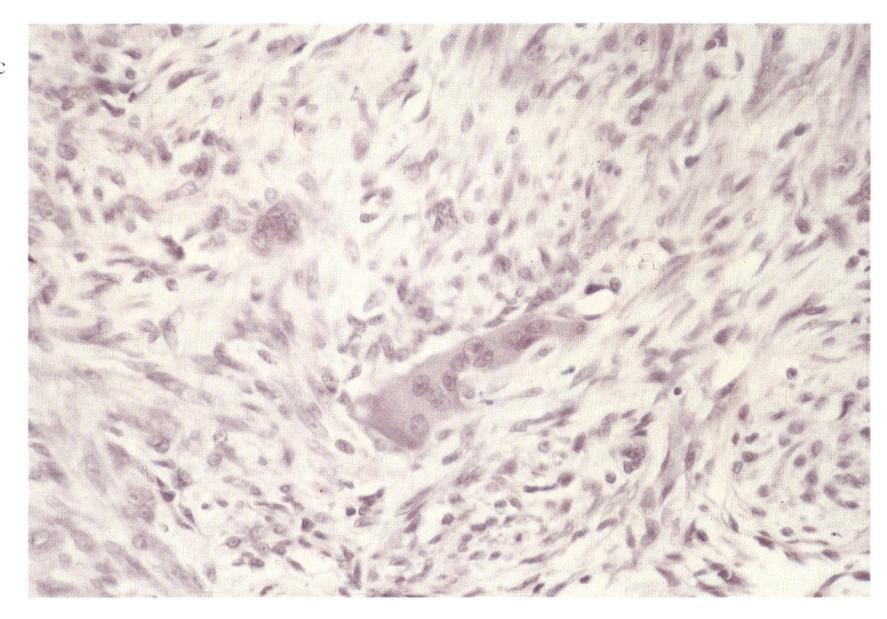

shoulder and the femur of young adults, children and even newborns. Occasionally, the progressively growing and sometimes painful lesion may affect the paramandibular soft tissue region[372, 431, 450, 496, 585]. There is no distinct sex preference.

Clinical aspects   The clinical features are not specific (Fig. 9-4). Diffuse swelling and destruction of the inferior border of the mandible characterize many cases[372, 563]. It is not always possible to clearly indicate whether the lesion arose from the paramandibular tissues or from the periosteum.

Radiographic aspects   The radiographic changes in fibromatosis may be very subtle or may show the picture of a periosteal reaction. In advanced cases an ill-defined osteolytic lesion may be observed.

Histologic aspects   Histologically, fibromatosis is characterized by a usually noncircumscribed proliferation of fibroblasts with a varying degree of cellularity. Cleft-like or cavernous vascular spaces may be present. Inflammatory cells are usually absent. In some cases the formation of cartilage can be observed[126]. Giant cells may also be present, making the distinction between fibromatosis and fibrous histiocytoma sometimes difficult (Fig. 9-5). This is also true with regard to the well-differentiated, low-grade fibrosarcoma and neurogenic lesions.

The histology of fibromatosis does not correlate with the clinical behavior and prognosis.

Treatment

Treatment, if possible at all, consists of wide surgical excision. In cases in which no radicality has been obtained, local recurrences are common, usually within the first year. Sometimes, recurrences are observed after five or more years. Fibromatosis rarely, if ever, gives rise to metastatic lesions.

Primary irradiation or postoperative irradiation after incomplete removal should be discouraged because of the risk of sarcoma eventually developing in irradiated bone.

Results of chemotherapy are rather disappointing.

Fibrosarcoma

Definition and epidemiology

A fibrosarcoma is a malignant fibrous tumor characterized by the formation by the tumor cells of interlacing bundles of collagen fibers, and by the absence of other types of histological differentiation, such as the formation of cartilage or bone[500].

Occurrence in the jaws is uncommon. The mandible is more often involved than the maxilla. Most reported patients have been in their third or fourth decades. There is no sex preference. In a series of 13 fibrosarcomas of the mandible collected from the Mayo Clinic, two appeared to have arisen in an ameloblastic fibroma and one in an irradiated patient with fibrous dysplasia[70]. Others also have reported that a fibrosarcoma may arise from malignant transformation of an ameloblastic fibroma[467], and also that a fibrosarcoma may be a radiation-induced neoplasm[386].

An infantile fibrosarcoma, that is when the tumor appears before the age of five years, apparently forms a more or less separate entity that rarely produces metastases[43].

Clinical aspects

The clinical symptoms consist of swelling, pain and loosening of the teeth[498]. A case of fibrosarcoma of the mandible has been reported presenting as a periodontal problem[248].

Radiographic aspects

Radiologically, a fibrosarcoma is depictured as an ill-defined radiolucency. It cannot be distinguished from other destructive lesions[348].

Histologic aspects

A fibrosarcoma is characterized by the formation by the tumor cells of interlacing bundles of collagen fibers, and by the absence of other types of histological differentiation, such as the formation of cartilage or bone. Often, a so-called herringbone pattern is present (Fig. 9-6)[500].

Fig. 9-6. Detail of fibrosarcoma. Notice the "herring-bone" pattern.

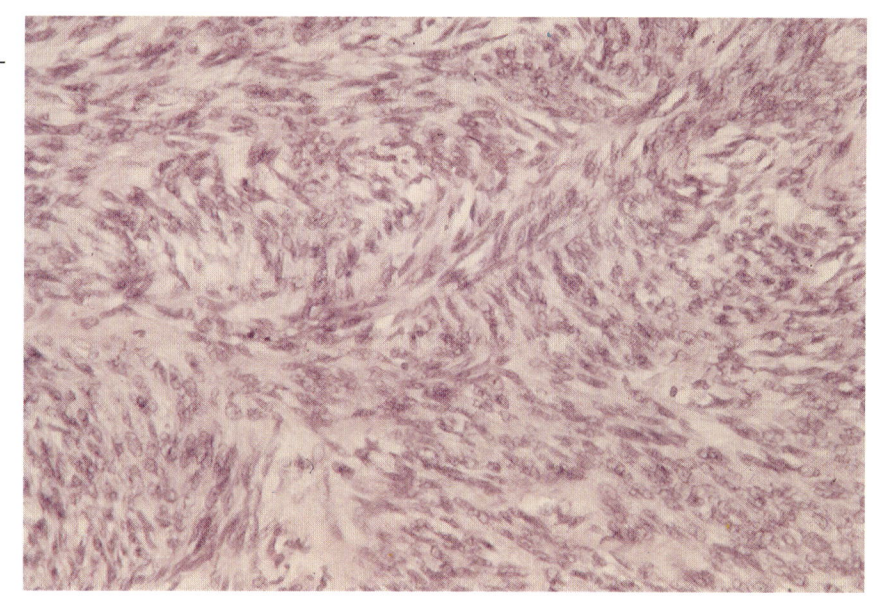

Treatment

Wide surgical removal is recommended as the treatment of choice. Metastases are rare and occur mostly in the lungs or in the bones elsewhere in the skeleton. Regional lymphnode involvement is uncommon.

Fibrous histiocytoma

Definition and epidemiology

A fibrous histiocytoma is a tumor or pseudotumor composed of cells that may differentiate to both fibroblasts and histiocytes.

Fibrous histiocytomas are found predominantly in the skin. In a study of 130 patients with malignant fibrous histiocytoma of bone, only 11 (8.5%) craniofacial sites were mentioned[283]. A number of cases of fibrous histiocytoma occurring in the jaws have been reported in recent years[3, 71, 100, 405]. Most lesions were located in the maxilla. Several cases have been reported as being malignant[29, 252, 513].

Clinical and radiographic aspects

There are no specific clinical and radiographic aspects.

Histologic aspects

One should realize that no uniform histologic criteria of malignancy are accepted. It has been suggested that those lesions exhibiting nuclear or cytoplasmic pleomorphism show a greater probability of being clinically aggressive or malignant[575]. Dahlin et al. emphasize that several other tumors, such as fibrosarcoma, dedifferentiated chondrosarcoma, osteosarcoma, and even metastatic carcinoma may greatly resemble a malignant fibrous histiocytoma[139]. In fibrous histiocytoma alpha-1-antitrypsin, alpha-1-antichymotrypsin and lysozyme can be demonstrated in addition to positive staining for vimentin[193]. In general, the immunoprofile of benign and malignant fibrohistiocytic tumors is not discriminative[465].

Treatment

Treatment consists of a combination of surgery, chemotherapy and radiotherapy. Especially the role of chemotherapy has been emphasized[262]. In a follow-up study of 26 patients with malignant fibrous histiocytoma, 14 recurrences were noted; metastatic lesions occurred in 16 patients, most commonly in the lungs[252].

Hemangioma

Definition and epidemiology

A hemangioma is a benign lesion consisting of newly-formed blood vessels, either of capillary or cavernous type[500]. The vertebrae and the skull are the sites of predilection.

A central hemangioma in the jaws is almost invariably due to an arteriovenous malformation. An arteriovenous malformation can be either congenital or acquired, e.g., the result of an accident.

The phenomenon appears to be present two to three times as often in women as in men and is usually found in the mandible[30].

Clinical aspects

The first sign of a central hemangioma may be persistent gingival bleeding or a gingivitis-like appearance (Fig. 9-7). There may also be some swelling of the bone (Fig. 9-8).

A central hemangioma in the maxilla is often of the cystic type and, therefore, usually causes more severe bleeding than a central hemangioma located in the mandible[23]. Several examples of a fatal outcome of the extraction of a tooth in an area involved by a central hemangioma have been reported.

Radiographic aspects

The radiographic aspect is not characteristic and may show a well-circumscribed or ill-defined lucency. A honeycomb structure is sometimes present, mimicking the features of a central giant cell granuloma, an aneurysmal bone cyst, an odontogenic keratocyst or an ameloblastoma. If a central hemangioma is suspected, arteriography should be performed[668]. Otherwise, the diagnosis results

Fig. 9-7a. Gingivitis-like appearance in the right part of the maxilla. The pulsatile nature was already clear from palpation of the alveolar ridge.

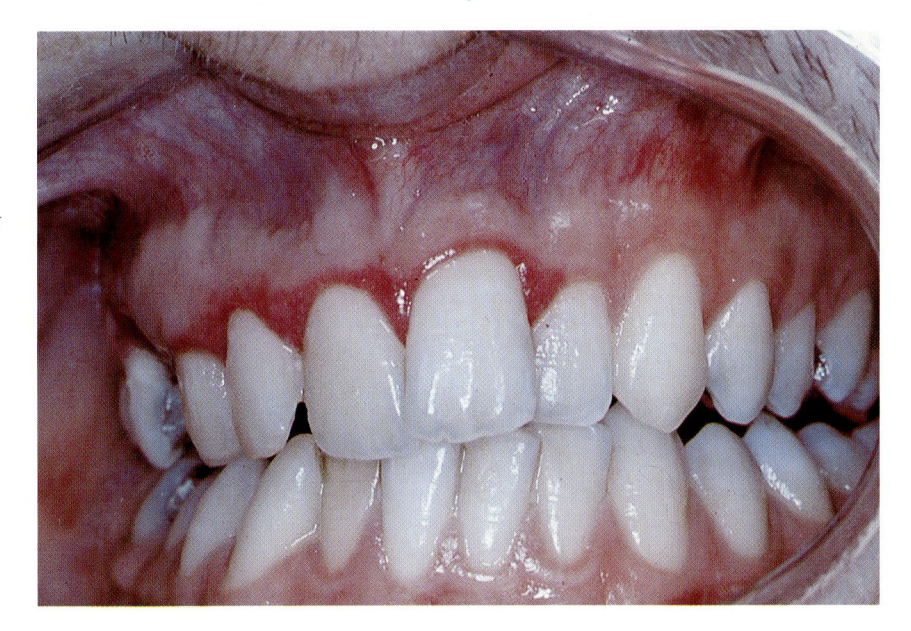

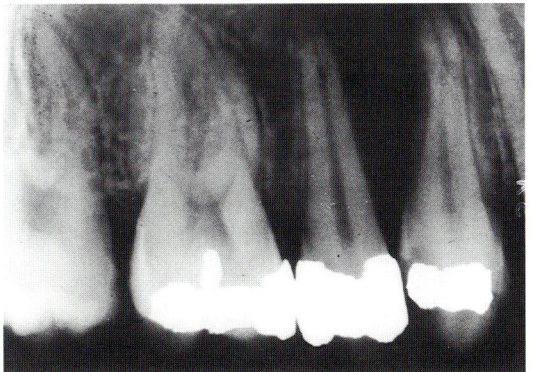

Fig. 9-7b. The periapical film shows an ill-defined lucency between 14 and 15, that also extends into the interradicular area of 15 and 16.

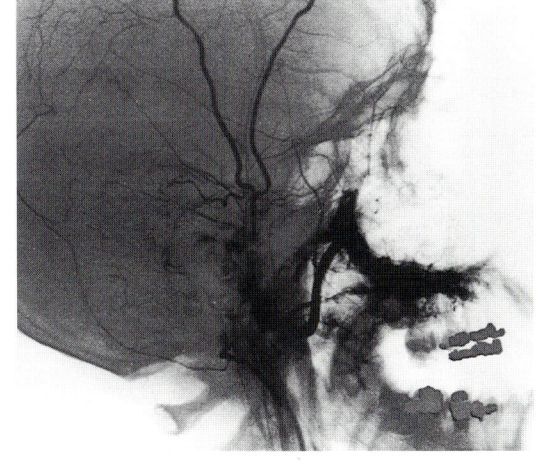

Fig. 9-7c. Arteriography demonstrated the extent of the vascular lesion in the maxilla. Repeated artificial embolization has been performed. (Courtesy Dr. E.R. Kraal, The Netherlands).

from a biopsy. When no strong arterial component is present, the biopsy procedure or even enucleation usually does not produce severe bleeding. On the other hand, a provisional diagnosis of central hemangioma is often erroneously made, based on the impression of the clinician when handling a vascular lesion, such as a central giant cell granuloma.

152 • Non-osseous, non-chondroid neoplasms

Fig. 9-8a.
Bony swelling caused by central hemangioma.

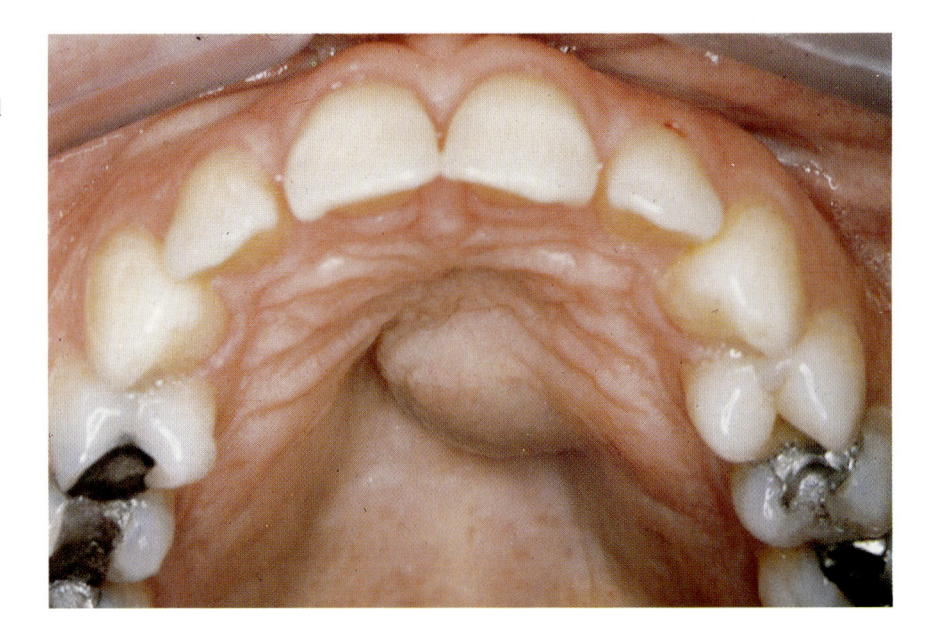

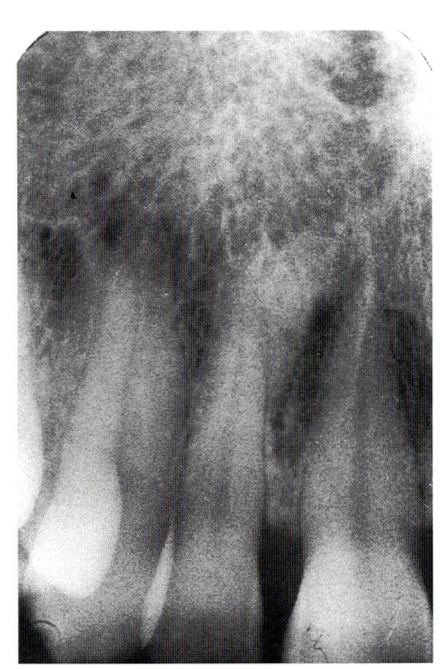

Fig. 9-8b.
The periapical film shows subtle, featherlike changes of the bone near the apices of 12 and 13.

Treatment   In a lesion which has a slow flow, evidenced by the lack of pulsatile quality or bruit and low vascular pressure on aspiration, consideration should be given to the use of sclerosing agents. The two most commonly used drugs are sodium morrhuate and sodium psylliate. Sodium morrhuate is available as a 5% aqueous solution

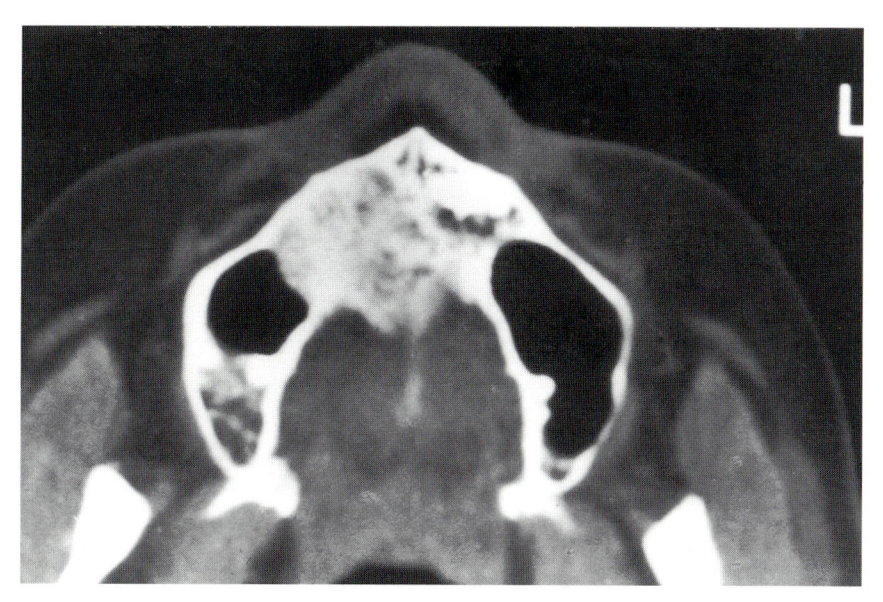

Fig. 9-8c. The CT-scan shows the extent of the lesion.

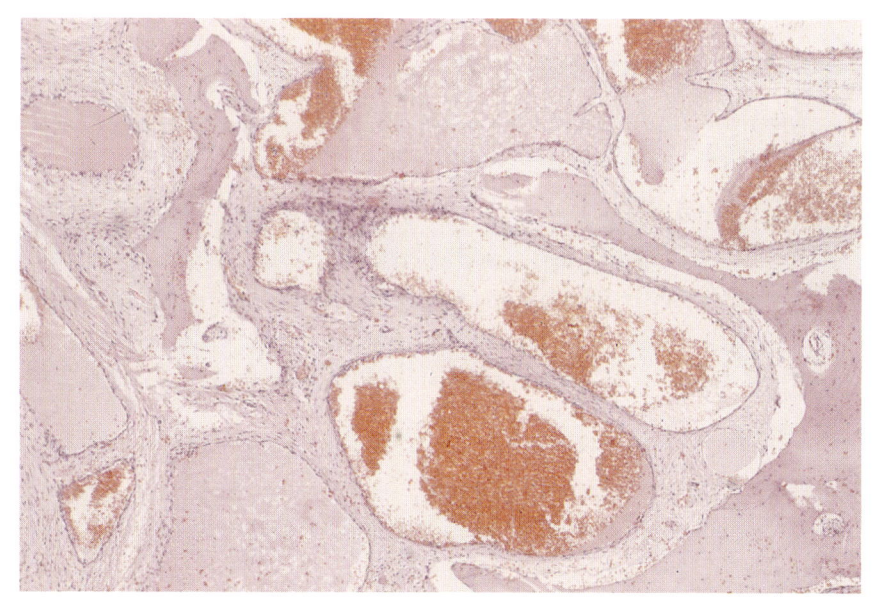

Fig. 9-8d. Histologic aspect of central nonpulsatile hemangioma, showing wide vascular spaces filled with erythrocytes.

containing 2% ethyl alcohol or benzyl alcohol as a preservative. The recommended technique is to inject 0.5 to 1.0 ml, via a 25-gauge needle, into the center of the lesion[109].

In recent years there has been an increasing interest in the application of artificial embolization, either as the only treatment modality[19,-524] or as a preoperative measure[484]. Various materials may be used such as radiopaque spheres of silicone and lyophilized dura[647]. In general, surgery is recommended in those circumstances within 24 hours after embolization. This treatment regimen significantly reduces peroperative bleeding. Others, however, prefer to perform surgery, if necesssary, seven to 14 days after embolization[200]. The latter authors drew attention to the fact that the preoperative embolization must not be so extensive as to interfere with postoperative wound healing or cause widespread ulceration.

A few cases have been reported in which the tumor was removed from the excised mandible, which was then sterilized and used in the immediate reconstruction of the surgical defect[606].

Angiosarcoma and hemangiopericytoma

An angiosarcoma, also called malignant hemangio-endothelioma or hemangio-endotheliosarcoma, is extremely uncommon[171, 658, 666]. It is known to develop as a primary tumor or from irradiated benign hemangioma. There are no specific clinical or radiologic features. Histologically, the tumor is characterized by the formation of irregular anastomosing vascular channels lined by one or more layers of atypical endothelial cells, frequently of immature appearance, and accompanied by solid masses of poorly differentiated or anaplastic tissue[500].

The best treatment consists of wide surgical excision. Prognosis is poor, mainly due to often occurring pulmonary metastases.

A hemangiopericytoma is a vascular tumor that typically occurs in the soft tissue of the extremities and trunk. In a series of 45 osseous hemangiopericytoma of the skeleton, four were located in the mandible[567].

Histologically, the tumor is characterized by a pattern of vascular spaces lined by a single layer of endothelial cells surrounded by zones of proliferating cells[500].

Treatment consists of wide surgical excision.

Leiomyoma and leiomyosarcoma

A few cases of (angio)leiomyoma of the mandible have been reported[369, 611]. It has been suggested that these lesions arise from the smooth muscles in the walls of blood vessels. The principal histologic differential diagnosis is venous hemangioma, which is defined as a vascular tumor in which the vessel walls contain smooth muscle cells. The determining feature that separates angioleiomyoma from the venous hemangioma appears to be the presence of smooth muscle in the stroma of the former[611].

The occurrence of leiomyosarcoma as a primary osseous jaw lesion is rare. Fewer than 10 such cases have been reported[2, 111, 185, 403]. The age varied from 18 to 73 years.

The prognosis is generally poor, due to widespread metastases.

Lipoma, lipoblastoma and liposarcoma

Lipomas centrally located in the jaws are rare[378]. Furthermore, a case has been reported of a parosteal lipoma[549], and of a lipoblastoma[411].

A few cases of intraosseous liposarcoma of the maxilla and mandible have been reported[28].

Lymphangioma

A lymphangioma is a benign lesion consisting of newly-formed lymph vessels, usually in the form of dilated spaces[500]. Lymphangiomas of the bone may occur in association with soft tissue lesions of the same type.

The intraossseous occurrence of a lymphangioma is extremely rare, with just two reported cases of mandibular involvement[170].

Lymphoreticular diseases

Malignant lymphoma (incl. Leukemia)

Definition and epidemiology

The malignant lymphoma comprises a group of tumors whose cells are derived from lymphoid tissue. Lukes defines the malignant lymphoma as a neoplastic proliferation of the lymphopoietic part of the reticuloendothelial system in which either the cells of the T- and B-lymphocytic system or histiocytes are involved in a homogeneous monoclonal population[346]. The pattern is either diffuse or nodular and the disease appears either localized or generalized. Lymphomas and leukemias of the lymphocytic and histiocytic type are, in essence, equal; possible differences in the number of peripheral blood cells are to be ascribed to the involvement of the bone marrow. The malignant lymphoma is subdivided into Hodgkin's lymphoma and non-Hodgkin's lymphoma. Hodgkin's lymphoma rarely affects the jaw bones. Approximately 10 cases have been reported[332]. This also holds true for jaw involvement by the rare reticulum cell sarcoma[306], and malignant histiocytosis (histiocytic medullary reticulosis)[105], if those entities still exist. Today, most pathologists regard them as being subtypes of non-Hodgkin's lymphoma.

In childhood leukemias osseous changes in the jaws have been reported in up to 62% of the cases[134]. Radiographic findings may consist of loss or thinning of the crypts of developing teeth and of the lamina dura of erupted teeth, and displacement of teeth (Fig. 9-9). Also bone destruction may be observed[616].

Clinical aspects

Non-Hodgkin's lymphoma may primarily be localized in the oral soft tissues or in the jaws[163, 208, 311, 474]. The clinical signs and symptoms may consist of anesthesia of one side of the lower lip or of localized, sometimes recurrent swelling (Fig. 9-10). Also the anesthesia may have a recurrent, and thereby misleading, character.

Radiographic aspects

There are no specific radiographic features. Actually, there is often the impression of some type of osteomyelitis, radiographically. Indeed, a low level of suspicion by the clinician probably allows many of these lesions to go undiagnosed until advanced stages of the disease[233]. Complementary CT-scans and scintigraphy may be of considerable help when a diagnosis of (lymphoreticular) malignancy is suspected.

Fig. 9-9a.
Periapical films of a 10-year-old and a 17-year-old boy affected by leukemia. Notice the loss of the crypt of the developing 45

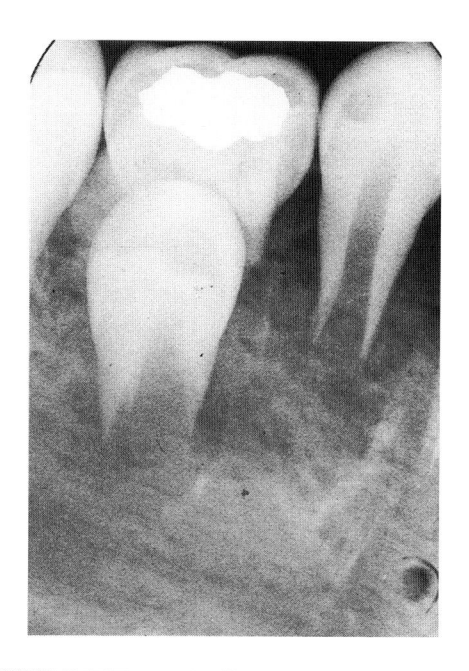

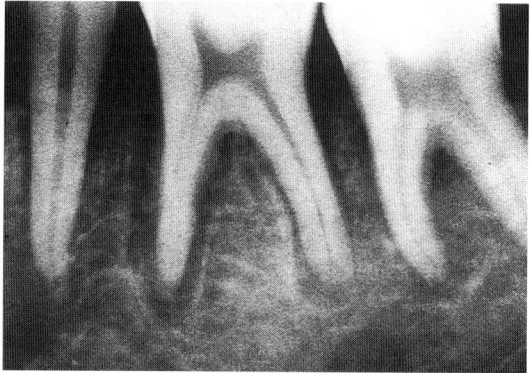

Fig. 9-9b.
and the loss of the lamina dura of 35, 36 and 37.

Histologic aspects

A number of different histologic classification systems of the non-Hodgkin's lymphomas has been used in the past, such as the so-called Rappaport classification. The presently used classification takes advantage of greatly increased knowledge in immunology. In the various stages of maturation of the T- and B-cells a blockade may take place, which is reflected to some extent in the prognosis. The malignant non-Hodgkin's lymphomas usually involve the T- and B-cell system and relatively seldom involve the histiocytic-monocytic system.

158 • Non-osseous, non-chondroid neoplasms

Fig. 9-10a. Swelling of the buccal aspect of the mandible caused by non-Hodgkin's lymphoma.

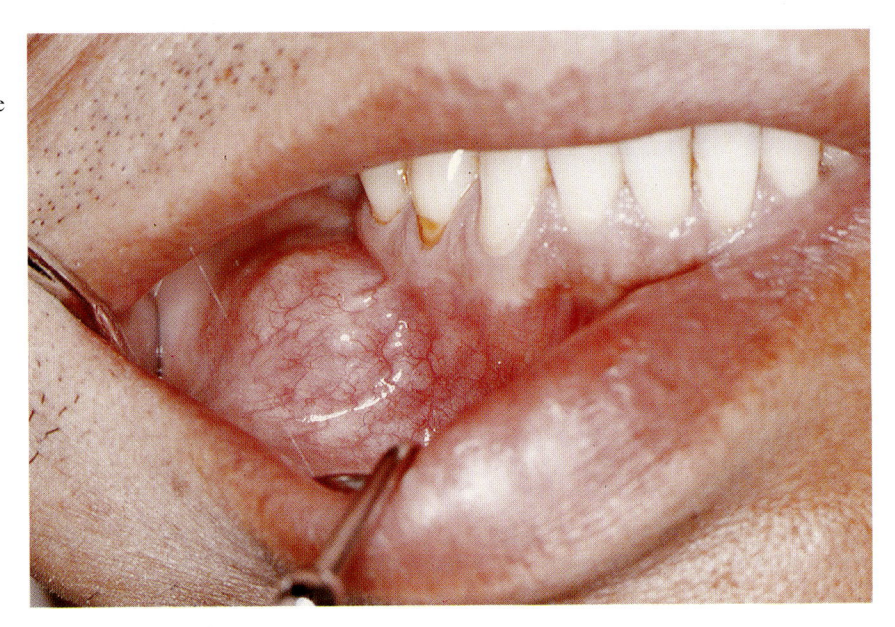

Table 9-1. Ann Arbor staging classification

Clinical staging

Stage I: Involvement of a single lymph node region (I) or of a single extralymphatic organ or site (I E).

Stage II: Involvement of two or more lymph node regions on the same side of the diaphragm (II) or localized involvement of an extralymphatic organ or site and 1 or more lymph node regions on the same side of the diaphragm (III E).

Stage III: Involvement of lymph node regions on both sides of the diaphragm (III) which may also be accompanied by localized involvement of the spleen (III S), extralymphatic site (III E), or both (III SE).

Stage IV: Diffuse or disseminated involvement of 1 or more extralymphatic organs or tissues with or without associated lymph node enlargement.

Fig. 9-10b.
The periapical film shows a subtle, ill-defined radiolucent change in the area distally to 44.

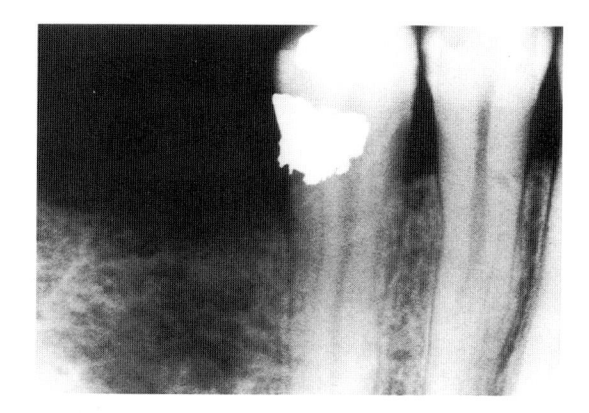

Fig. 9-10c. Low-power view of intraosseous non-Hodgkin's lymphoma.

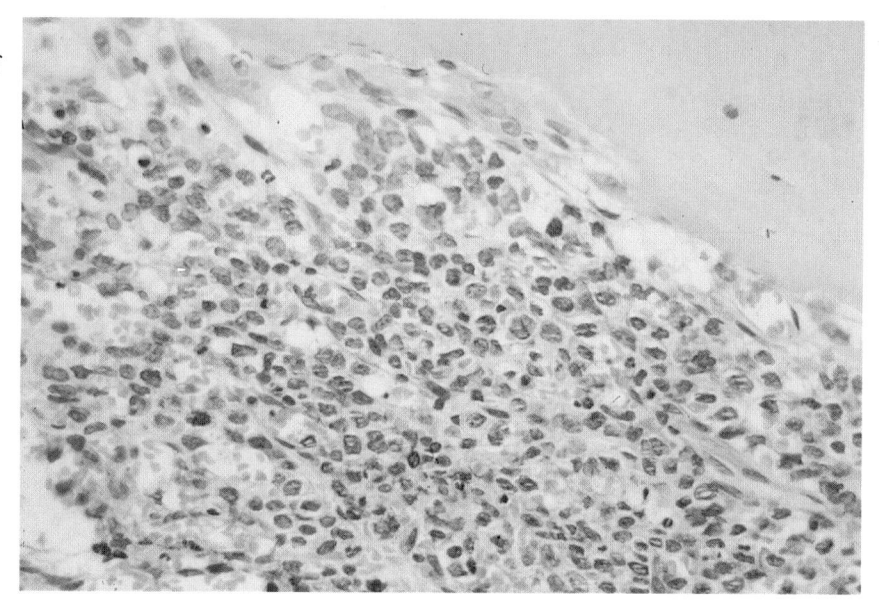

Staging A staging procedure must be carried out before instituting any type of treatment. In general the Ann Arbor staging classification is used (Table 9-1).

Treatment Treatment usually consists of a combination of chemotherapy and radiotherapy. The prognosis is largely determined by the histologic type and the extent of the disease.

Fig. 9-11a. Swelling of right side of maxilla and left side of mandible in patient suffering from Burkitt's tumor.

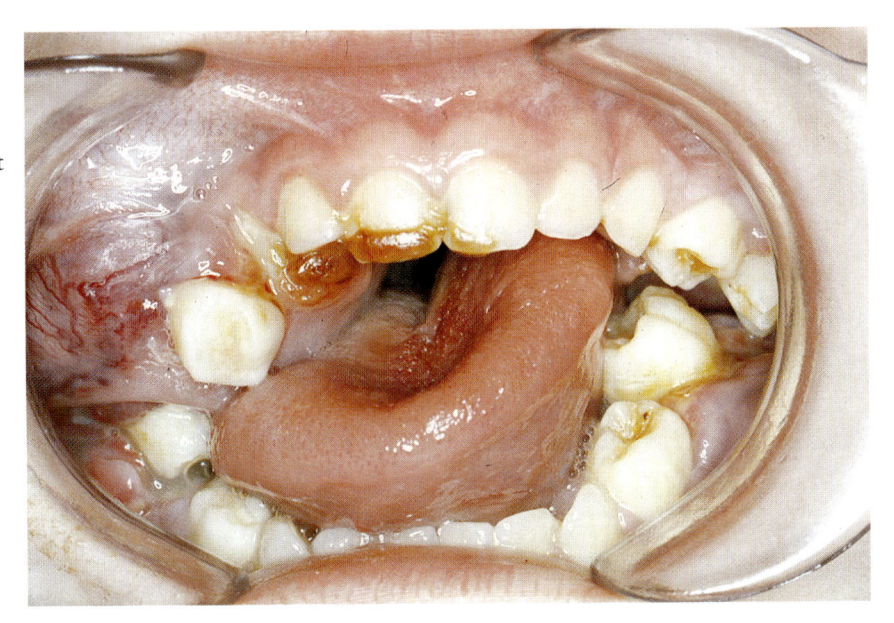

Burkitt's tumor (African jaw tumor)

Definition and epidemiology

Burkitt's tumor appears particularly in the jaws of children in Central Africa. The lesion has also been reported in other parts of the world, especially in North America[495]. It is almost certain that a herpes-like virus, the Epstein-Barr virus, plays a role in the etiology. When the presence of Epstein-Barr virus cannot be demonstrated, the term non-Hodgkin's lymphoma, Burkitt's type, may be used. The literature also refers to a malignant lymphoma that has been designated "Middle East" jaw lymphoma[320].

The African jaw tumor appears almost always in children between two and 14 years of age, in contrast to the American variant, which also may affect adults. There is no sex preference, except for a group of 22 patients reported from South Africa and Namibia in which a male predominance was found[267].

In a study from Lagos a predilection of the tumor for the mandible was observed[18].

Clinical aspects

The lesion appears chiefly as a rapidly growing tumor of the jaws with destruction of bone, anesthesia or paresthesia of the mental nerve, and increased mobility of the teeth (Fig. 9-11)[129].

Radiographic aspects

Radiographically, the cortex surrounding the tooth crypts is at first attenuated and ultimately destroyed, as is the lamina dura around developing or erupted teeth. The teeth and tooth buds become

Lymphoreticular diseases • 161

Fig. 9-11b. No suitable radiograph available. Low-power view of Burkitt's tumor extending close to the epithelium of the oral mucosa. Notice the "starry sky" appearance.

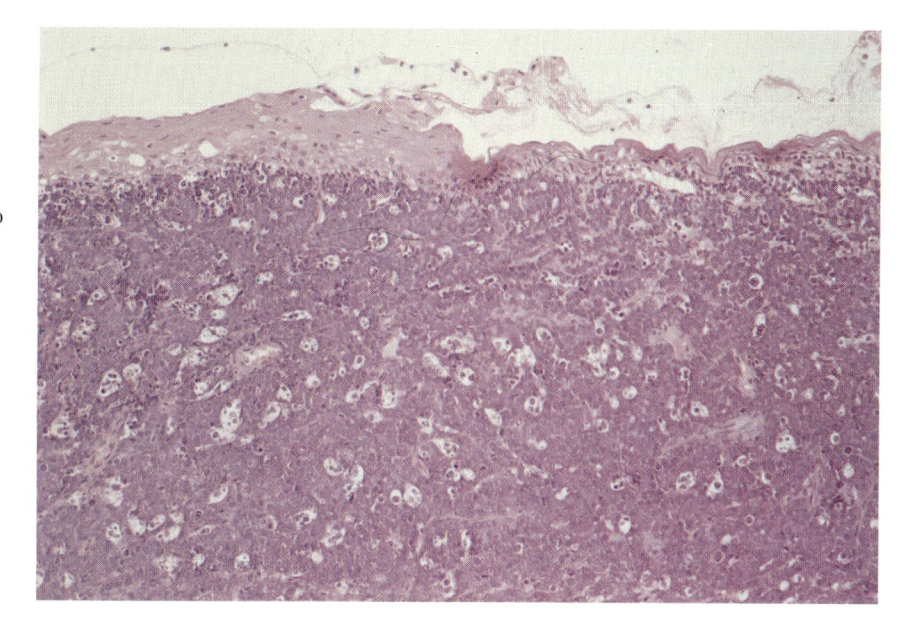

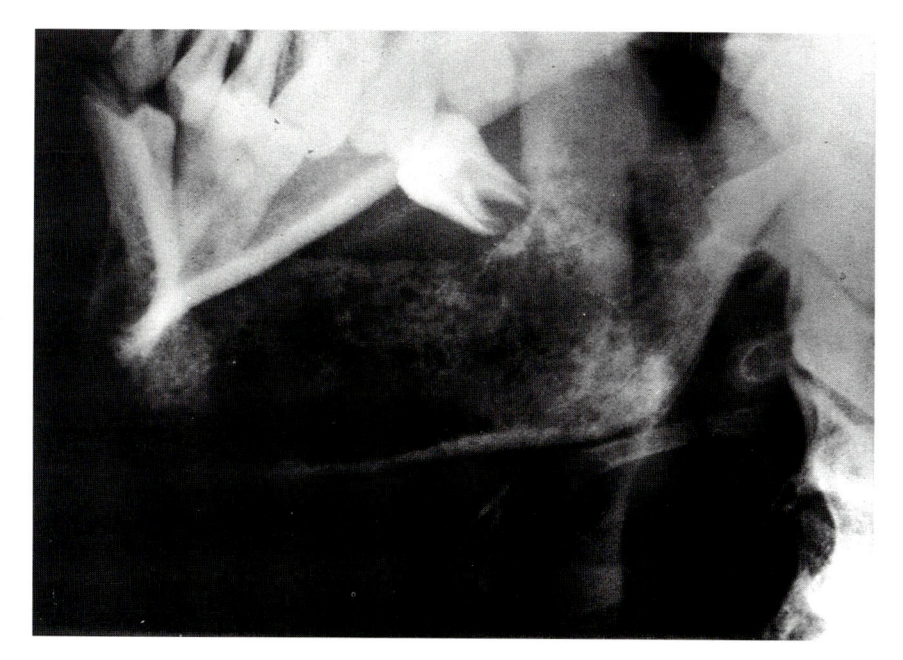

Fig. 9-12. Diffuse destruction of mandible caused by Burkitt's tumor, producing the impression of "teeth floating in air".

displaced, and the tooth follicles enlarge. Finally, there may be so much loss of the bone supporting the teeth that it gives the impression of "teeth floating in air" (Fig. 9-12)[281].

Histologic aspects   The microscopic aspect is characterized by the presence of undifferentiated monomorphic lymphoreticular cells. In general a high mitotic activity can be observed. There are many macrophages with a clear cytoplasm that result in a "starry sky" appearance. This appearance is not pathognomonic, but is at least suggestive of the diagnosis Burkitt's tumor.

Treatment   In general a Burkitt's tumor reacts well to cytostatic drugs. However, insufficient data are available to comment on long-term survival rates.

Solitary plasma cell myeloma

The solitary plasma cell myeloma, also called plasmacytoma, is a rare lesion. It occurs most frequently in the vertebrae, femur and pelvis. The maximum incidence occurs in the fifth to seventh decades. There is a 2:1 male-female ratio. According to some authors this entity is not related to multiple myeloma. Others, however, warn that one should approach the diagnosis of "solitary myeloma" with suspicion, as the majority of cases progress to generalized myelomatosis[500].

Occasionally, the lesion has been reported to occur in the bone of the mandible or maxilla, sometimes even with multiple, bilateral lesions[341].

The clinical presentation can be a non-tender swelling, often slow-growing.

In a German paper, the value of measuring the serum level of the immunoglobulin produced by the tumor is emphasized[554].

The presenting radiological feature can be a defined destructive or multilocular lesion (Fig. 9-13).

Treatment consists of surgical removal or irradiation. The prognosis is favorable. Occasionally, a local recurrence has been reported[115].

Fig. 9-13.
Solitary plasmacytoma of the ascending ramus of the mandible.
Notice the somewhat scalloped outline.
(Courtesy Drs. H. Storch and G. Löwicke, Germany).

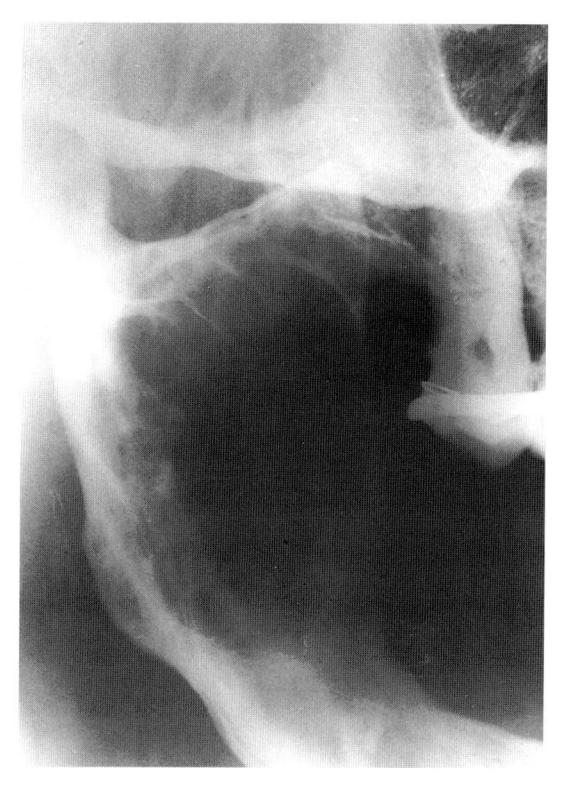

Multiple myeloma
(Kahler's disease)

Definition and epidemiology

Multiple myeloma, also referred to as myelomatosis or Kahler's disease, is characterized by neoplastic proliferation of a clone of plasma cells capable of synthesizing and secreting immunoglobulins or their subunits[456]. In rare instances one may be dealing with a non-secretory myeloma.

Usually several bones are involved at the same time, which may indicate both a multicentric and a metastasizing process.

The skeletal lesions are usually confined to areas of red marrow and are located in the ribs, flat bones, vertebrae, pelvis, skull, clavicles, sternum, femur and humerus[661].

The disease appears twice as often in men as in women, most often between the ages of 40 and 70 years. The first symptoms consist of pain, swelling, or a fracture.

Clinical aspects

Often the mandible, particularly the molar region and the angle of the mandible, is involved[159, 387]. This may result in anesthesia or

164 • Non-osseous, non-chondroid neoplasms

Fig. 9-14a.
Diffuse destructive, lytic changes of mandible in patient suffering from multiple myeloma.

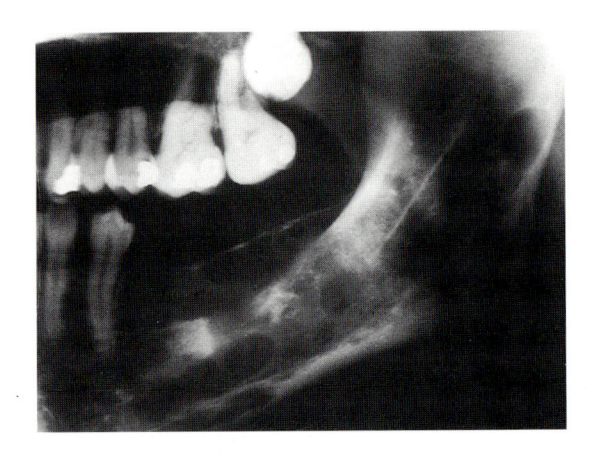

Fig. 9-14b. Histologic section of multiple myeloma. There is some cellular and nuclear pleomorphism.

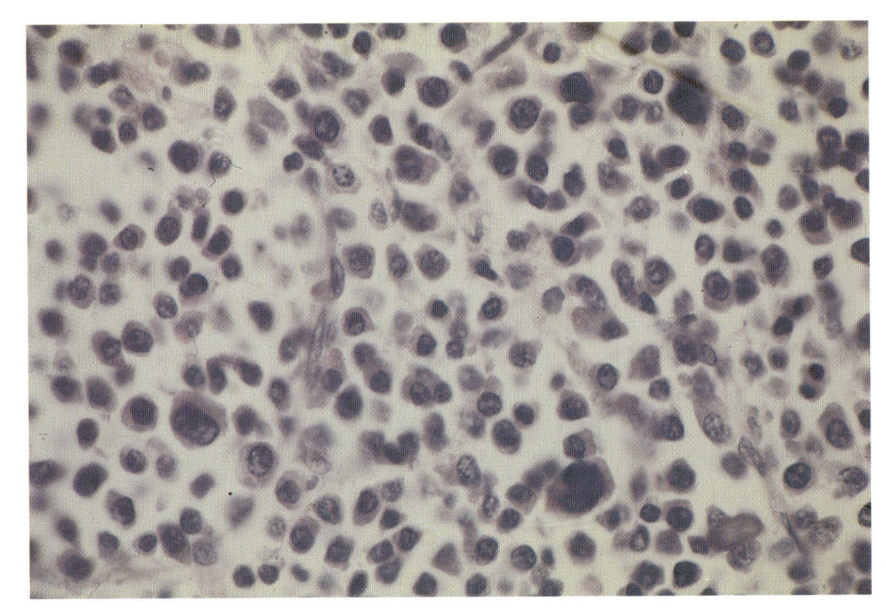

paresthesia of the lower lip. Lesions are rarely present in the maxilla[457]. In a series of 193 patients with multiple myeloma 5% had typical osteolytic alteration of the mandible whereas the maxilla was never involved[326].

Radiographic aspects The radiographic aspect of the involved bone may show either a rather well-demarcated or a diffuse, destructive lytic lesion (Fig. 9-14). Occasionally, external root resorption has been reported[175].

Laboratory findings On laboratory examination, hyperglobulinemia and hypercalcemia, anemia, an increased sedimentation rate and low levels of factor VIII are often seen. In the urine, Bence Jones protein may appear.

Histologic aspects

On microscopic examination aggregates of plasmacytoid cells are observed. These are monoclonal plasmacellular proliferations, which can further be determined with immunoperoxidase techniques[633]. In most cases Russell's bodies, conglomerates of globulins, are present.

Treatment

Treatment can only be palliative and consists of irradiation and/or treatment with cytostatic drugs. The survival time is seldom longer than a few years.

Myelofibrosis

Myelofibrosis is usually a chronic disease of the bone marrow, characterized by progressive fibrosing of the marrow, extramedullary blood production, and leukoerythroblastic anemia. The disease has rarely been observed in the oral cavity[486, 671].

Waldenström's disease

Waldenström's macroglobulinemia is a rare immunoproliferative disease of lymphocytes and sometimes also of plasma cells. Involvement of the mandible is exceptional[523].

Myelosarcoma (chloroma)

Definition and epidemiology

Myelosarcoma or granulocytic sarcoma, also referred to as chloroma due to the green coloration of the tumor, is a rare localized neoplasm of the myeloid cells, usually found in subperiosteal or soft tissues. In most cases the patient is already known to suffer from myeloid leukemia. The disease usually occurs in young and middle-aged adults. The sacrococcygeal region is the site of preference, followed by the spheno-occipital area. There is a slight male predilection. All ages may be affected.

Involvement of the jaw bones is exceptional[466, 486, 577]. A case has been reported of oral soft tissue involvement which developed 15 months before the peripheral blood and bone marrow exhibited evidence of myeloid leukemia[189].

Fig. 9-15. Maxillary swelling caused by melanotic neuro-ectodermal tumor of infancy. (Courtesy Prof.dr. J.J. Pindborg, Denmark).

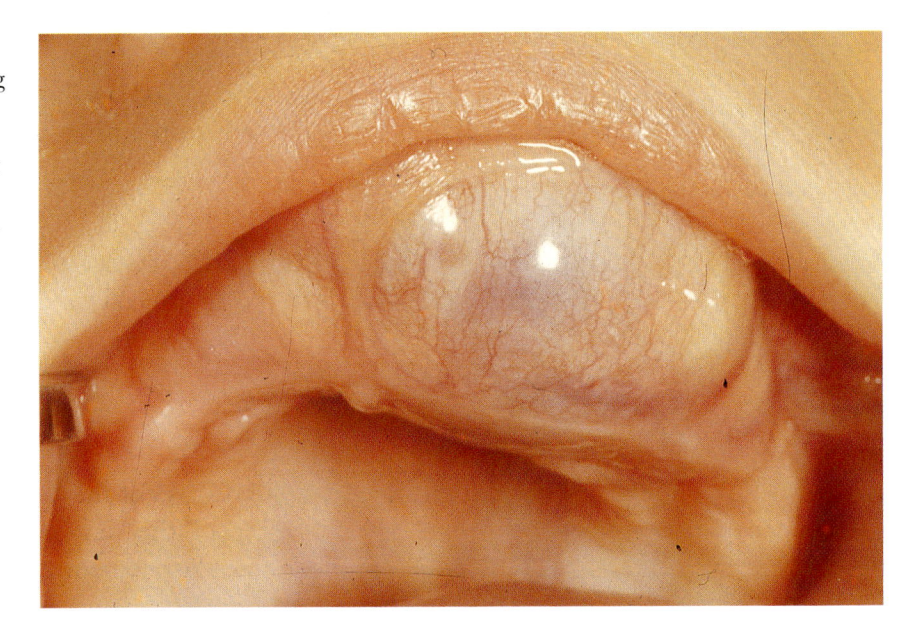

Melanotic neuroectodermal tumor of infancy

Definition and epidemiology

The melanotic neuroectodermal tumor, also referred to as progonoma, appears in infants, as often in boys as in girls[282]. The tumor is usually benign and is most often located in the maxilla. There are also reports of location elsewhere in the body[296]. It is generally assumed that the tumor cells are derived from the neural cyst[402].

Because of a rather strong preference for occurrence in the jaws, the tumor has been classified in the past as an odontogenic tumor.

Clinical aspects

The tumor is rapidly growing, nonulcerative, and may be dark-colored (Fig. 9-15). In a review of the literature, in which 160 cases were described, only a very few appeared to be malignant[135]. A rare case of multicentric distribution has been reported[548].

Laboratory findings

The urine of patients with a melanotic neuroectodermal tumor contains large quantities of vanillylmandelic acid, which is also seen in patients with pheochromocytomas and neuroblastomas.

Radiographic findings

The radiograph usually shows a poorly delineated lucency of the bone (Fig. 9-16). One or more developing teeth may be pushed aside.

Histologic aspects

The melanotic neuroectodermal tumor of infancy consists of two cell types - epithelium-like cells, often arranged in strands, and

Fig. 9-16a.
Ill-defined radiolucency in a 10-year-old patient. Histopathologic diagnosis: melanotic neurectodermal tumor.

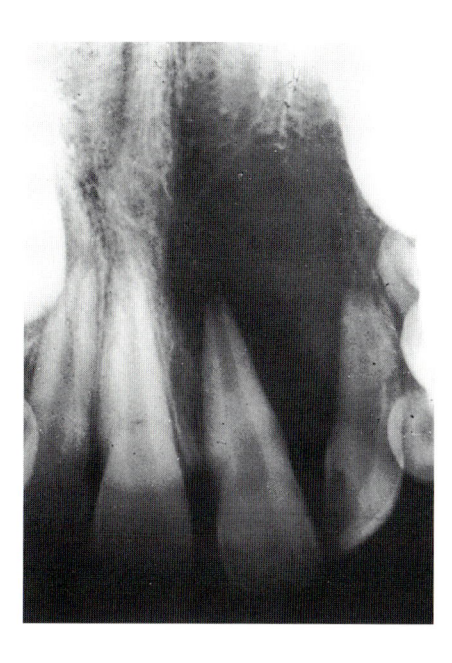

Fig. 9-16b.
Low power view of melanotic neuro-ectodermal tumor. (Courtesy Dr. P.J. Slootweg et al., The Netherlands).

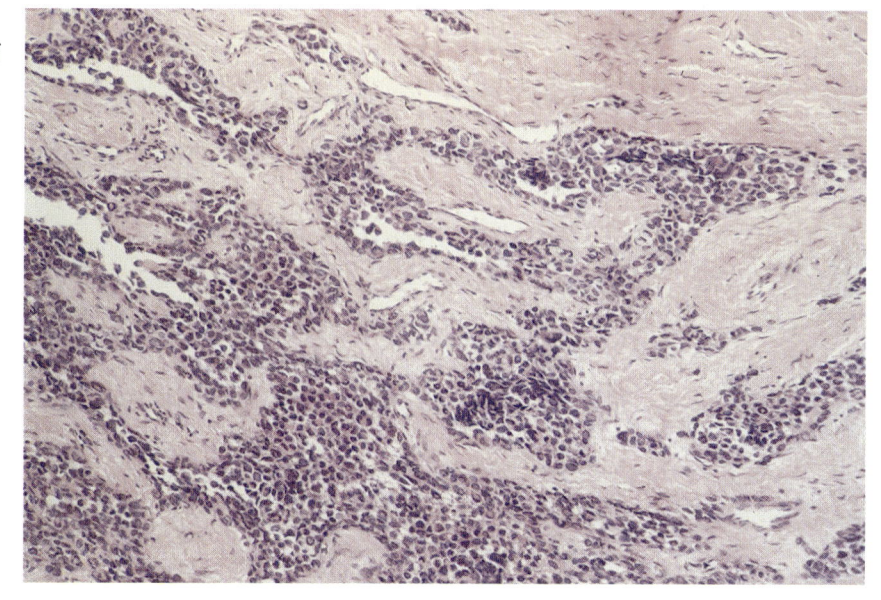

small darkly-staining lymphocyte-like cells – in a cellular fibrous stroma (Fig. 9-16). Melanin is found within the epithelium-like cells, and to a lesser extent within the lymphocyte-like cells[437]. In most cases the tumor is not encapsulated.

Immunohistochemical study of the tumor seems to have little diagnostic significance.

168 • Non-osseous, non-chondroid neoplasms

Fig. 9-17a. Metastatic tumor of the mandible. The history revealed the removal of breast cancer four years previously.

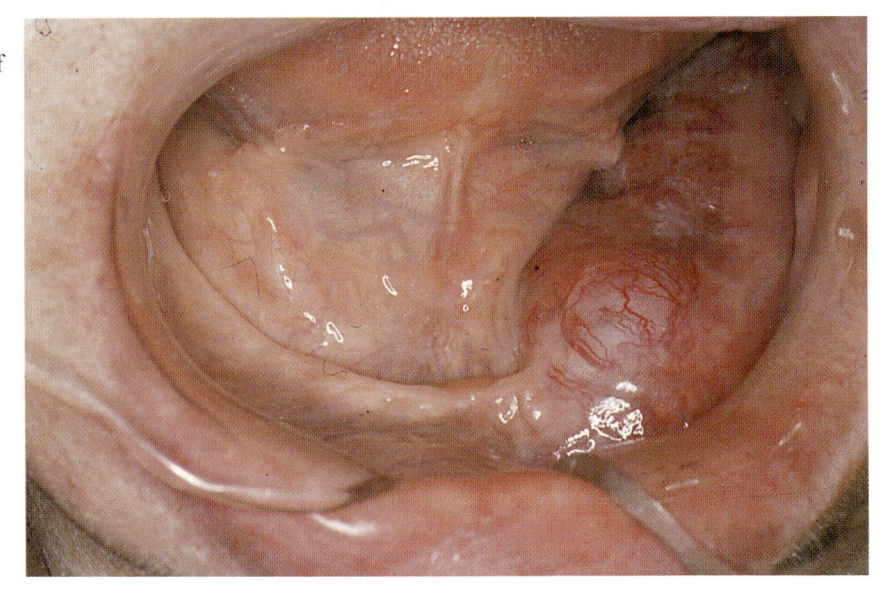

Treatment

Treatment consists of conservative surgical removal, although some clinicians advocate a more aggressive type of surgery, with or without postoperative radiotherapy[279, 537]. Recurrences are rare.

Metastatic tumors

Definition and epidemiology

Metastases in the jaws are relatively uncommon. The following criteria are used for accepting a lesion in the jaws to be a metastasis[120]:

1. The lesion must be a true metastasis localized to the bone tissue, as distinguished from direct invasion by a primary tumor, and from metastasis to the surrounding soft tissue;
2. It must be a microscopically verified tumor;
3. The location of the primary must be known. It should be added that the primary and the lesion under discussion must show identical histologic features.

In a series of 408 malignant tumors of the oral cavity, jaws and face just over 3% metastatic tumors from a distant primary site were recorded[559]. In most cases the mandible is involved, particularly the angle. In a series of 97 cases, collected from the literature from 1884 to 1961, there were 33 cases in which the discovery of a metastasis led to the detection of a primary neoplasm located elsewhere in the body[120].

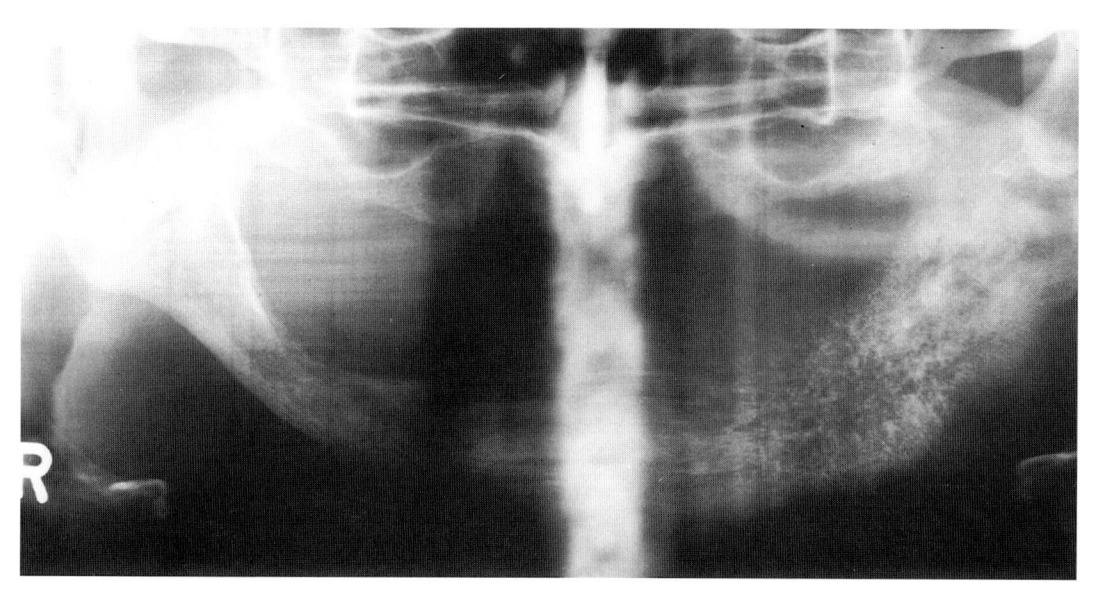

Fig. 9-17b. The radiograph showed a diffuse destruction across the midline. Notice the periosteal reaction in the left side of the mandible. No metastases elsewhere in the body were detected.

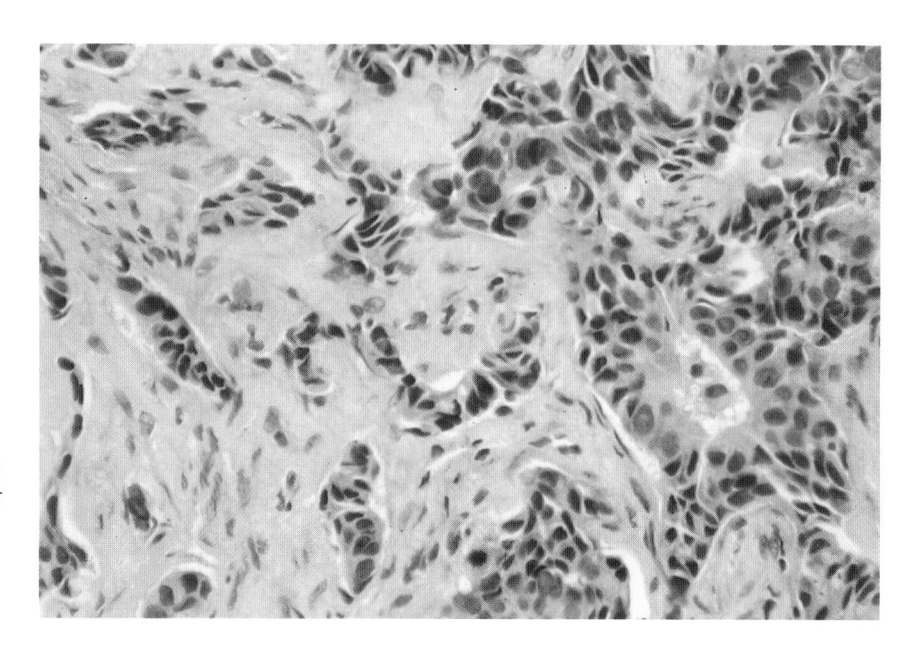

Fig. 9-17c. The biopsy of the mandibular tumor showed the same histologic picture as was seen in the breast.

Location of the primary

The primary is usually, in descending order, to be localized in the breast[639], the lungs[462], the prostate[345], the kidneys[194], colon[361] and rectum[221]. Rare primary sites are the thyroid gland[404], the stomach, the esophagus[297,544,576], the skin[396], the testes[325], the bladder, the liver[588], the cervix, the ovary, and pancreas[205].

Fig. 9-18.
Radiolucency in the angle of the mandible caused by a metastasis of an adenocarcinoma.

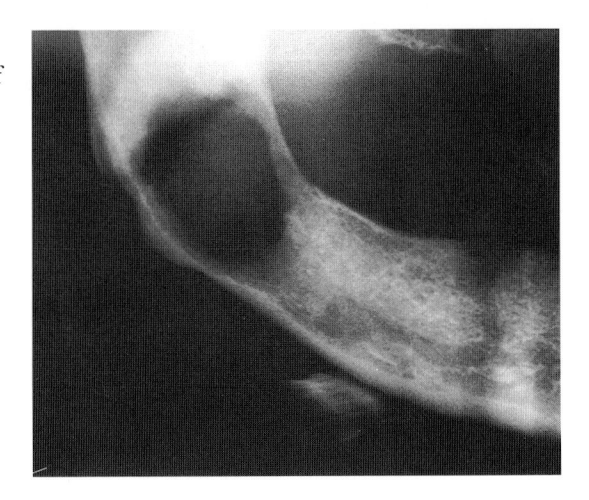

Osteogenic sarcomas of the jaws as a metastasis of primary osteogenic sarcoma located elsewhere in the skeleton are a rarity[556]. This also holds true for metastases of primary neoplasms occurring at an early age, such as retinoblastoma[427], medulloblastoma[182, 473], neuroblastoma[102], chordoma[228,530], and angiosarcoma[399, 511].

A number of patients with metastases of seminomas to the jaws have been described in the literature. It has been pointed out, however, that some or perhaps all of the patients suffered from a malignant lymphoma[57].

In a study of 62 mandibles from autopsied carcinoma deaths, in which none involved a primary carcinoma of the oral region, metastases were confirmed histologically as an incidental finding in 10 cases[258].

In a number of patients with skeletal metastases the primary remains unknown[528]; this is also the case in some jaw metastases.

Clinical aspects

Metastases in the jaws, in rare instances even occurring bilaterally, or simultaneously in the mandible and maxilla, may cause an asymptomatic swelling (Fig. 9-17). On the other hand, anesthesia or paresthesia of the lower lip may be seen. Another sign of a metastatic lesion may be increased mobility of one or more teeth.

A number of cases of metastasis of carcinoma of the lung by implantation in tooth sockets have been reported[367]. Metastasis to the jaw sometimes resembles periodontal or periradicular diseases[400].

Radiographic aspects

On the radiograph a metastasis usually appears as a lucent lesion (Fig. 9-18). Sometimes, however, a radiopaque appearance may be seen as well, in particular in a metastasis of a prostate carcinoma or a carcinoma of the breast, as has been shown already in Fig. 9.17. The radiographs may be negative at the initial stage of a metastasis to the jaw.

Treatment

Only when the primary is under control and in proven absence of metastasis elsewhere in the body is a surgical approach of a curative nature warranted. In most cases treatment can only be of a palliative nature, either due to the extent of the jaw metastasis or due to multiple metastases elsewhere in the body. As has been mentioned earlier, in some cases no primary can be detected, especially when dealing with an adenocarcinoma.

Neuroblastoma

Definition and epidemiology

A neuroblastoma develops from primitive sympathetic neural tissue. It is the most common malignant tumor in infants. The majority of the tumors is located within the abdomen, derived from the adrenal medulla or from the adjacent symphatic chain.

The occurrence of primary neuroblastomas in the jaws is exceptional[36, 96]. Metastatic neuroblastomas to the jaws are slightly more common[102].

Neurofibroma and neurilemmoma

Definition and epidemiology

The terms neurofibroma and neurilemmoma (Schwannoma) are sometimes used as synonyms. There is at least a distinction with regard to the encapsulation, a neurofibroma being almost always unencapsulated. Furthermore, neurofibromas can be a manifestation of Recklinghausen's disease, also referred to as neurofibromatosis[590].

With regard to location in the jawbones the two entities are often grouped together by applying the term "benign neural sheath neoplasm"[169] or benign neurogenic tumors[659]. These tumors occur predominantly in females, under 45 years of age.

Clinical aspects

Reviews of the literature revealed approximately 30 cases of a neurilemmoma located centrally in the mandible[336, 497]. A case of neurilemmoma of the inferior alveolar nerve in association with the organ of Chievitz has been reported[507]. Occurrence in the maxilla is rare[418]. A review of solitary neurofibromas of the mandible also disclosed approximately 30 cases[439].

In a series of 38 patients with neurofibromatosis, 92 % of the sample had at least one intraoral or radiographic sign of the disease[140].

Swelling of the involved site of the bone is the most common symptom. Pain and paresthesia have also been described. In neurofibromatosis also mandibular deformities and enlargement of the mandibular foramen may be observed (Fig. 9-19)[516].

Radiographic aspects

Radiographically, both neurilemmoma and neurofibroma appear as a unilocular or multilocular lesion that may give rise to resorption of teeth (Fig. 9-20)[589].

Histologic aspects

The histologic features of a neurilemmoma are classically described as consisting of two cell types, Antoni type A and Antoni type B. The A cells have an elongated nucleus and form a palisade pattern. The B cells do not show such a pattern. Verocay bodies are another characteristic finding. They are small hyalinelike structures, situated between the Antoni type A cells. The tumor is usually well-encapsulated, the latter feature being the most obvious one with regard to the possible distinction between a neurilemmoma and a neurofibroma.

Treatment

Neurofibromas tend to recur more often than neurilemmomas when treated by conservative excision[271].

Ganglioneuroma

Only three cases of a so-called ganglioneuroma of the mandible have been reported. In one of the cases the jaw lesion possibly represented a metastasis from an unknown primary site[112].

Neurogenic sarcoma

Malignant tumors of peripheral nerves, in general referred to as neurogenic sarcomas, are rare and may be the result of malignant transformation of benign tumors of the nerve sheath or may arise *de novo*[632]. Such malignancies can occur in patients suffering from neurofibromatosis, but also prevail isolated[301].

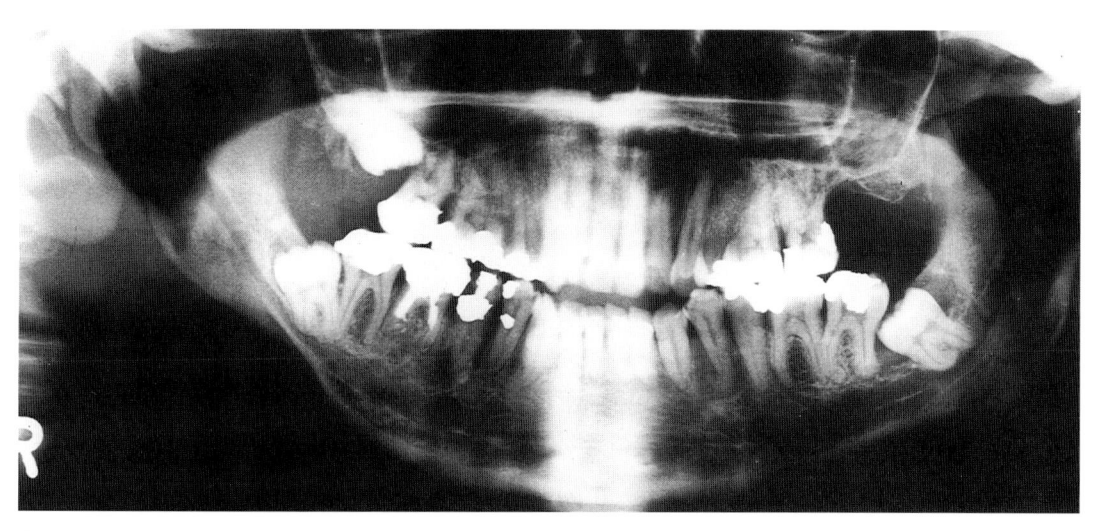

Fig. 9-19. Mandibular deformity at the right side in patient with neurofibromastosis.

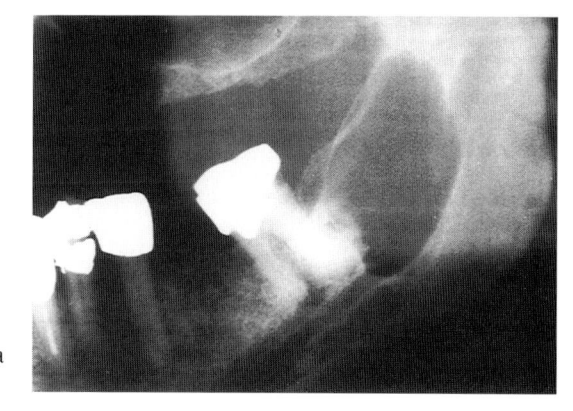

Fig. 9-20. Well-circumscribed radiolucency in left ascending ramus caused by a solitary neurofibroma.

Rhabdomyosarcoma

Rhabdomyosarcomas of the jaw bones are rare[428, 617]. There are no characteristic clinical or radiographic features.

The prognosis is generally poor, due to widespread metastases.

Fig. 9-21a.
Multilobular radiolucency in the angle of the mandible. A biopsy revealed the presence of a muco-epidermoid carcinoma.

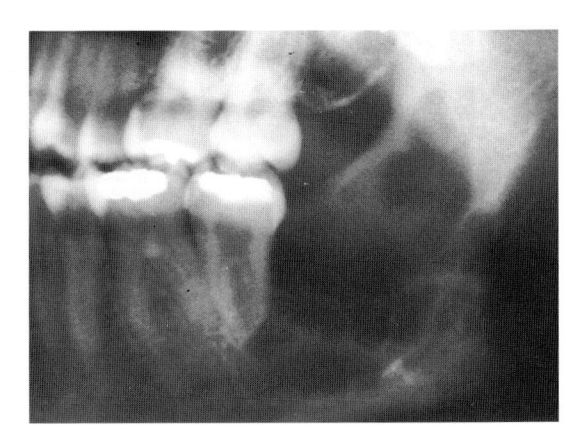

Salivary gland neoplasms

Salivary gland neoplasms developing centrally in the jaws, in particular the mucoepidermoid tumor, are extremely rare[222]. When such a tumor appears, the question arises as to whether the tumor in fact originates primarily in the bone.

The possible presence of salivary gland tissue in the bone could be attributed to a developmental disturbance, in which salivary gland tissue is enclosed within the bone. Also the possibility of mucous metaplasia of the lining epithelium of odontogenic cysts has been considered. The proposal has been made to include the most commonly reported intraosseous salivary gland tumor, the mucoepidermoid carcinoma, in the group of primary intraosseous carcinoma[602] (See chapter 10, p. 232). Primary central adenoid cystic carcinomas are rare[275], and may mimic an ameloblastoma and even a metastatic basal cell carcinoma.

Radiographically, intraosseous salivary gland tumors may resemble an ameloblastoma or an odontogenic cyst. The radiographic aspect may also consist of diffuse, opaque changes (Fig. 9-21).

Treatment consists of surgical removal.

Salivary gland neoplasms • 175

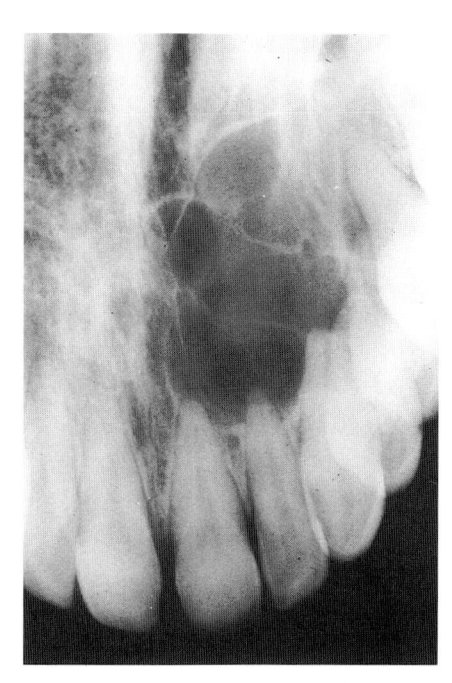

Fig. 9-21b. A somewhat similar radiographic aspect of a mucoepidermoid carcinoma in the maxilla.

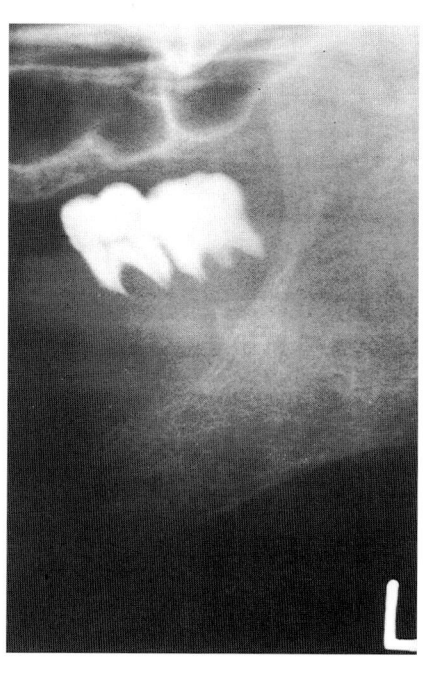

Fig. 9-21c. Diffuse radiopaque changes in the mandible caused by an intraosseous adenoid cystic carcinoma. Note the "floating in air" impression of the two molars. (Courtesy Drs. K.G.H. van der Wal et al., The Netherlands).

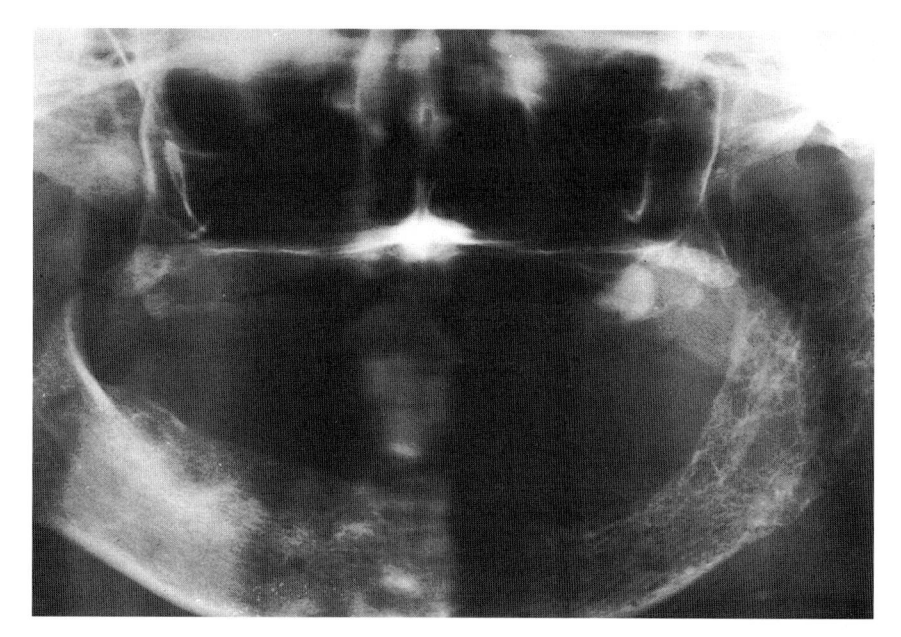

Fig. 9-21d. Another example of the radiographic changes of the left side of the mandible caused by an intraosseous adenoid cystic carcinoma.

Teratoma

A teratoma, defined as a neoplasm composed of several tissue types, rarely occurs in the oral cavity, either in the soft tissues or in the bones.

In the literature an exceptional case of a malignant teratoma involving the mandible has been reported[280]. The patient was a 14-year-old girl. The tumor was located around an impacted lower wisdom tooth and had extended through both the buccal and lingual cortical plates.

Another case of a teratoma has been reported to occur in the maxilla of an 11-year-old Malayan boy[215].

CHAPTER 10

Odontogenic tumors

Odontogenic tumors involve one or more of the dental tissues. Some of them are to be considered developmental disturbances.

Various classifications of odontogenic tumors have been proposed. The discussion here will be based on a modified version of the classification proposed by the World Health Organization[437] (Table 10-1). The main clinical, radiographic, and histologic aspects of both benign and malignant central (intraosseous) odontogenic tumors and their treatment will be discussed.

Table 10-1. Classification of odontogenic tumors (WHO)[437], modified

Benign odontogenic tumors
  Benign ameloblastoma
  Squamous odontogenic tumor
  Calcifying epithelial odontogenic tumor
    (Pindborg tumor)
  Ameloblastic fibroma
  Ameloblastic fibro-dentinoma
    ("Dentinoma")
  Ameloblastic fibro-odontoma
  Odontoameloblastoma
  Adenomatoid odontogenic tumor
  Calcifying odontogenic cyst (Gorlin cyst)
  Odontoma (compound, complex)
  Fibroma (odontogenic, central and
    peripheral)
  Myxoma (odontogenic)
  Cementum containing lesions
  – Cementoblastoma ("True cementoma")
  – Fibro-osseous cemental lesions
  – Ossifying and cementifying fibroma

Malignant odontogenic tumors
  Odontogenic carcinomas
  – Malignant ameloblastoma and
    ameloblastic carcinoma
  – Primary intraosseous carcinoma
  – Other carcinomas arising from
    odontogenic epithelium
  – Clear cell odontogenic tumor/
    carcinoma
  Odontogenic sarcomas
  – Ameloblastic fibrosarcoma
    (ameloblastic sarcoma)
  – Ameloblastic odontosarcoma

Fig. 10-1a.
Profile of patient with a histologically benign ameloblastoma of the mandible. The swelling was of at least 10 years duration.

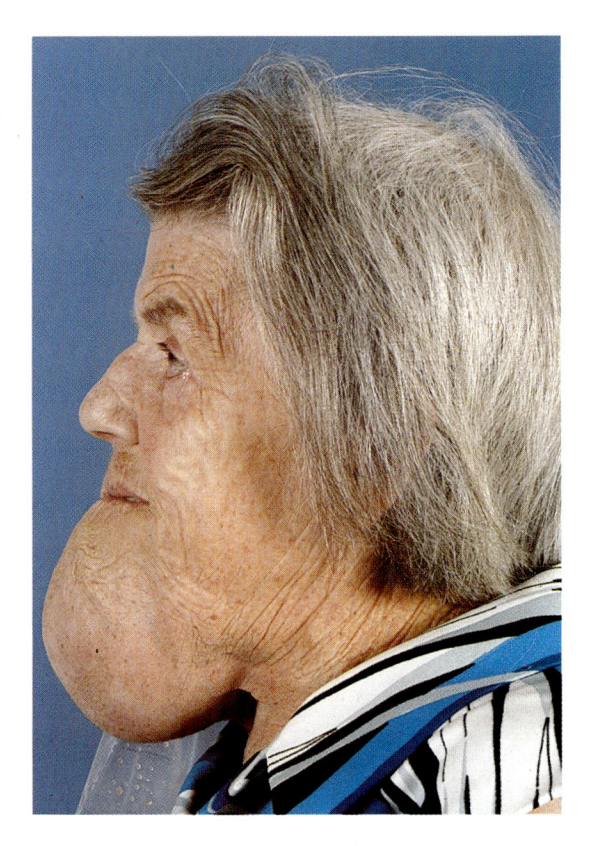

Benign neoplasms

Benign ameloblastoma

Definition — The benign ameloblastoma has in the past been called "adamantinoma". Today, the term ameloblastoma is widely accepted. It is a benign, but locally invasive neoplasm consisting of proliferating odontogenic epithelium lying in a fibrous stroma[437]. It is beyond the scope of this chapter to discuss the so-called adamantinoma of long bones[307].

The tumor cells resemble ameloblasts, but there is no enamel production. The majority of ameloblastomas are located within the bone. In rare instances an ameloblastoma apparently arises from the basal cells of the oral mucosa, being referred to as an extraosseous or peripheral ameloblastoma[33].

Epidemiology — No exact data are available on the incidence of ameloblastoma. Presumably it is about 1 per million population per year. There are

Fig. 10-1b.
Intraoral view.

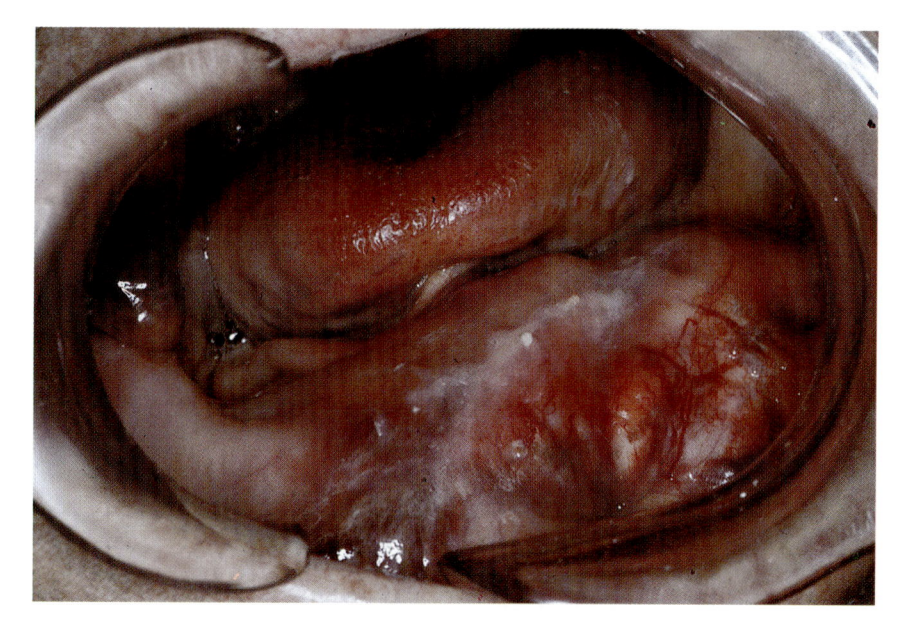

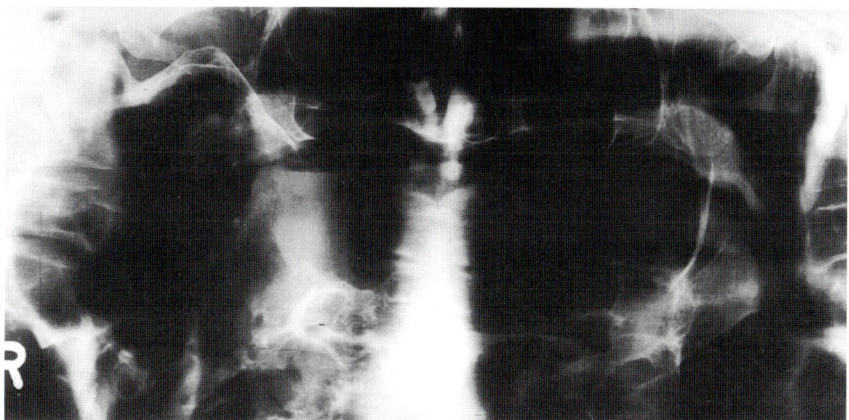

Fig. 10-1c. The panoramic view revealed the involvement of almost the entire mandible.

possibly some slight geographic differences. There is no distinct preference for either sex.

The usual age at the time of diagnosis is about 20 to 30 years. The age at the time of diagnosis for the ameloblastoma in the maxilla is generally higher.

Clinical aspects   Most ameloblastomas are localized in the mandible, especially in the molar region[302]. The neoplasm may appear as a swelling of varying consistency (Figs. 10-1, 10-2). The overlying mucosa remains intact. Complaints of pain are rare. Even with very large ameloblas-

Fig. 10-2a. Ameloblastoma of the maxillary tuberosity with secondary ulceration due to a partial denture.

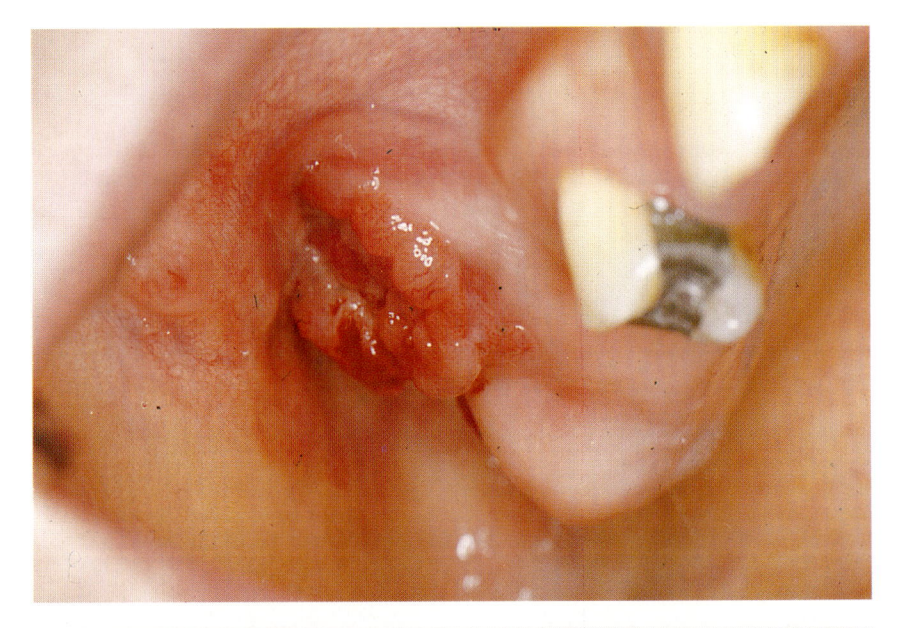

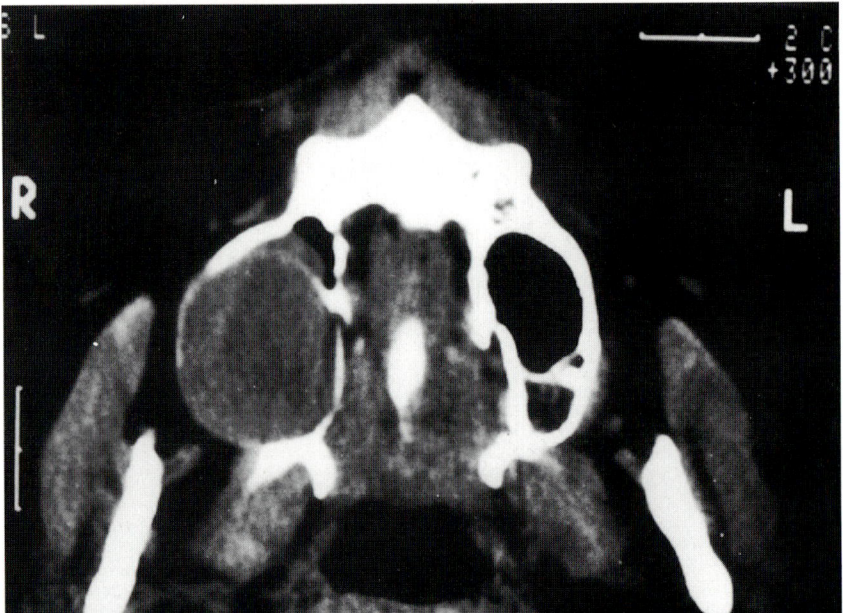

Fig. 10-2b. Notice the involvement of the right maxillary sinus. (Courtesy Prof.dr. J. Valk, The Netherlands).

tomas, localized in the mandible, the alveolar nerve remains undisturbed. An ameloblastoma rarely, if ever, gives rise to trismus. Although a considerable resorption of the apices of the teeth may appear, it is relatively uncommon that these teeth become mobile.

Radiographic aspects

The radiographic aspect of an ameloblastoma may vary considerably. It may be a uni- or a multilobular lucency, with or without an associated impacted tooth. The tumor is usually well-circumscribed. Expansion of the cortical plates may be observed. The cortical plates can sometimes be perforated by the tumor cells, which may or may not be visible on radiographs. In some instances resorption of the apices of the adjacent teeth has taken place (Figs. 10-3 to 10-5).

In unicystic or cystogenic ameloblastomas six radiographic patterns have been identified: pericoronal unilateral, extensive pericoronal unilocular, pericoronal scalloped, periapical unilocular, interradicular, and multilocular[180]. It should be realized that the radiographic impression of a cystic lesion can be false and may be based on a solid (ameloblastomatous) tumor.

In the radiographic differential diagnosis a number of odontogenic cysts and tumors should be considered, as well as central giant cell granuloma, fibrous dysplasia or ossifying/cementifying fibroma, or solitary bone cyst, and aneurysmal bone cyst.

Magnetic resonance images (MRI) of ameloblastomas have been compared with computed tomographic (CT) images. In spite of some improvements gained from MRI, familiarity with CT dictates that the MRI evaluation complements, and does not substitute for, the CT evaluation[266].

Histologic aspects

Based on the histologic features of an ameloblastoma, various subclassifications can be made, such as follicular and plexiform. In a study of 97 cases of mandibular ameloblastomas, the plexiform type was more common in young patients while the follicular type was more common in patients older than 20 years of age[583].

The tumor cells of a follicular ameloblastoma are arranged in follicles; the outer row of cells forms a characteristic palisade arrangement. Palisading is an accentuation of the basal cell layer of the epithelium with a linear arrangement of the centrally located nuclei which have an increased basophilia[443]. The cells more centrally situated in the follicles may be somewhat vacuolated and resemble cells of the stellate reticulum of a developing tooth (Fig. 10-6). Differentiation toward squamous epithelium may appear centrally in such islands of a follicular ameloblastoma. This may lead to further histologic subtyping and be called "acanthomatous" ameloblastoma. If the cytoplasm of the epithelial tumor cells also show granular changes, the term granular cell ameloblastoma may be ap-

Fig. 10-3.
Well-circumscribed radiolucency suggestive of dentigerous cyst. The "cyst", however, is extending well beyond the enamel-cemental junction, which warrants suspicion. Histopathologic diagnosis: ameloblastoma.

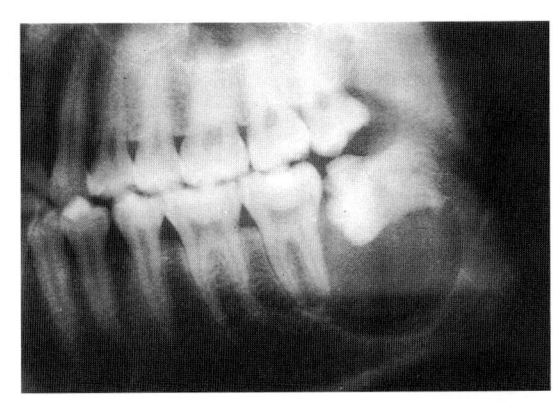

Fig. 10-4.
Rather well-circumscribed radiolucency between 45 and 46. No symptoms. The radiographic picture is not diagnostic. Histopathologic diagnosis: ameloblastoma.

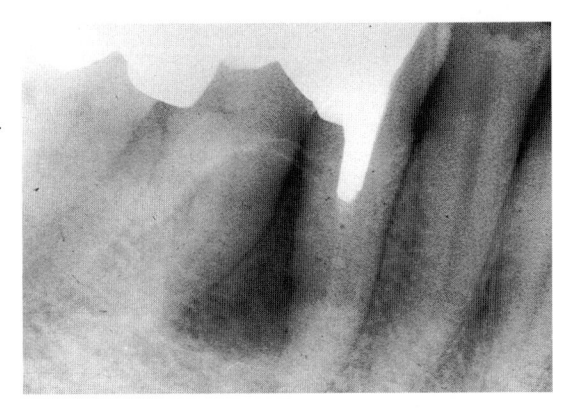

Fig. 10-5.
Well-circumscribed radiolucency. The 46 and 47 were vital. Notice the resorption of the apices. Ameloblastoma.

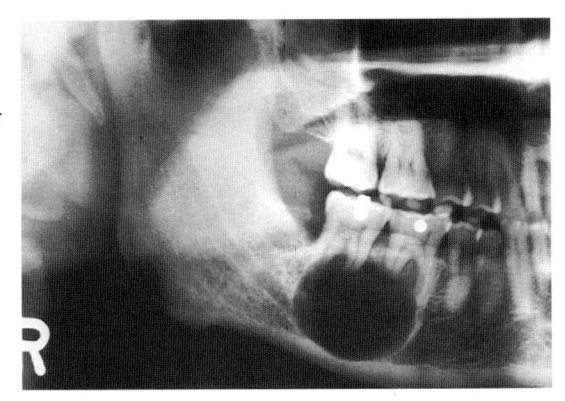

plied[641]. Another possible histologic feature of a follicular ameloblastoma is the cystic degeneration that occasionally may take place in the epithelial islands.

The plexiform ameloblastoma consists of anastomosing fields and strands of tumor cells without the distinct palisading of the outer cell layer that is characteristic of the follicular ameloblastoma.

Fig. 10-6. Follicular ameloblastoma. Palisade arrangement of the outer row of cells of the follicles.

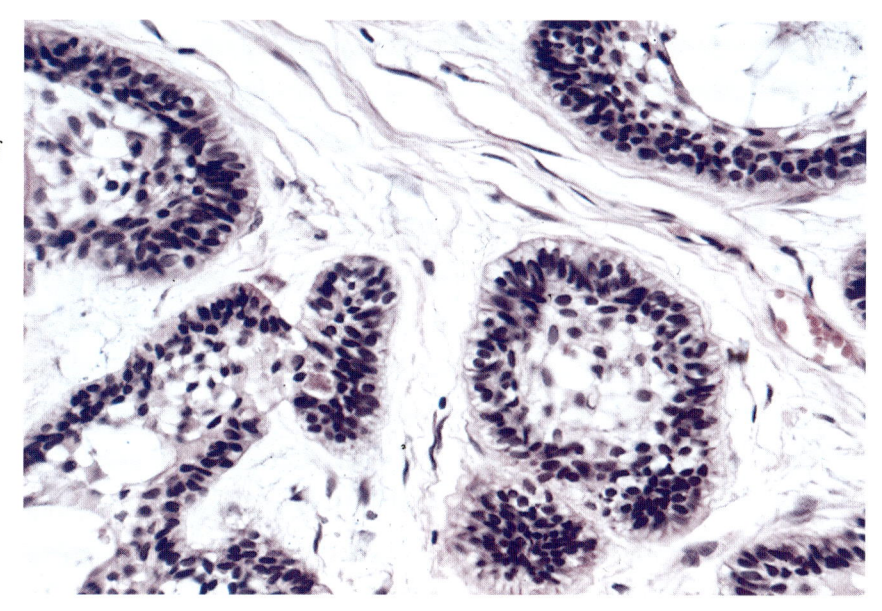

Fig. 10-7. Plexiform ameloblastoma. Cystic changes in the stromal part of the tumor.

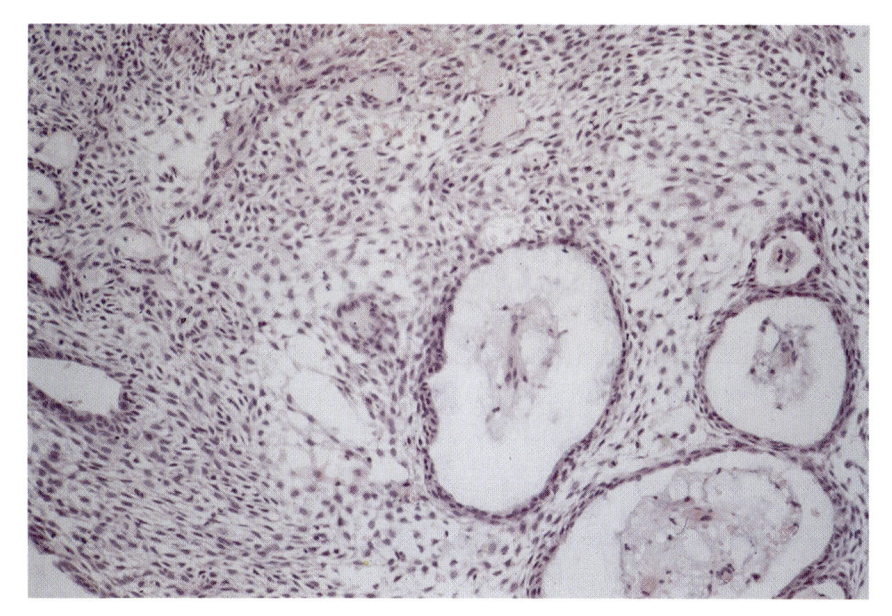

The plexiform ameloblastoma also lacks the stellate reticulum-like changes. Cystic changes may occur in the stromal part of the tumor (Fig. 10-7).

Histologically, neither the follicular nor the plexiform type of ameloblastoma is clearly encapsulated, which in itself is no proof of malignancy. The cellular and nuclear polymorphism and the number of mitoses of a benign ameloblastoma are low.

Fig. 10-8. Part of the wall of a unicystic "luminal" ameloblastoma.

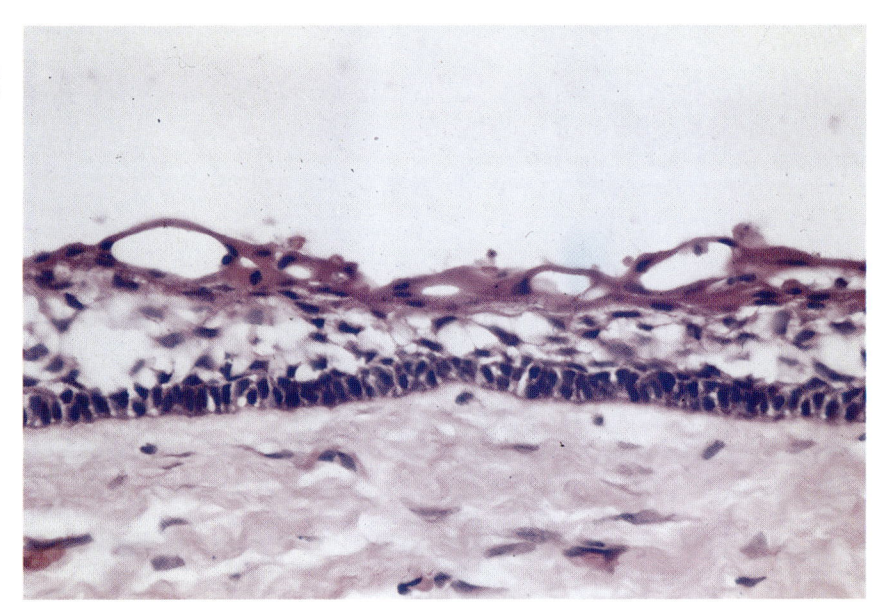

The connective tissue of an ameloblastoma is often rich in collagen. Hyalinization is sometimes seen around the tumor fields. Such hyaline changes may also be seen in other odontogenic lesions. In a study of 116 ameloblastomas, the phenomenon of desmoplasia has been described in the connective tissue of ameloblastoma in 14 cases[598]. Occasionally, bone formation may be observed[415].

Special consideration should be given to the unicystic ameloblastoma. Macroscopically and microscopically it is a cystic lesion that could be mistaken for an odontogenic cyst. On histologic examination the epithelial cells of the cyst lining have an ameloblastomatous appearance, characterized by palisading of the basal cells, a distinct vacuolization of the cells of the spinal layer, and a squamous cell-like superficial layer toward the lumen (Fig. 10-8). This variant of the ameloblastoma is sometimes called "luminal" ameloblastoma. Occasionally, ameloblastic proliferations extend either into the lumen or into the surrounding "cyst" wall ("mural") (Fig. 10-9). Unfortunately, the terms unicystic, luminal, and mural ameloblastomas are not always used in the same way throughout the literature. Luminal proliferation can be defined as proliferation of the lining epithelium into the cystic cavity, whereas proliferation of the lining epithelium into the fibrous capsule can be called "mural"[443].

In tooth follicles of impacted teeth, proliferations of odontogenic

Fig. 10-9. Part of the wall of a unicystic "mural" ameloblastoma.

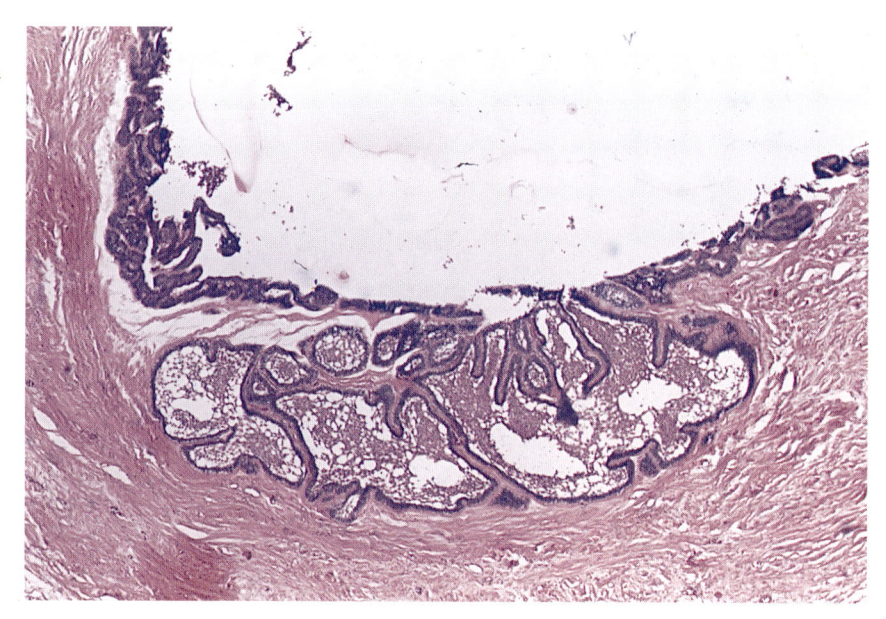

Fig. 10-10. Epithelial nests in a normal tooth follicle, not to be mistaken for an ameloblastoma.

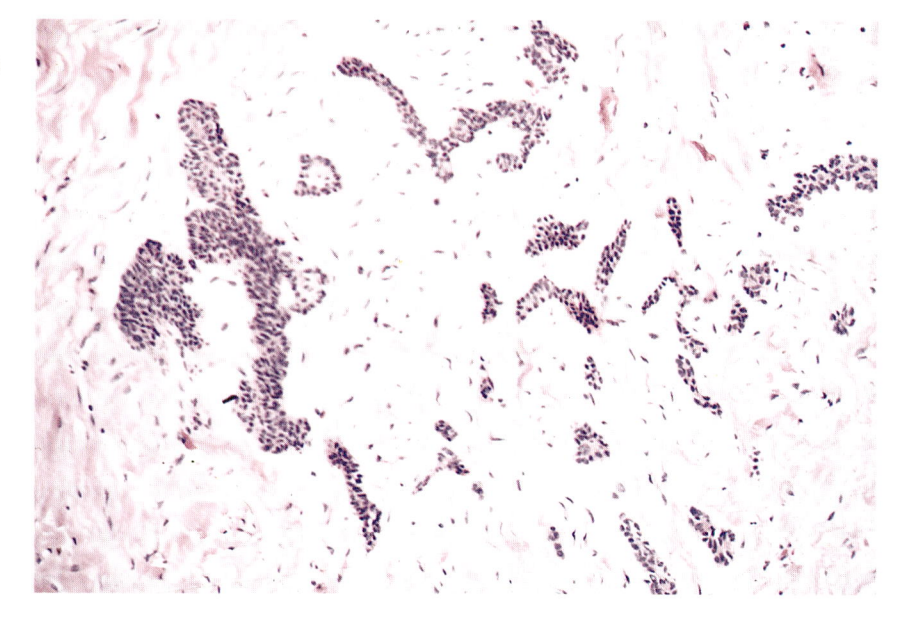

epithelium are often encountered that, on histologic examination, may be mistaken for ameloblastic tumor cells (Fig. 10-10). In that case the clinical and radiographic data are of utmost importance in arriving at a correct diagnosis. On the other hand, the histologic differential diagnosis of a benign (or malignant) ameloblastoma includes, apart from other odontogenic tumors such as the ameloblastic fibroma and the squamous odontogenic tumor, the rare intraosseous adenoid cystic carcinoma and the even more rare metastasis of a basal cell carcinoma of the skin.

Treatment

The treatment of an amelobastoma consists of wide surgical removal, except in case of a unicystic ameloblastoma, to be discussed later. If there is any doubt about possible spreading into the soft tissues, a wide excision of the involved mucosal area should be performed at the same time. As to the radicality in the bone, it appears justified to allow a margin of 1 cm around the tumor. This means, in practice, that only small ameloblastomas of the mandible may be removed by a segmental resection, leaving the continuity intact. For an ameloblastoma of the maxilla it is unanimously accepted that an aggressive surgical approach is required in all instances.

In a study from Japan it was shown that in ameloblastomas that have been treated conservatively the recurrence rate was significantly higher in the follicular type than in the plexiform type; besides, recurrence was seen more frequently in the multilocular than in the unilocular type, and patients under age 20 had a better prognosis[582]. Others, too, have reported a low rate of recurrence following enucleation or curettage of unicystic ameloblastoma[329]. It should be realized, however, that the unicysticity of the tumor can not be predicted preoperatively from the radiograph.

In practice the clinician often is not aware of the possibility of an ameloblastoma before or even during treatment. This is understandable since the clinical and radiographic features of an ameloblastoma are not pathognomonic. The question then arises whether the lesion has been removed completely or whether additional surgery is required. In many such cases a wait-and-see policy is favored, especially in case of localization in the mandible, and even more so when one has been dealing with a unicystic ameloblastoma.

Although few data are available, it is generally assumed that an ameloblastoma is not radiosensitive. This may not apply to a small volume of tumor cells left behind after a surgical procedure[88]. Yet, favorable results have been described with primary irradiation of extensive ameloblastomas in the maxilla and the maxillary sinus[38]. Nevertheless, radiotherapy does not appear to be the appropriate primary treatment for an operable ameloblastoma[211].

The most significant problem in the treatment of the benign ameloblastoma is the chance of local recurrence. Such recurrences usually appear within five years[392], but may in rare cases become manifest after as long as 25 years. Recurrences that develop in a bone transplant used for reconstruction are not uncommon. Furthermore, a benign ameloblastoma may change into a malignant one after incomplete removal. In all, more than enough reasons exist to follow a patient who has been treated for an ameloblastoma both clinically and radiographically for at least 10 years. At first, this should take place twice a year and, thereafter, once a year or once every two years.

Squamous odontogenic tumor

Definition and epidemiology

At the time the WHO classification was proposed, the squamous odontogenic tumor (SOT) had not yet been described as a separate entity in the literature. It is a benign tumor, presumably arising from epithelial rests of Malassez.

The tumor appears as often in the maxilla as in the mandible, occasionally in multiple sites or bilaterally, and is usually seen in young or middle-aged patients. Also familial occurrence has been reported[330].

Clinical aspects

No characteristic clinical aspects are present.

Radiographic aspects

Radiographically, the tumor characteristically has been described as a triangular or circular radiolucency adjacent to the root of an erupted tooth[447].

Histologic aspects

Histologically, the SOT consists of islands of odontogenic epithelium which lack the palisading of the outer cell layer that is seen in ameloblastoma. No signs of induction around the epithelial nests are present in the connective tissue. Often, intraepithelial calcifications appear. On the one hand, the SOT may be confused with a well-differentiated squamous cell carcinoma. On the other hand, an acanthomatous ameloblastoma may erroneously be diagnosed as a SOT, which may lead to inadequate treatment.

Treatment

In general, conservative surgical removal seems the treatment of choice, but a more radical approach is perhaps indicated when dealing with a SOT in the maxilla. Some authors have mentioned a malignant variant, without giving their criteria for malignancy.

Calcifying epithelial odontogenic tumor
(Pindborg tumor)

Definition and epidemiology

The calcifying epithelial odontogenic tumor (CEOT), also referred to as Pindborg tumor, is an uncommon epithelial odontogenic tumor. It is a locally invasive epithelial neoplasm characterized by the development of intra-epithelial structures, probably of an amyloid-like nature, which may become calcified and which may be liberated as the cells break down[437].

The epithelial cells are presumably derived from the stratum intermedium of the dental organ. In a review of the literature, more than 100 patients have been described[202]. The average age in men is 25 and in women approximately 50 years.

Clinical aspects

The tumor appears particularly in the mandible. The premolar-molar regions are the sites of preference. Most CEOT's are situated intraosseously. A few extraosseous peripheral CEOT's have been reported. The tumor usually is manifested as a nonpainful swelling.

Radiographic aspects

Radiographically, CEOT's may vary widely. They may be well-circumscribed lesions, but also diffuse ones that often have a mixed opaque-lucent appearance (Fig. 10-11). In half the cases there is an associated impacted tooth.

Histologic aspects

Microscopically, the CEOT is characterized by the presence of epithelial cells, often arranged in nests, resembling to some extent the features of an adenocarcinoma. The cellular outlines are usually not very distinct. There is an eosinophilic, slightly granular cytoplasm. The nuclei are often polymorphic. Giant cells may be present. The presence of amyloid-like structures is characteristic. Another characteristic finding is the presence of calcifications in the amyloid-like material.

Treatment

Some investigators suggest treating the calcifying epithelial odontogenic tumor in the same way as an ameloblastoma, while others advocate a less aggressive approach. True malignant behavior is uncommon.

Fig. 10-11a.
Mixed opaque-lucent aspect of CEOT in the maxillary tuberosity.

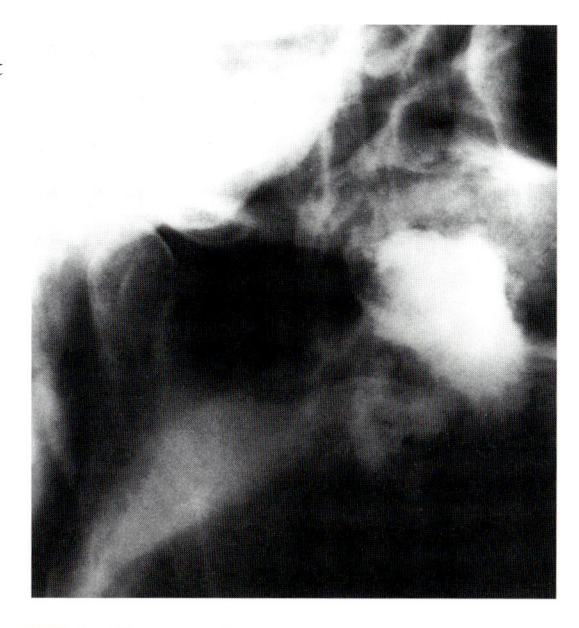

Fig. 10-11b. Histopathologic aspect. Notice the nuclear pleomorphism.

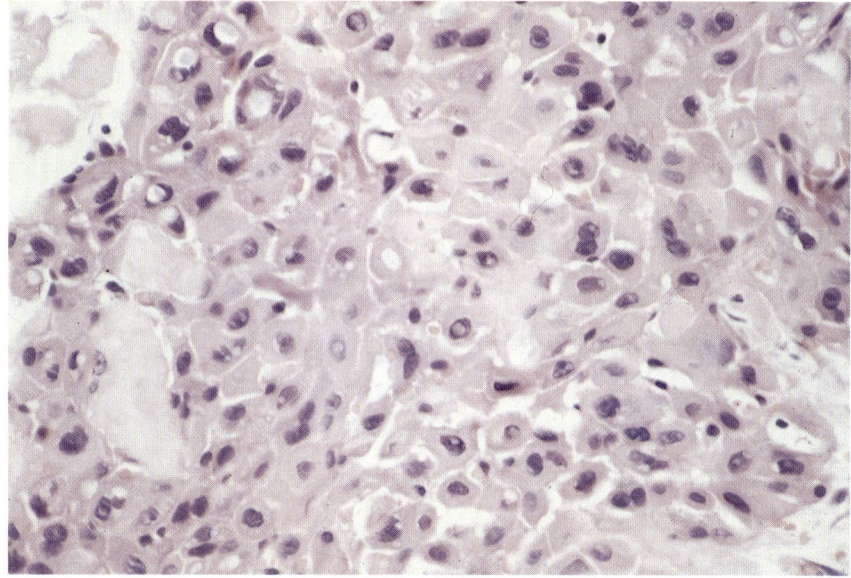

Ameloblastic fibroma

Definition and epidemiology

The ameloblastic fibroma, also referred to as one of the mixed odontogenic tumors[533], is a neoplasm composed of proliferating odontogenic epithelium embedded in a cellular mesodermal tissue that resembles the dental papilla, but without the formation of odontoblasts[437].

A distinction must be made between hamartomatous proliferations that may be encountered in tooth follicles or in peripheral epulislike swellings of the gingiva and a true intraosseous ameloblastic fibroma with neoplastic properties.

The ameloblastic fibroma is a rare tumor. The lesion occurs in men twice as often as in women. The average age of the patients is about 15 years.

Clinical and radiographic aspects

The tumor is usually located in the molar regions of the mandible. Clinically and radiographically the tumor cannot be clearly distinguished from an ameloblastoma. In some cases there is an associated impacted tooth.

Histologic aspects

The microscopic aspect is characterized by islands of odontogenic epithelium in various configurations, strongly resembling an ameloblastoma. There is usually no distinct stellate reticulum. The most significant feature is the appearance of the connective tissue showing the structure of the dental papilla, the primitive pulp (Fig. 10-12). Occasionally, some hyalinization can be observed around the epithelial islands. There have been a few reports of a granular cell ameloblastic fibroma; the granular changes appeared in cells of the mesodermal component. Perhaps the granular cell ameloblastic fibroma should be designated as central odontogenic fibroma, granular cell variant[522]. There have also been descriptions of melanin pigmentation in an ameloblastic fibroma.

Fig. 10-12. Ameloblastic fibroma. Notice the appearance of the stromal part, which resembles the dental papilla.

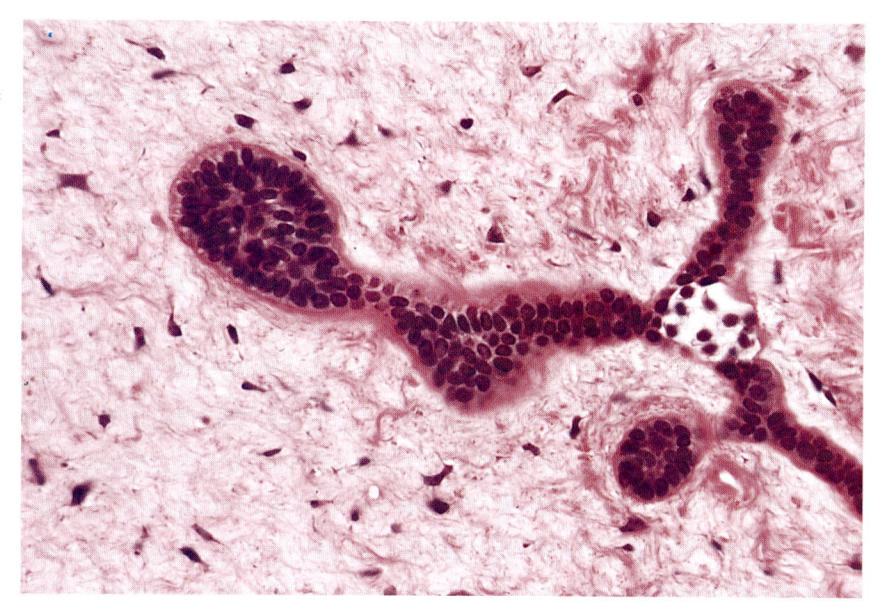

If formation of both enamel and dentine is observed, the term ameloblastic fibro-odontoma should be applied (See p. 193). Some investigators simply consider both the ameloblastic fibroma and the ameloblastic fibro-odontoma to be stages in the development of an odontoma. In the presence of only (dysplastic) dentine, the term ameloblastic fibro-dentinoma ("Dentinoma") is used (see p. 192). One may question whether or not the distinction between ameloblastic fibroma, ameloblastic fibro-dentinoma and ameloblastic fibro-odontoma is of any clinical relevance.

Treatment

Treatment of an ameloblastic fibroma consists of surgical removal. It is usually possible to separate the tumor from the surrounding bone. The literature contains no reliable data on the recurrence rate. In a rare case malignant changes into an ameloblasic fibrosarcoma may take place[467].

Fig. 10-13. Part of central ameloblastic fibro-dentinoma.

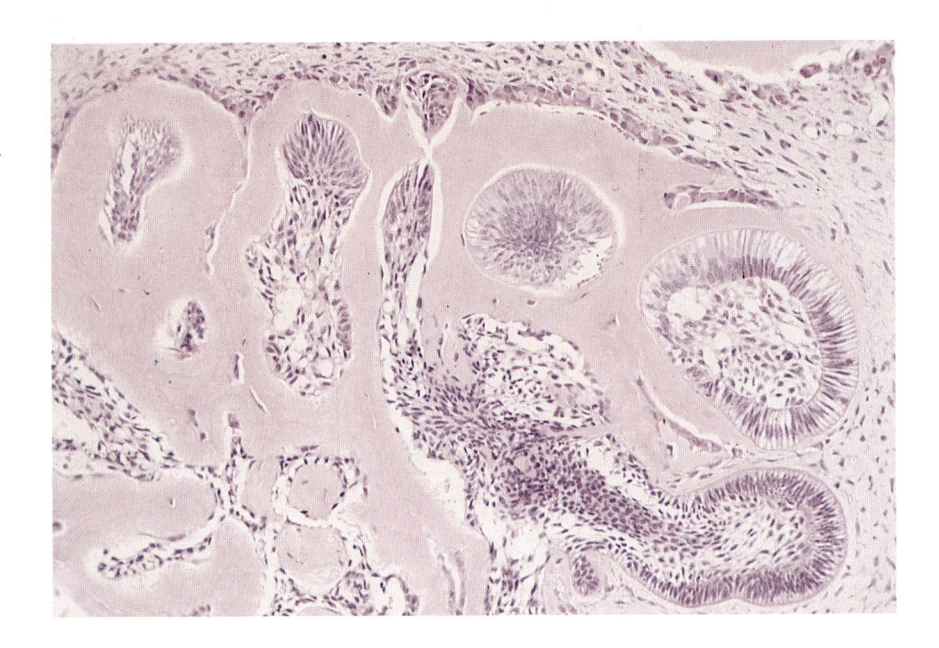

Ameloblastic fibro-dentinoma ("Dentinoma")

The ameloblastic fibro-dentinoma, also referred to as dentinoma, is a controversial, rare neoplasm composed of odontogenic epithelium and an immature connective tissue, in which the formation of dysplastic dentine can be observed[437]. The connective tissue has the same appearance as in ameloblastic fibroma (Fig. 10-13). In case of a peripheral lesion associated with an erupting tooth one is most likely dealing with a hemartomatous proliferation.

Some authors have suggested that this diagnosis is only justified when, in the mineralized substance, similar dentinal tubules are seen as appear in the dentine of a normal tooth[468].

Clinically, there are no characteristic features. The lesion may even be an incidental finding on the radiograph[347]. Radiographically, it may vary from an opaque to a lucent lesion[31]. It is questionable whether the distinction between ameloblastic fibroma, ameloblastic fibro-dentinoma and ameloblastic fibro-odontoma is of clinical importance.

Treatment consists of surgical removal.

Fig. 10-14.
Radiographic aspect of an ameloblastic fibro-odontoma. Notice the scattered calcified structures.
(Courtesy Dr. L.A. Bergsma, The Netherlands).

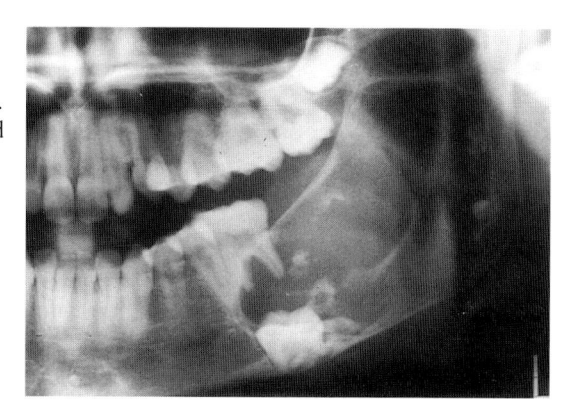

Ameloblastic fibro-odontoma

The ameloblastic fibro-odontoma is a quite uncommon lesion that usually appears in association with an impacted tooth. It is a neoplasm having the general features of an ameloblastic fibroma but containing dentine and enamel[437]. Possibly, a number of ameloblastic fibro-odontomas described in the literature should be regarded as developmental lesions arising in tooth follicles, especially when dealing with peripheral, epulislike lesions.

This lesion is often an incidental finding with no characteristic clinical features to be noted[69].

Radiographically it is usually a well-circumscribed lucent lesion with opaque structures (Fig. 10-14). The differential diagnosis may include odontogenic lesions with mixed radiolucency and radiopacity, and fibro-osseous lesions[260].

The microscopic aspect resembles that of an ameloblastic fibroma but, additionally, shows the presence of tooth structures. One cannot always clearly recognize odontoblasts, and the dentine or dentinoid material may not show a tubular architecture[532]. When no enamel matrix is present, a diagnosis of ameloblastic fibro-dentinoma should be considered.

Treatment consists of conservative surgical removal. There has been an occasional report of malignant transformation of an ameloblastic fibro-odontoma into an ameloblastic fibrosarcoma.

Odontoameloblastoma

The rare odontoameloblastoma is a neoplasm, characterized by the presence of enamel, dentine, and an odontogenic epithelium resembling that of an ameloblastoma both in structure and in behavior[437].

There are no characteristic clinical aspects. The tumor may present as a painless swelling. Loosening of the teeth has been reported[237].

Radiographically, an odonto-ameloblastoma is sometimes indistinguishable from an ordinary odontoma.

On histologic examination the characteristics of both an odontoma and an ameloblastoma are seen. Therefore, the possibility of an odonto-ameloblastoma should be considered in case of an apparent odontoma. For that reason the tissue of an odontoma should be sent for microscopic examination of both the calcified structures and the soft tissues.

Adenomatoid odontogenic tumor

Definition and epidemiology

The adenomatoid odontogenic tumor (AOT), in the past called an adenoameloblastoma, is generally believed not to be a neoplasm. It is defined as a tumor of odontogenic epithelium with duct-like structures and with varying degrees of inductive change in the connective tissue. The tumor may be partly cystic, and in some cases the solid lesion may be present only as masses in the wall of a large cyst[437]. The etiology of the AOT is unknown.

Some 200 cases have been reported in the literature. The lesion appears more often in men than in women. The average age at which the tumor is diagnosed is about 18 years[130].

Clinical aspects

The AOT is seen more often in the maxilla than in the mandible. The tumor is seldom located distally to the premolar region. In the majority of cases there is an associated impacted tooth, often a canine. The AOT may appear as a nonpainful swelling. The tumor is usually located within the bone, but there have been reports of peripheral extraosseous lesions.

Radiographic aspects

Radiographically, the tumor may appear as a rather well-circumscribed lucency that is often indistinguishable from a follicular or a residual cyst (Fig. 10-15). Radiopaque foci are sometimes seen in the lucent lesions. Quite often an impacted tooth is present.

Fig. 10-15.
Rather well-defined radiolucency between 23 and 24, caused by an adenomatoid odontogenic tumor. (Courtesy Dr. R.F. van Hoof, The Netherlands)

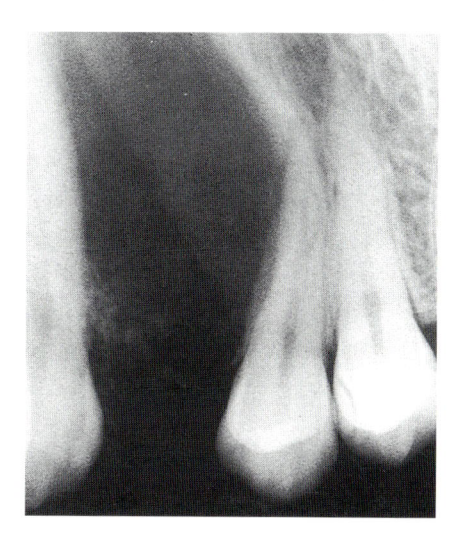

Fig. 10-16.
Low power view of an adenomatoid odontogenic tumor. Notice the ductlike structures and the presence of some calcified configurations.

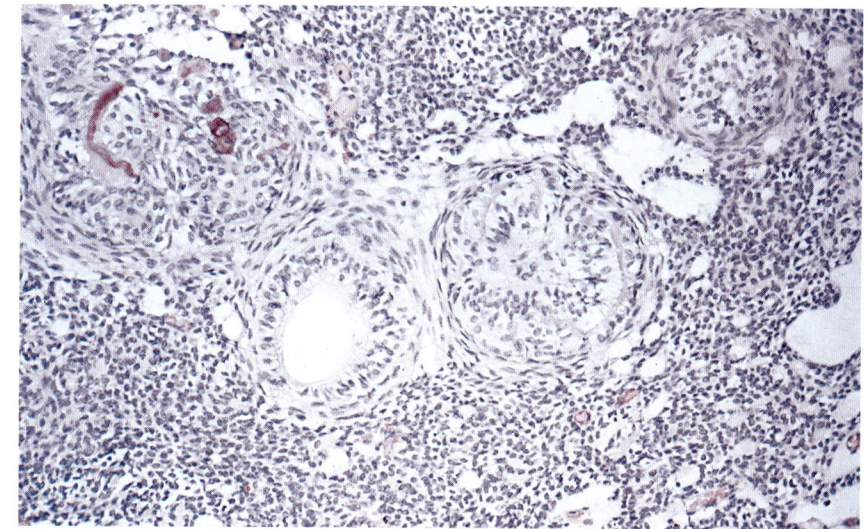

Histologic aspects

The tumor is composed of epithelial cells. In general there is little stroma. The epithelial cells may be arranged in a widely varying pattern. Ductlike structures may be found in which an eosinophilic coagulum may be observed. Mitoses are extremely scarce. Calcifications may be encountered; these have been interpreted by several investigators as dysplastic dentine (Fig. 10-16). The tumor is usually well encapsulated. In an ultrastructural study degenerative changes of the blood vessels were found, affecting both the endothelial lining and the perivascular connective tissue[168].

Treatment

Treatment consists of conservative surgical removal. Recurrences are uncommon.

Calcifying odontogenic cyst

Definition and epidemiology

The World Health Organization has defined the calcifying odontogenic cyst (COC), also called Gorlin cyst, as a non-neoplastic cystic lesion in which the epithelial lining shows a well-defined basal layer of columnar cells, an overlying layer that is often many cells thick and that may resemble stellate reticulum, and masses of "ghost" epithelial cells, that may be in the epithelial cyst lining or in the fibrous capsule. The "ghost" epithelial cells may become calcified. Dysplastic dentine may be laid down next to the basal layer of epithelium[437]. Some investigators classify the lesion as an odontogenic cyst, whereas others make a distinction between cystic and neoplastic types, as will be discussed later. Malignant transformation is rare[287]. Many of the COC's are associated with an odontoma; also the association with a dentigerous cyst has been mentioned[515].

The COC, as presented in a review of the literature, appears as often in men as in women and does not show a strong preference for any age[331]. In a Japanese study of 23 patients the mean age was 21 years[397].

Clinical aspects

Most of these lesions are located within the bone. Only a few cases of peripheral COC's have been reported[515]. There are no typical clinical features except for a slowly increasing swelling.

Radiographic aspects

The radiograph shows a rather well-circumscribed lucency with or without an associated impacted tooth. Occasionally spotty opaque structures are observed throughout the lesion (Fig. 10-17). Root resorption of adjacent teeth is not uncommon. In a rare case the radiograph picture resembles an odontoma. Based on a review of the literature it was noticed that root resorption was one of the most important radiographic findings, if the adjacent teeth were involved[568].

Histologic aspects

On microscopic examination the lining of the cystic lesion appears to consist of cylindric or cubic cells. The architecture sometimes strongly resembles that of an ameloblastoma. Characteristic is the presence of keratinizing cells of which the cell borders are still vaguely recognizable (Fig. 10-18). These are the so-called ghost or shadow cells that have been defined as pale eosinophilic swollen epithelial cells that have lost the nucleus but show a faint outline of the cellular and the nuclear membrane[443]. These cells are some-

Fig. 10-17.
Occlusal view of calcifying odontogenic cyst with impacted upper canine. Notice some spotty calcifications.
(Courtesy Dr. C.A. Bertheux, The Netherlands).

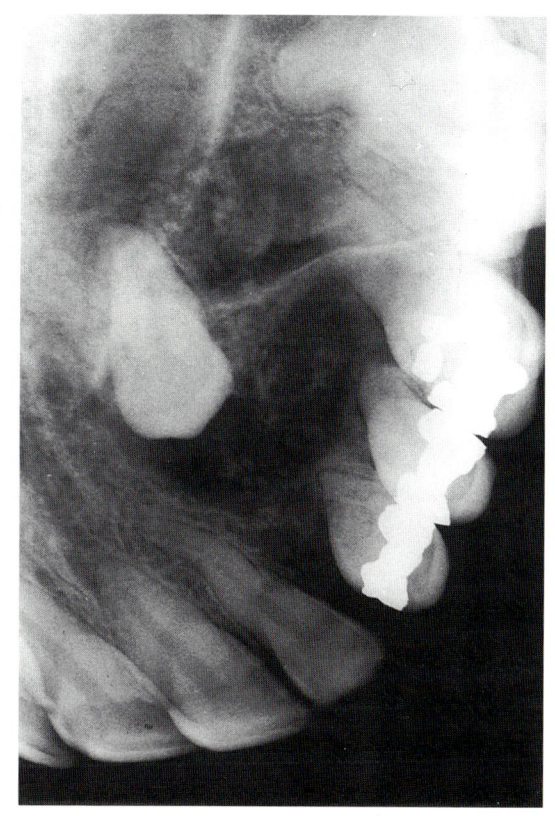

Fig. 10-18. Calcifying odontogenic cyst. Note the so-called ghost or shadow cells in the middle of the ameloblastomalike cells.

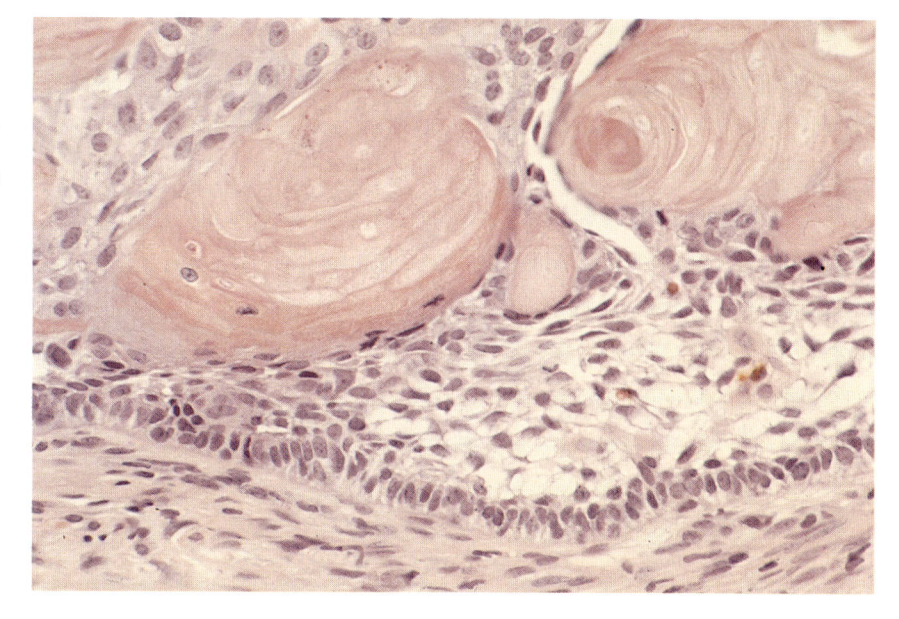

times completely calcified. The presence of dentine or osteodentine, usually juxtaepithelially, has also been reported. Often another odontogenic tumor, such as an odontoma or an ameloblastic fibroma or fibro-odontoma, is seen in association with a COC. The question then arises whether the COC should be regarded as a separate entity or as a developmental stage of another odontogenic tumor.

In a study of 16 COC's, Praetorius et al. divided them into two groups, cysts and neoplasms[443]. Three variants were distinguished among the cysts: 1. A unilocular cyst with mural proliferation of epithelium and little or no dentinoid (dysplastic dentine). This cyst could appear at any age; 2. A unilocular cyst that forms an odontoma in its lumen or that shows the presence of an ameloblastic fibroma in the cyst wall. This cyst appears most often between the ages of 10 and 30 years; 3. A unilocular cyst with extensive ameloblastoma-like proliferations both toward the lumen and into the cyst wall. Praetorius et al. considered the neoplasm to be a totally different lesion, with ameloblastoma-like strands and islands of odontogenic epithelium that grew invasively in a collagen-rich connective tissue. In the epithelium varying numbers of ghost cells were observed. At the same time varying amounts of dentinoid material were seen adjacent to the odontogenic epithelium. They suggested using the term "dentinogenic ghost cell tumor". This tumor most often appears in later life. Other investigators have suggested the term "cystic calcifing odontogenic tumor", or "dentinogenic ghost-cell ameloblastoma"[509].

Treatment

Treatment consists of surgical removal. Not enough data are available to report on the possible recurrence rate, particularly in view of the division into cysts and neoplasms.

Odontoma (compound; complex)

Definition and epidemiology

Strictly speaking the term odontoma can be used for any benign neoplasm of odontogenic origin. In practice, however, the term is only used for a non-neoplastic lesion in which both epithelial and mesenchymal odontogenic cells have fully differentiated, leading to the formation of enamel, cementum, and dentine.

Relatively few data are available about the incidence or prevalence of odontomas. At the time of the diagnosis the average age is under 20 years. The lesion is seen more often in men than in women.

The etiology of an odontoma is unknown. Trauma possibly plays a role. In some cases an odontoma is associated with a calcifying odontogenic cyst (See p. 196).

Clinical aspects

An odontoma is nearly always located within the jaws and may appear both in the maxilla and in the mandible. There may be a slight expansion of the bone. Otherwise, an odontoma is asymptomatic and is usually discovered as an incidental finding on a radiograph. An odontoma may cause a delayed eruption of a tooth, usually a permanent tooth rather than a primary one. With Gardner's syndrome multiple odontomas can be found in the jaws (See chapter 7 p. 113). There have been reports on the presence of multiple odontomas (odontomatosis), without the other characteristics of Gardner's syndrome.

Radiographic aspects

The radiograph usually shows a radiopaque, irregular structure, in which the outline of one or more teeth may be distinguished (Fig. 10-19). Around the odontoma a narrow lucent band can be observed, representing follicular tissue.

Histologic aspects

It is striking that on microscopic examination most of the odontomas in the anterior region appear to be of the compound type and those in the molar region of the complex type. The prefix "compound" is used when the odontogenic structures are more or less recognizable as a normal tooth. In the absence of such recognizable architecture, the prefix "complex" is applied (Fig. 10-20). In treatment and prognosis there is no difference between complex and compound odontomas. For that reason they are discussed together here although the WHO classifies them separately.

The odontoma may show such a regular architecture that no distinction can be made between a (compound) odontoma and a normal tooth. In some cases it is as correct to speak of supernumerary teeth as of an odontoma. The significance of the microscopic examination lies particularly in the verification of the surrounding follicular tissue. As has already been mentioned, an odontoma and an ameloblastoma may in rare instances develop simultaneously. In that case the lesion should be treated as an ameloblastoma.

Sometimes ghost cells can be observed in an odontoma, with or without the simultaneous occurrence of a calcifying odontogenic cyst.

Treatment

When the diagnosis of odontoma seems more or less proven on the basis of the radiographic features there is no strong indication to biopsy the lesion or to insist on removal. Of course, when the need is felt for a more secure diagnosis one should not hesitate to perform a biopsy or to remove the entire lesion. Another consideration for removal is the chance of secondary infection when the oral mucosa is broken. If the odontoma occurs in association with a tooth in a normal position, the tooth need not be removed.

Fig. 10-19.
Periapical film showing a picture which is more or less diagnostic of an odontoma.

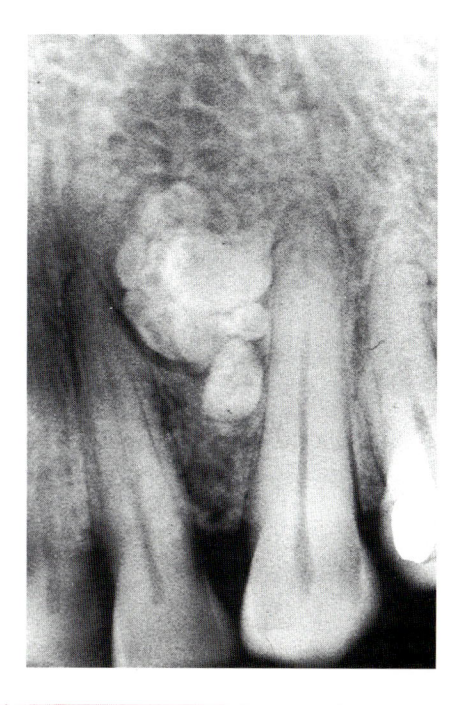

Fig. 10-20.
Decalcified section of odontoma, showing remnants of enamel and dysplastic dentine in a disorderly pattern ("complex").

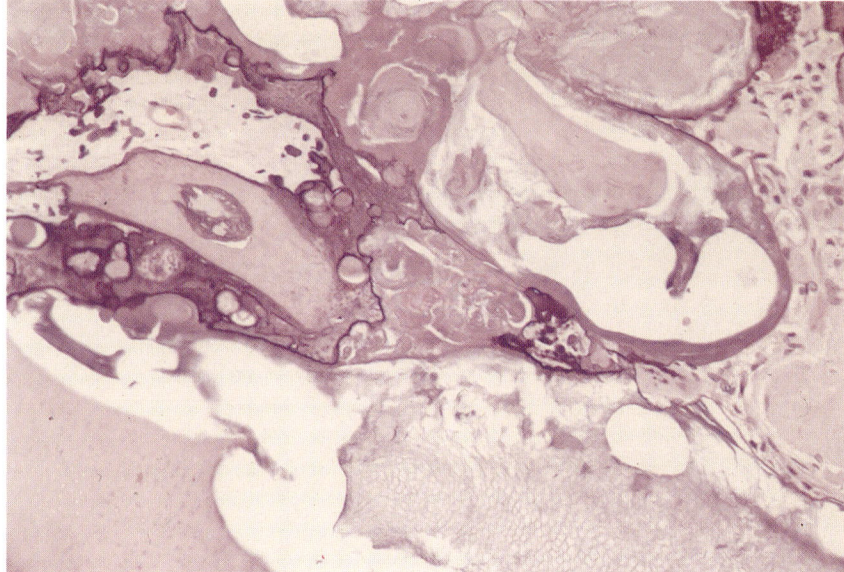

Fibroma (odontogenic), central and peripheral

Definition and epidemiology

A central fibroma, located within the bone, is rare. It is difficult to prove whether such a fibroma is, in fact, of odontogenic origin, or belongs to the group of benign fibro-osseous lesions, e.g. ossifying fibroma[210]. Perhaps some of these fibromas are variants of odontogenic myxomas. Several of the reported cases of central odontogenic fibroma may actually represent hyperplastic dental follicles.

Clinical aspects

Clinically, the central odontogenic fibroma does not present characteristic findings apart from a non-painful, localized swelling[512].

Radiographic aspects

Radiographically, the lesion appears as a well-defined radiolucent area that may be associated with unerupted or displaced teeth (Fig. 10-21).

Histologic aspects

Histologically, the lesions show primarily mature collagen interspersed with fibroblasts. Inactive odontogenic epithelium in strands and nests may be present. Various amounts of a cellular, cementumlike particles may be present. Some authors distinguish a simple type and a so-called complex (WHO) type[156, 210]. The simple type has a histologic appearance similar to that of a dental follicle, while the complex type consists of fibrous connective tissue with varying amounts of odontogenic epithelium, dentine and/or cementumlike material (Fig. 10-22). Furthermore, a so-called granular cell variant of central odontogenic fibroma has been proposed in the literature[522]. In a case with florid osseous metaplasia the term "ossifying odontogenic fibroma" has been used[298].

At the ultrastructural level, the tumor cells may contain large numbers of fine filaments with focal densities similar to those described in smooth muscle cells[605].

Treatment

Treatment consists of surgical removal. The recurrence rate is probably low.

Fig. 10-21.
Well-defined radiolucency of central odontogenic fibroma. The tumor has probably developed from the tooth-bud of 37. The partly formed and displaced tooth germ in the ascending ramus most likely represents 38. (Courtesy Dr. G.J.P. Albrecht, The Netherlands).

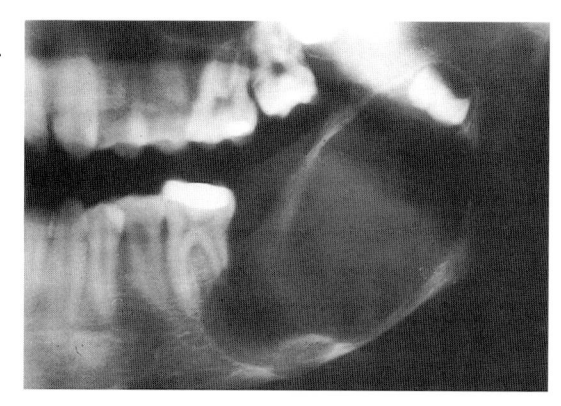

Fig. 10-22. Histologic section of central odontogenic fibroma of the so-called complex (WHO) type.

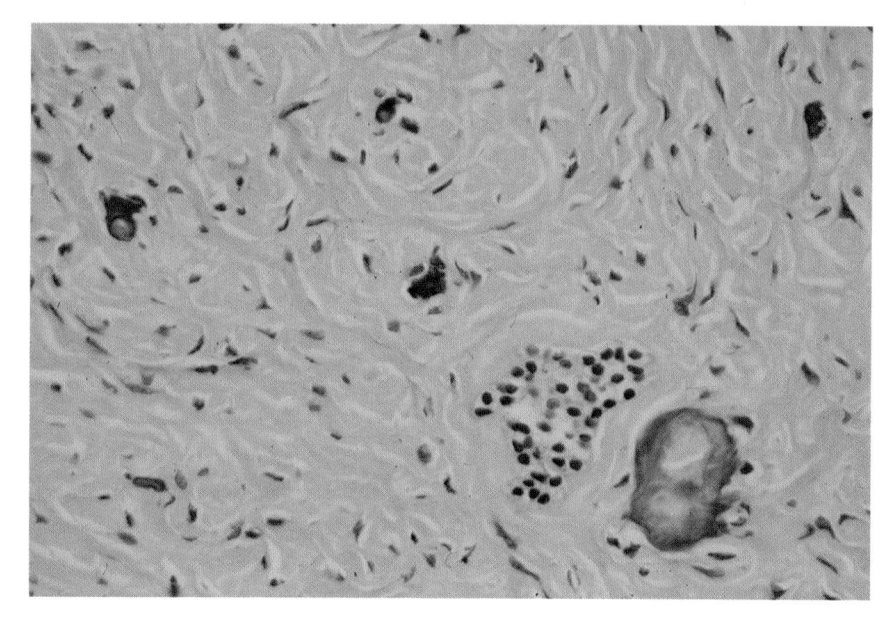

Myxoma (odontogenic)

Definition and epidemiology

The odontogenic myxoma, sometimes referred to as myxofibroma, is a locally invasive neoplasm consisting of rounded and angular cells lying in an abundant mucoid stroma[437].

The tumor is believed to originate from the mesenchyme of a developing tooth or from the periodontal ligament. Yet, uncertainly exists as to whether it is an odontogenic lesion at all. One argument in favor of an odontogenic origin is that myxomas are rarely found in other parts of the skeleton. Myxomatous tumors in other bones appear to be myxoid variants of other types of tumors. Also in the jaws, the possibility of myxoid changes in a Schwannoma, a connective tissue tumor, or a fibro-osseous lesion should be considered. Some authors believe the myxomas to be (odontogenic) fibromas that have undergone myxomatous changes.

The odontogenic myxoma is a quite rare, intraosseous neoplasm. The tumor is usually diagnosed between the ages of 20 and 30, as often in men as in women.

Clinical aspects

The tumor is seen more often in the mandible than in the maxilla. Expansion of the bone may take place. In general, the tumor tends to grow extremely slowly[4].

Radiographic aspects

Radiographically, the odontogenic myxoma appears as a uni- or a multilobular lucency. Often a honeycombed aspect is seen (Fig. 10-23). In many cases there is an associated impacted tooth. Myxomas in the maxilla may spread into the maxillary sinus.

Histologic aspects

The microscopic aspect is characterized by loose tissue that is not actually encapsulated and that usually consists of spindle and stellate cells. Cellular and nuclear polymorphism is rare, as is mitotic activity (Fig. 10-24). Numerous capillaries may be present. Nests of odontogenic epithelium may be present as well. Occasionally, such islands show a stellate reticulum-like aspect. Myxoid changes in tooth follicles can be misinterpreted as being part of a myxoma[58].

In an immunohistochemical study of two cases vimentin, neuron-specific enolase, glial fibrillary acidic protein, neurofilament, desmin, factor VIII-related antigen and antibody against S-100 protein showed a strong positive reaction in the cytoplasm of the tumor cells[342].

Benign neoplasms • 205

Fig. 10-23.
Multilobular radiolucency produced by an odontogenic myxoma. Notice the honeycombed appearance.

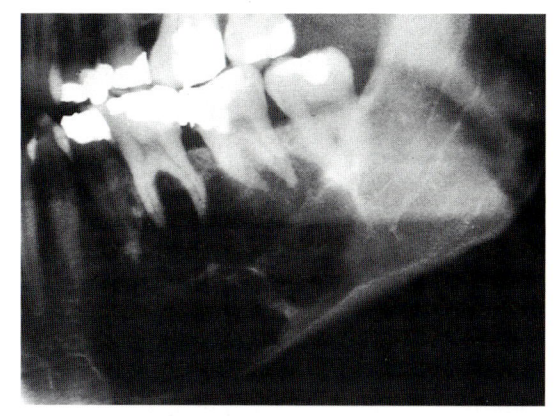

Fig. 10-24a.
Section through mandibular odontogenic myxoma.

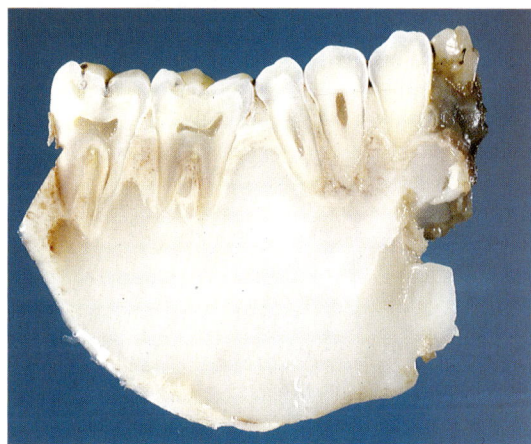

Fig. 10-24b.
Low power view of odontogenic myxoma. (Courtesy Dr. R. Martatko, Indonesia).

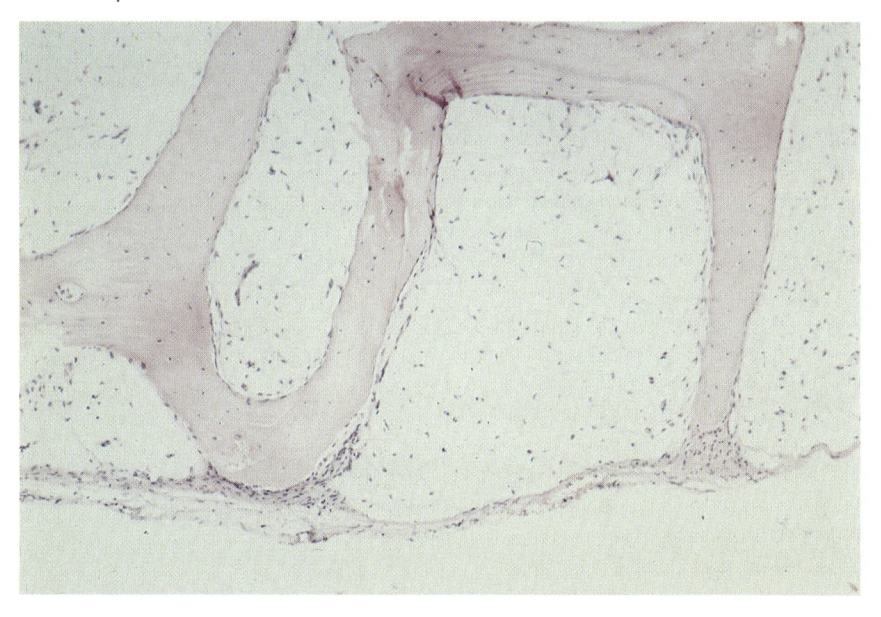

Treatment Treatment consists of wide surgical removal. It is sometimes difficult to remove the neoplasm completely. Several reports have mentioned a recurrence rate after curettage of approximately 35%. Some clinicians, therefore, prefer to treat the odontogenic myxoma in the same way as an ameloblastoma.

Cementum containing lesions (CCL)

The hypothesis has been formulated that lesions that arise from the periodontal ligament contain cells which may form cementum, bone and fibrous tissue[247, 597, 599, 600]. Some authors refer to these lesions as fibro-osseous cemental lesions of periodontal ligament origin. Furthermore, the presence of dentine, dentinoid or osteodentine has been observed in fibro-osseous cemental lesions[98].

It has been generally accepted that the distinction between bone and cementum may be difficult, if not impossible, to make from histologic observation[220]. The occurrence of so-called cementomas in the long bones further questions the justification for the distinction between cementum- and bone-containing lesions[12].

The heading "Cementum containing lesions" is therefore somewhat contradictory. Furthermore, as a consequence of the previous discussion one could question the odontogenic nature of this group of lesions. It would, indeed, be possible to classify some or perhaps all of these lesions as "related to fibrous dysplasia" or just as "fibro-osseous lesions".

In this text three subgroups of cementum containing lesions will be discussed.

Cementoblastoma ("True cementoma")

Definition The cementoblastoma has been defined as a neoplasm characterized by the formation of sheets of cementum-like tissue, which may contain a very large number of reversal lines and be unmineralized at the periphery of the mass or in the more active growth areas[437]. In the WHO classification the prefix "benign" is used.

Epidemiology The estimated incidence is less than 1 case per million population per year, without preference for age or sex.

Clinical aspects In the reported cases the main clinical feature consisted of an expansile, bony hard lesion[5]. The tumor is usually found around the

Fig. 10-25.
Cementoblastoma attached to temporary lower central incisor (Courtesy Dr. E. Cataldo, U.S.A.).

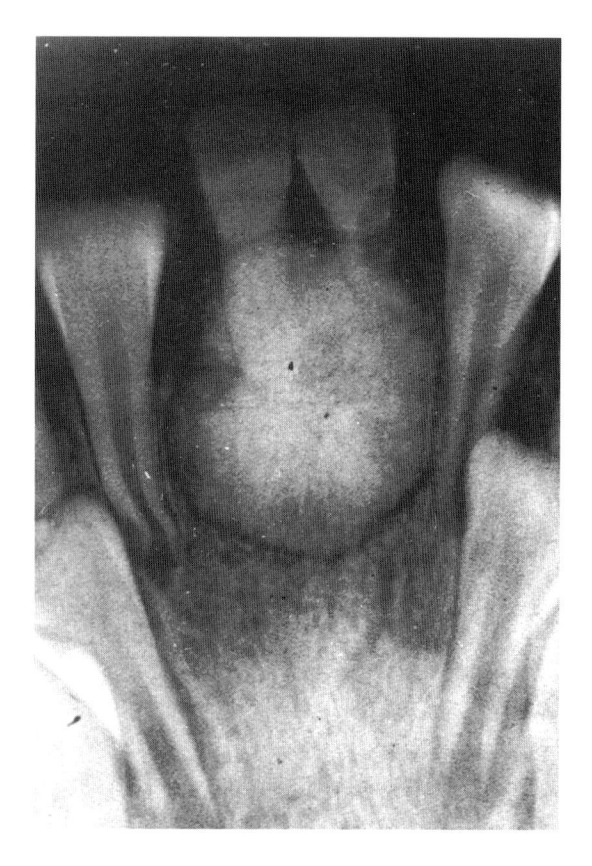

root of a premolar or molar tooth in the mandible. Occurrence in the deciduous dentition is exceptional (Fig. 10-25)[424].

Radiographic aspects

As stated in the WHO monograph, the tumor is radiographically well-defined. The main radiopaque part is commonly surrounded by a radiolucent zone of uniform width[437]. Root resorption may be evident.

Histologic aspects

Usually, dense masses of cementumlike material are seen with a fibrous, sometimes rather vascular stroma. The cementoblastoma is regarded by some authors as the cementum analogue of an osteoblastoma. Others have stated that peripheral radiating columns of cementum rimmed by large cementoblasts are pathognomonic of a cementoblastoma and thus assist in distinguishing it histologically from osteoblastoma and osteoid osteoma[125]. The most reliable parameter, however, remains the true connection with the surface of the root of a tooth[207].

208 • Odontogenic tumors

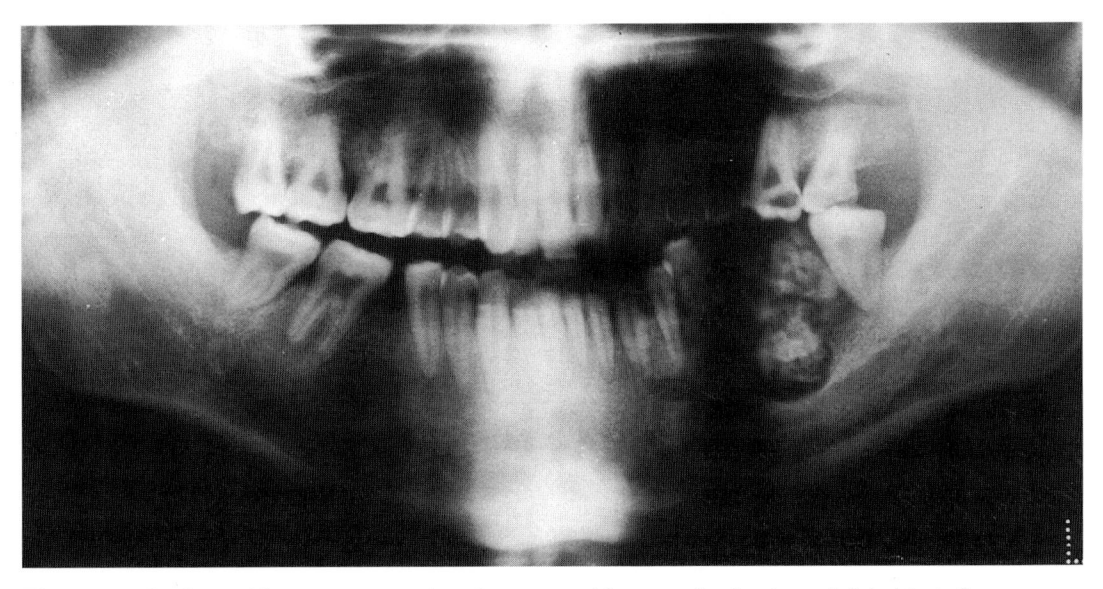

Fig. 10-26a. Radiographic aspect suggestive of a cementoblastoma that has been left behind after extraction of 36.

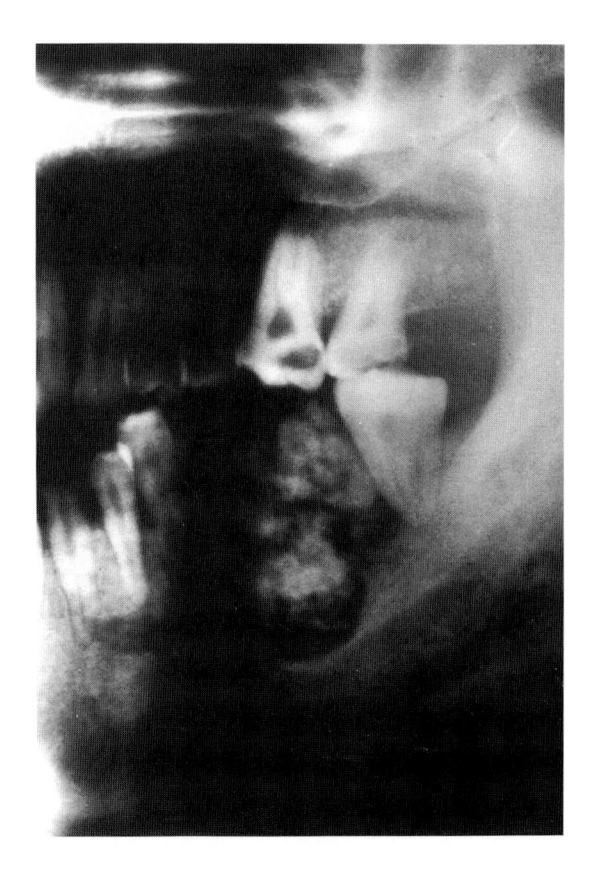

Fig. 10-26b. Detail.

Fig. 10-26c. The peripheral radiating columns seem to support a diagnosis of cementoblastoma. (Courtesy Prof.dr. C. Lekkas, The Netherlands).

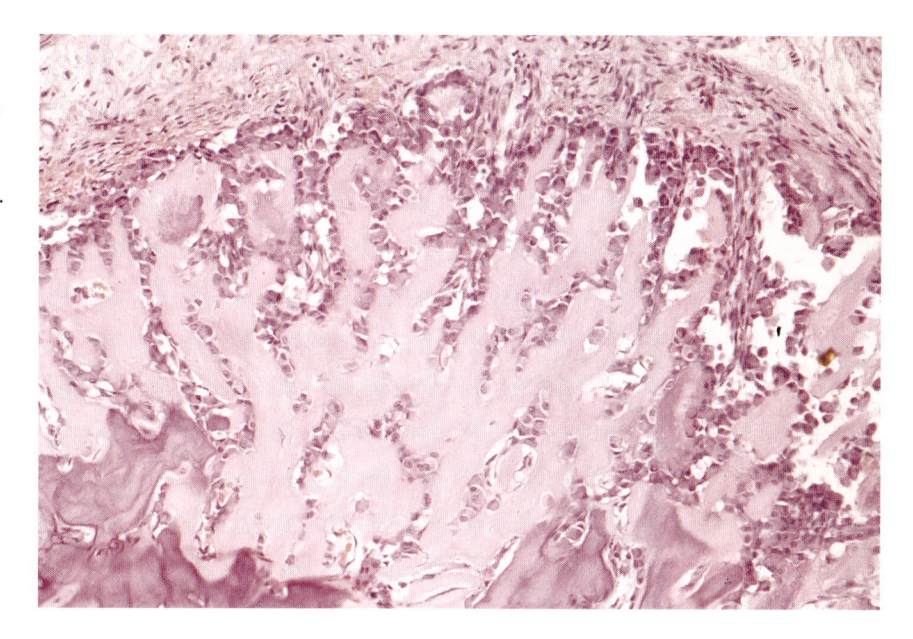

Treatment — Extraction of the involved tooth is recommended, in which case the tumor apparently remains attached to the root. In a rare case part of the cementoblastoma may be left behind, requiring additional surgical enucleation (Fig. 10-26). The tumor does not show a tendency to recur[437].

Fibro-osseous cemental lesions (FOCL)
(Incl. Periapical cemental dysplasia, gigantiform cementoma, sclerotic cemental masses, and florid osseous dysplasia)

Terminology

In the 1972 WHO classification the entity of *periapical cemental dysplasia* is defined as "A lesion similar in structure to the cementifying fibroma. It is mainly fibroblastic in its early stages and contains increasing amounts of cementum-like tissue, occasionally interspersed with trabeculae of woven bone"[437].

The use of the prefix "periapical" seems somewhat questionable since a number of radiologically and histologically similar lesions are not really located at the apex of a tooth, but may be present halfway to the root or may even not be related to a tooth at all (Fig. 10-27). When present in an edentulous part of the jaw one may only speculate that the lesion has been left behind after the extraction of the tooth with such a periapical lesion (Fig. 10-28).

For fibro-osseous cemental lesions, not located in a periapical position and present in multiple quadrants of the mandible and maxilla, the term *"gigantiform cementoma"* has been used in the 1972 WHO classification, being defined as "A lobulated mass of dense, highly calcified, almost acellular cementum typically occurring in several parts of the jaws"[437]. In that classification the term "familial multiple cementomas" has been added in parentheses. A strict distinction between single and multiple lesions would require the availability of full-mouth radiographs or a panoramic view of the patient. Such a requirement does not seem feasible in daily practice. In only few cases of gigantiform cementoma has a familial occurrence been reported[104, 654]. Considering the relatively harmless nature of these lesions, it would often not be a reasonable requirement to ask for full-mouth radiographs of one or more members of the patient's family. Finally, the adjective "gigantiform" is used by some authors only to describe a single giant or monstrous cementum-containing lesion, which further contributes to the confusion of the terms "gigantiform cementoma" and "familial multiple cementomas".

In the past, the term *"sclerotic cemental masses of the jaws"* has been used, which included, among others, chronic sclerosing osteomyelitis, sclerosing osteitis, multiple enostosis, and gigantiform cementoma[601]. It should be noted, however, that sclerosis is not al-

Fig. 10-27.
Fibro-osseous cemental lesion not really located at the apex of 34 and 35. (Courtesy Dr. N.P.J.B. Sieverink, The Netherlands).

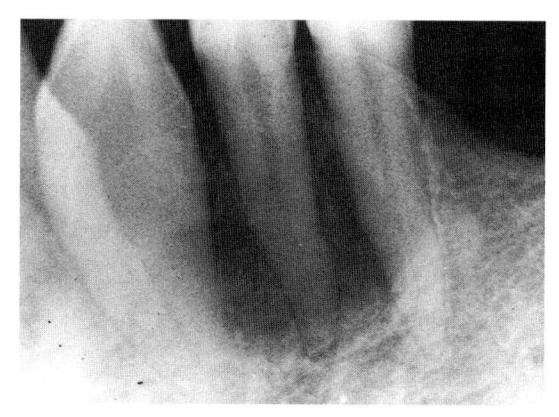

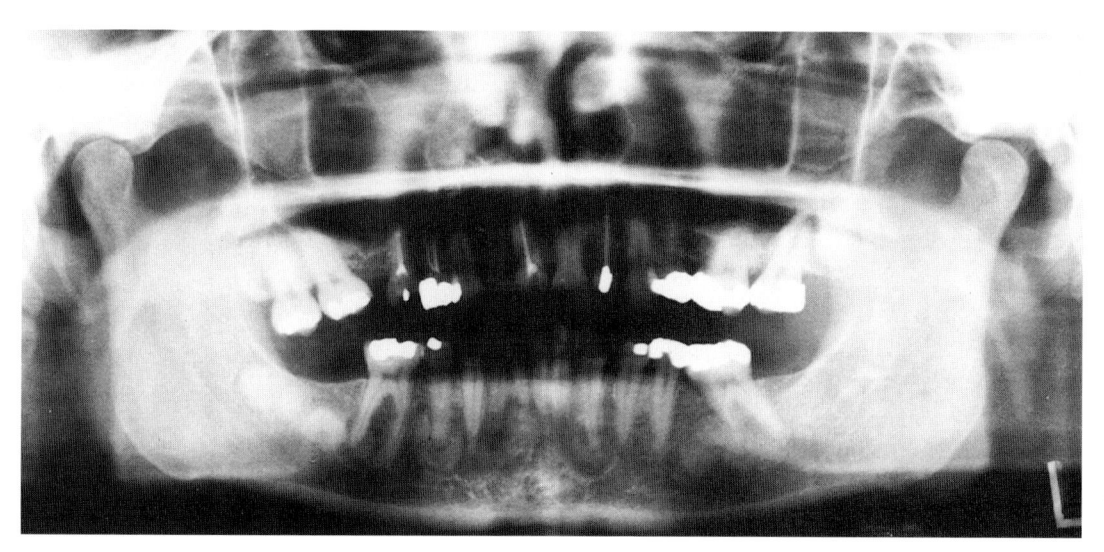

Fig. 10-28a. Periapical and non-periapical fibro-osseous cemental lesions.

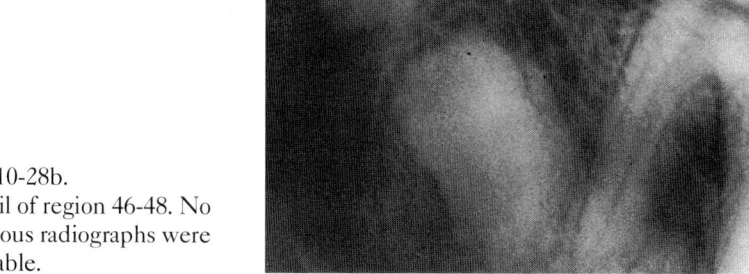

Fig. 10-28b. Detail of region 46-48. No previous radiographs were available.

ways the main feature in the FOCL. The occasional presence of inflammatory cells in FOCL seems in most cases to be of a secondary nature, although it has to be admitted that that hypothesis is difficult to prove scientifically.

Melrose et al. introduced the term *"florid osseous dysplasia"*, referring to active growth of dysplastic lesions, involving more than one jaw quadrant, which mainly were found in Negro women[373]. Since no prediction can be made on clinical, radiologic or histologic grounds as to which lesions will behave in an active fashion and which will not, the term florid osseous dysplasia can only be used in retrospect. Interestingly, Melrose et al. reported 17 solitary bone cysts in the affected quadrants of 14 of their 34 patients. Only one case of familial occurrence has been reported[395].

In view of the previous discussion preference is given to the term "fibro-osseous cemental lesion" (FOCL), which includes both single and multiple lesions, either being at a periapical or a nonperiapical location, and being either familial or nonfamilial. It is questionable whether there is room for a separate entity of ossifying and cementifying fibroma, as is further discussed on p. 225. Rarely, if ever, does confusion arise with regard to the distinction between a cementoblastoma and FOCL.

Epidemiology   No statistics are available of the prevalence of FOCL. In general, it is assumed that the lesion has a preference for middle-aged women, especially in Negroes.

Etiology   The etiology of FOCL is unknown. In most cases heredity does not seem to play a major role. In some instances the lesion seem to be the result of a trauma, e.g. the extraction of a tooth (Fig. 10-29).

Waldron used the term "localized, solitary, fibro-osseous cemental lesion" for a lesion that most likely was of a reactive nature in spite of the histologic resemblance to the group of fibrous dysplasia-like lesions (Fig. 10-30)[597].

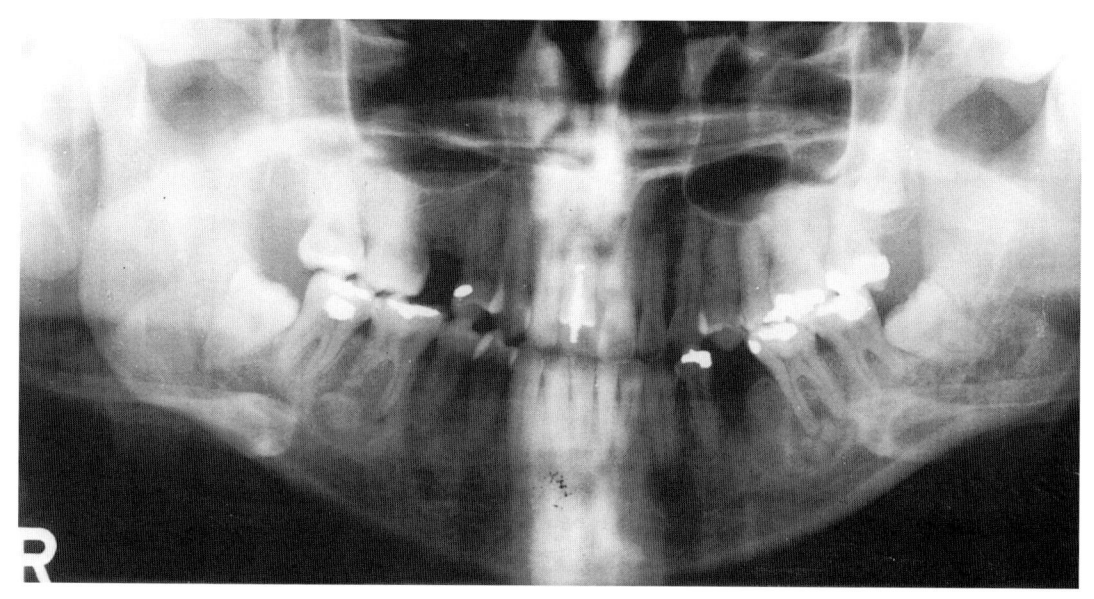

Fig. 10-29a. Multiple FOCL's, best visible at apices of 36 and 46.

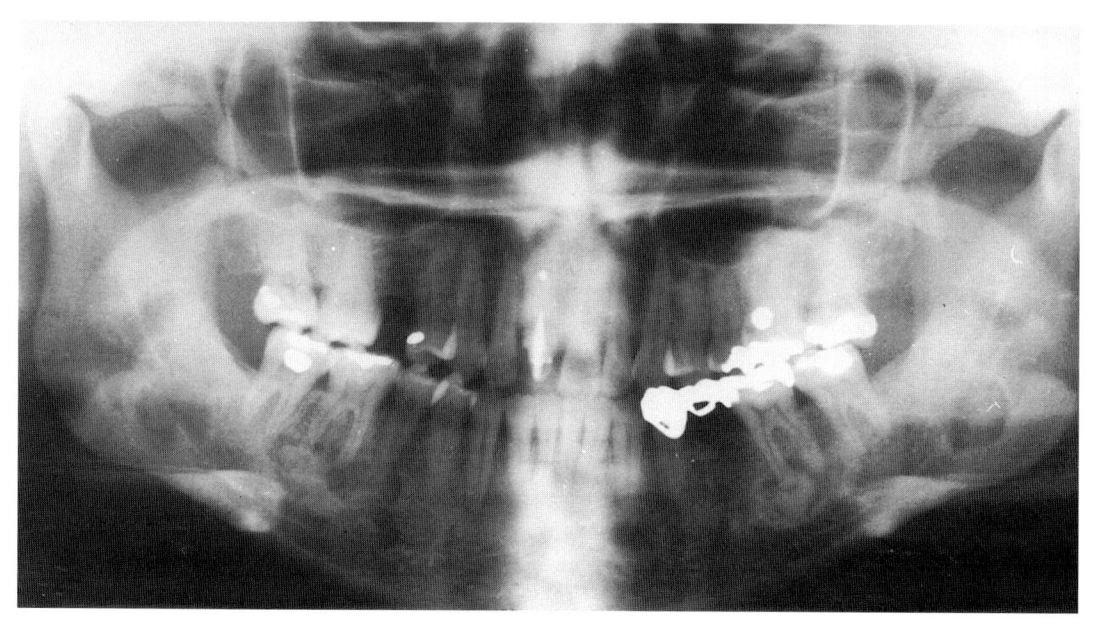

Fig. 10-29b. Two years after the removal of the impacted 38 and 48 new lesions were seen at the apical level of the removed wisdom teeth.

214 • Odontogenic tumors

Fig. 10-30a. Solitary sclerotic lesion in the maxillary tuberosity region as an incidental finding on an otherwise normal panoramic view in an edentulous patient.

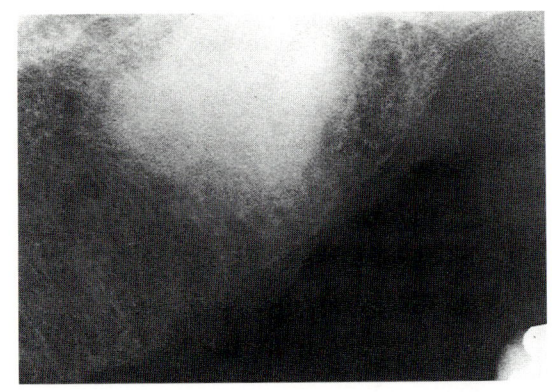

Fig. 10-30b. The histologic aspect is compatible with a fibro-osseous cemental lesion. Reactive ?

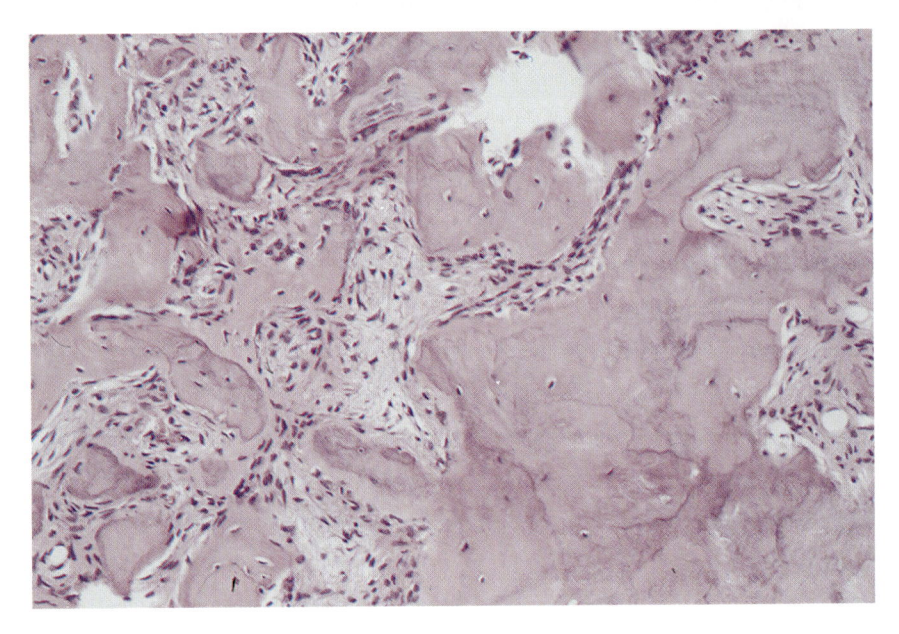

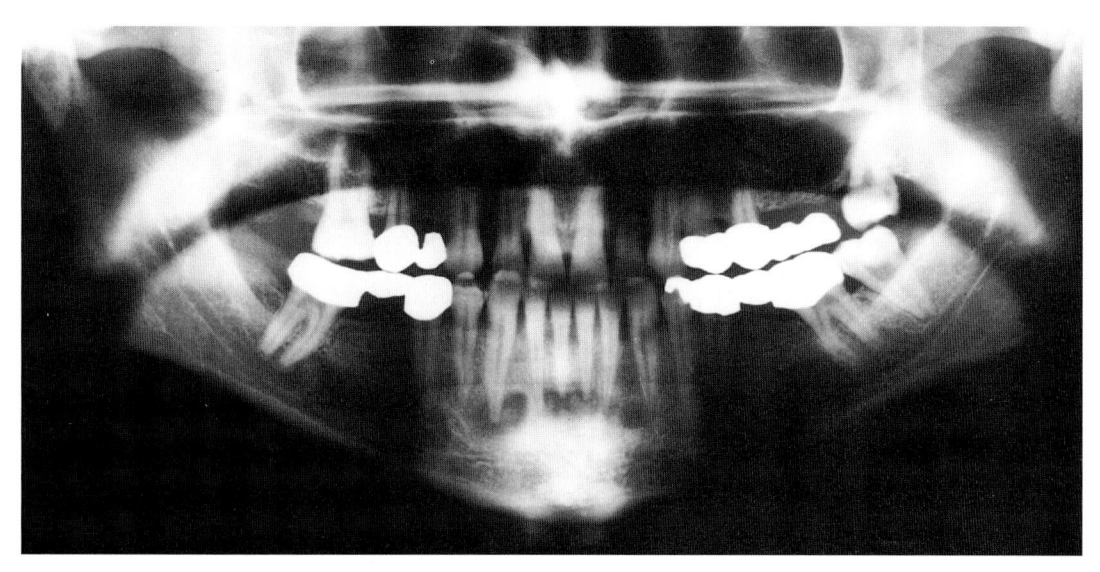

Fig. 10-31. Incidental finding on a panoramic view, more or less diagnostic of (periapical) FOCL of the lower anterior teeth.

Clinical aspects   Often there is a location at the apices of one or more lower incisors (Fig. 10-31). In a study from Japan the premolar-molar regions were the site of predilection[566]. In many cases there is a symmetrical distribution between the right and the left side. Interestingly, periapical location of FOCL's is more or less limited to the lower dentition. Maxillary lesions are perhaps often overlooked. In case of periapical location the vitality of the tooth remains undisturbed.

The majority of FOCL's are asymptomatic, being detected during a radiographic examination for other purposes. Swelling is rare and, if present, points to an active growth, which sometimes may even be rather progressive[448]. Such active growth may occur both in patients having their own dentition and in edentulous patients (Figs. 10-32, 10-33)[621].

216 • Odontogenic tumors

Fig. 10-32a. Expansion of upper alveolar ridge. Note secondary ulceration.

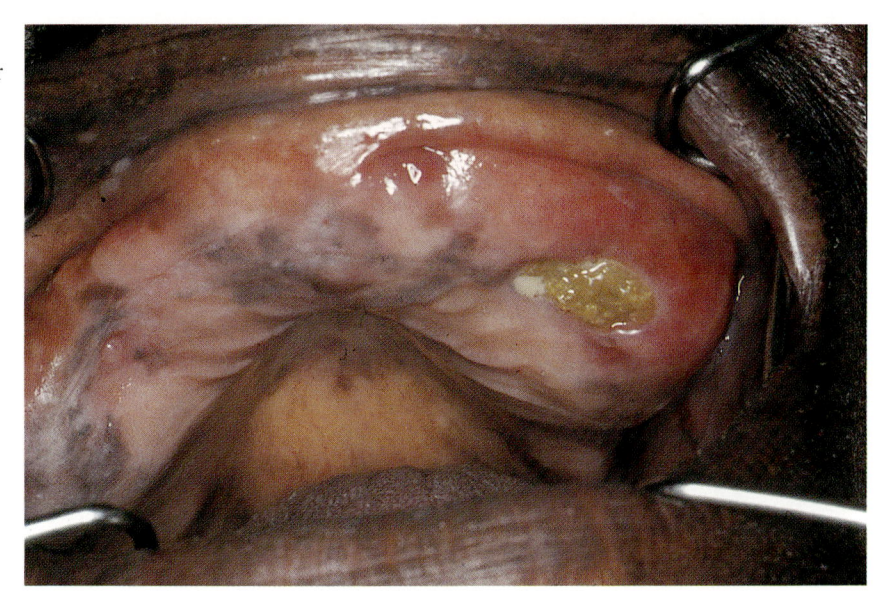

Fig. 10-32b. Expansion of lower alveolar ridge.

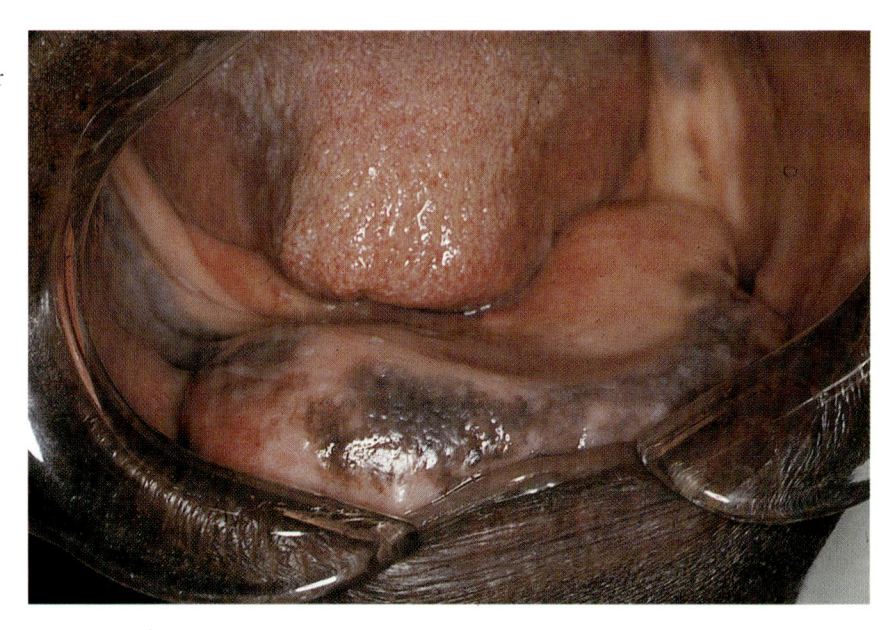

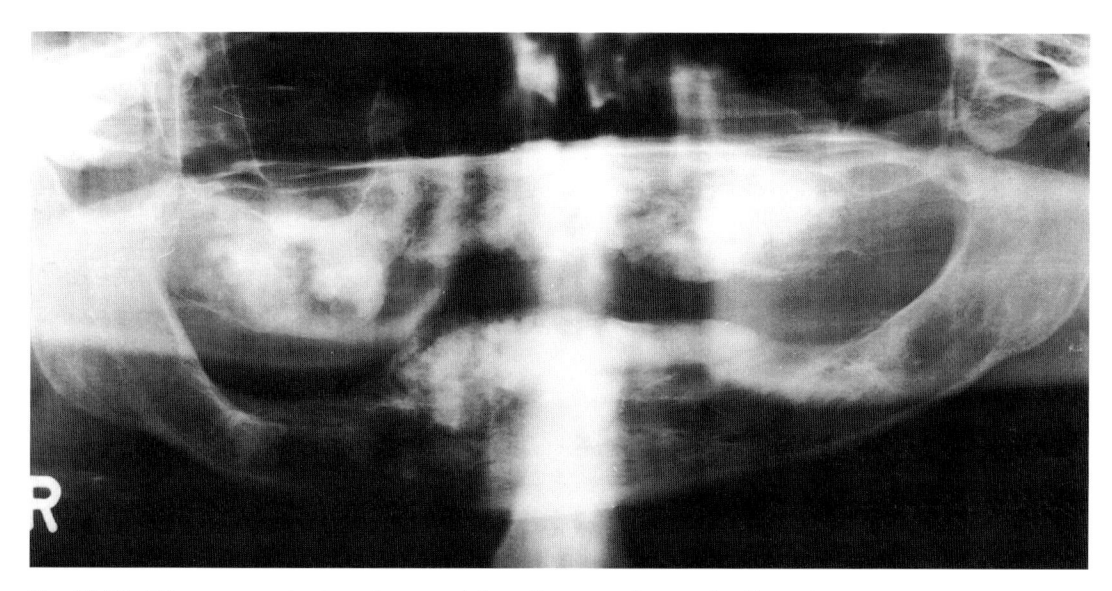

Fig. 10-32c. The panoramic view shows mainly radiopaque changes in all quadrants.

Fig. 10-32d.
The occlusal view of the anterior part of the mandible gives another impression of the extent of the lesion. The biopsy is shown in Fig. 10-36d.

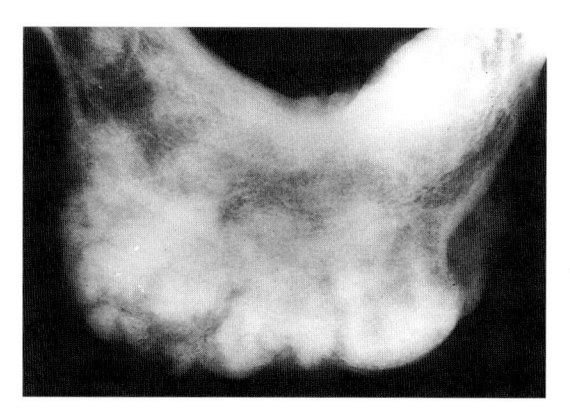

218 • Odontogenic tumors

Fig. 10-33a. Slight, bony hard swelling of left side of the maxilla in a Caucasian man.

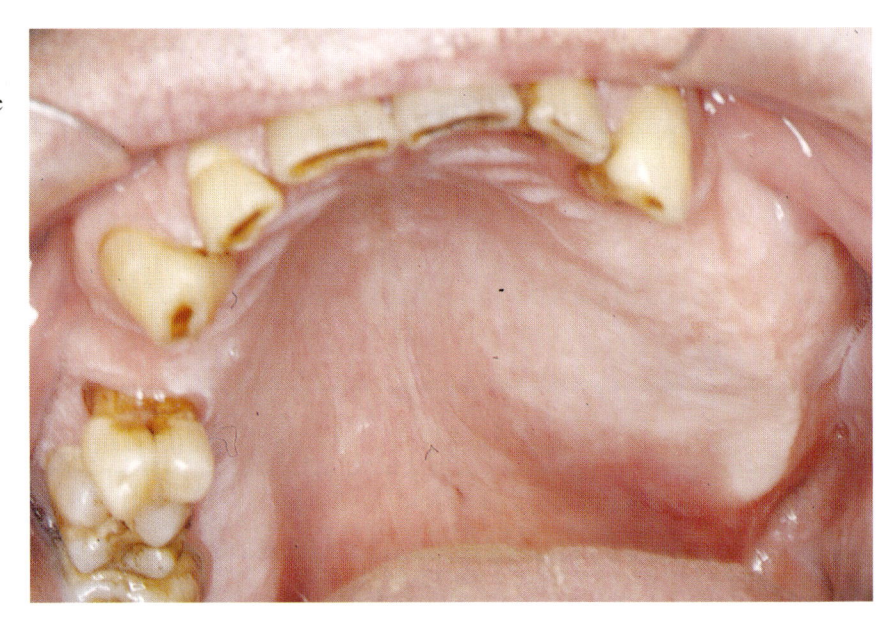

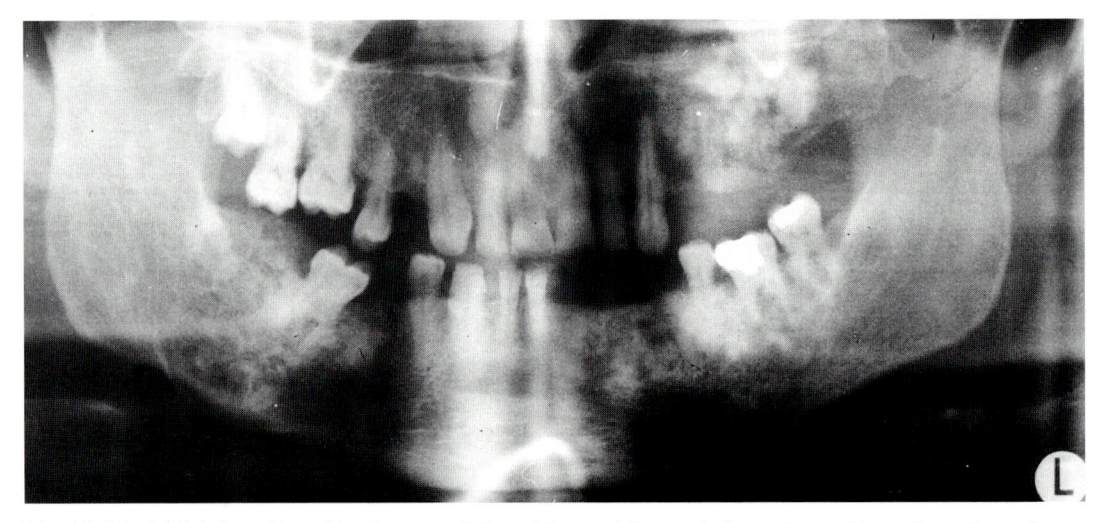

Fig. 10-33b. Multiple radiopacities in upper left and lower right and left quadrant. There is perhaps also a lesion at the extraction site of 14. Note expansion of right mandibular border. The biopsy is shown in Fig. 10-36c.

Radiographic aspects

In the initial stage FOCL produces a rather ill-defined radiolucent area. At this stage a solitary lesion can, radiographically, barely be distinguished from a periapical granuloma (Fig. 10-34). With time, central calcification takes place, finally resulting in a dense opaque

Fig. 10-34.
Periapical radiolucency at apex of vital 42, more or less diagnostic, in the absence of signs or symptoms, of a fibro-osseous cemental lesion.

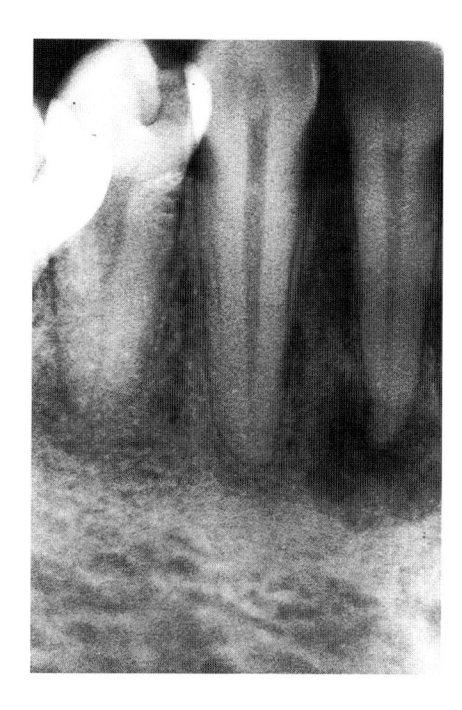

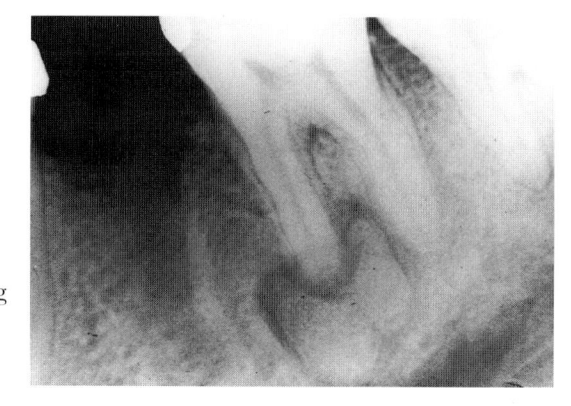

Fig. 10-35.
Detail of Fig. 10-29, showing central calcification and peripheral radiolucency at apex of vital 36.

lesion often with a radiolucent periphery, which is of help in differentiating the lesion from focal chronic sclerosing osteomyelitis (Fig. 10-35). In the non-periapical FOCL such a periapical lucent zone is often missing. FOCL usually does not cause resorption of apices.

In the radiographic differential diagnosis, not only the possibility of a reactive lesion, e.g. osteomyelitis, but also an osteosarcoma should be included.

Fig. 10-36a. Histologic aspect of periapical and non-periapical fibro-osseous cemental lesions. Low-power view of radiolucent lesion, showing a fibrous dysplasia-like architecture.

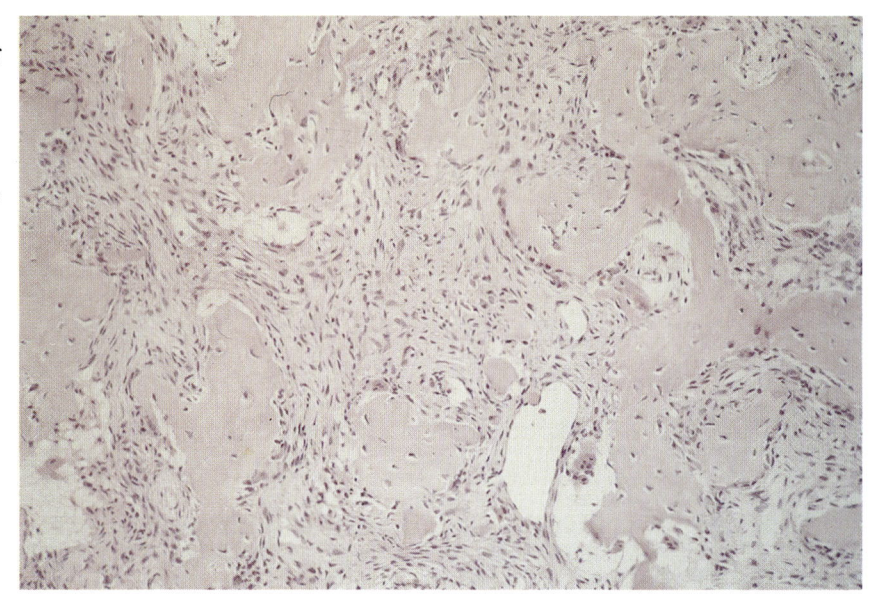

Fig. 10-36b. Detail from another lesion showing osteoclastic activity.

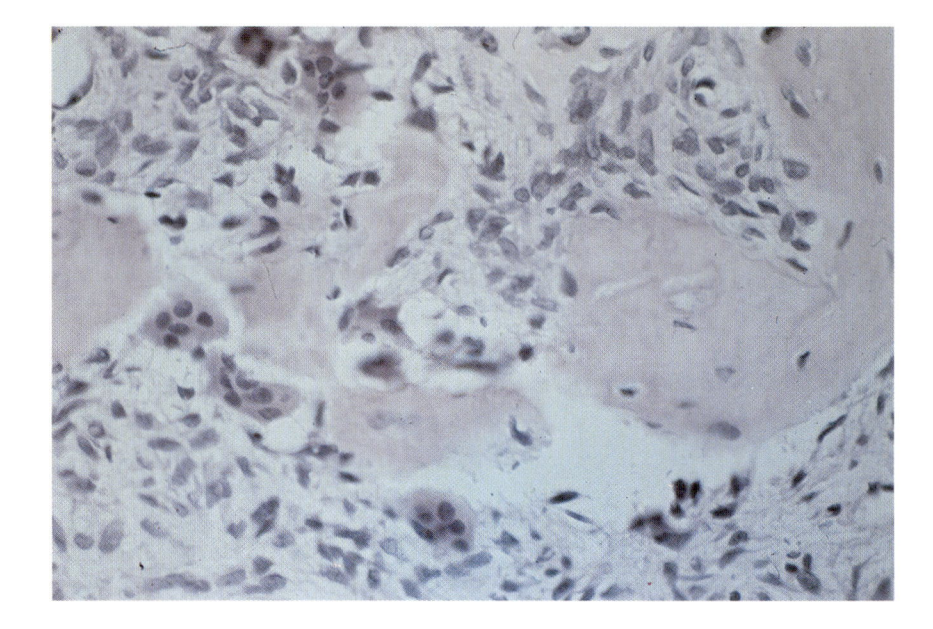

Histological aspects

When no clinical signs or symptoms are present the taking of a biopsy is in most instances not necessary and is actually contraindicated. Occasionally, however, one may feel the need for a biopsy, especially in order to rule out other diseases.

As has been mentioned already in the WHO definition of periapical cemental dysplasia the FOCL is fibroblastic in its early

Fig. 10-36c. In some areas lamellar bone can be seen.

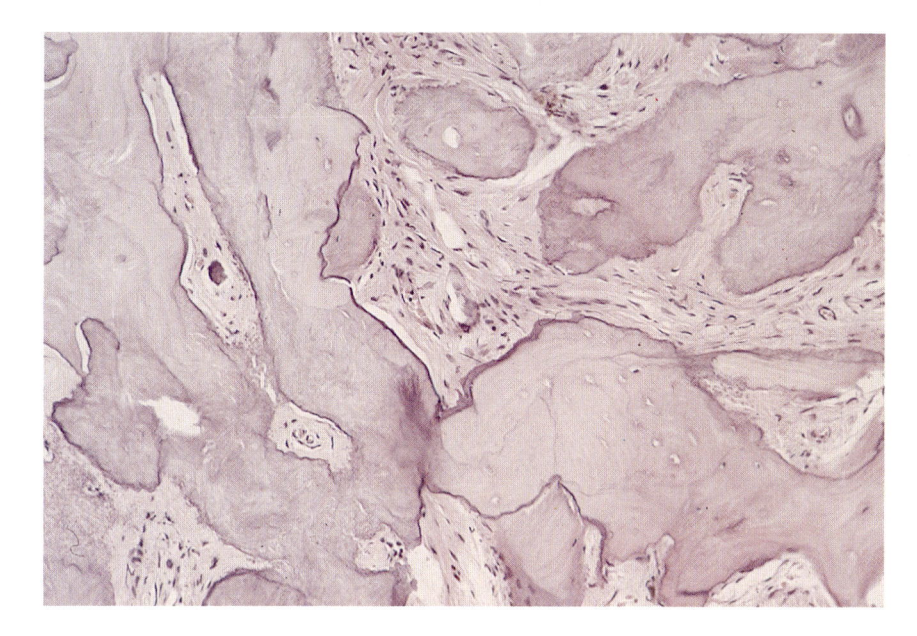

Fig. 10-36d. A (secondary?) inflammatory infiltrate may be encountered.

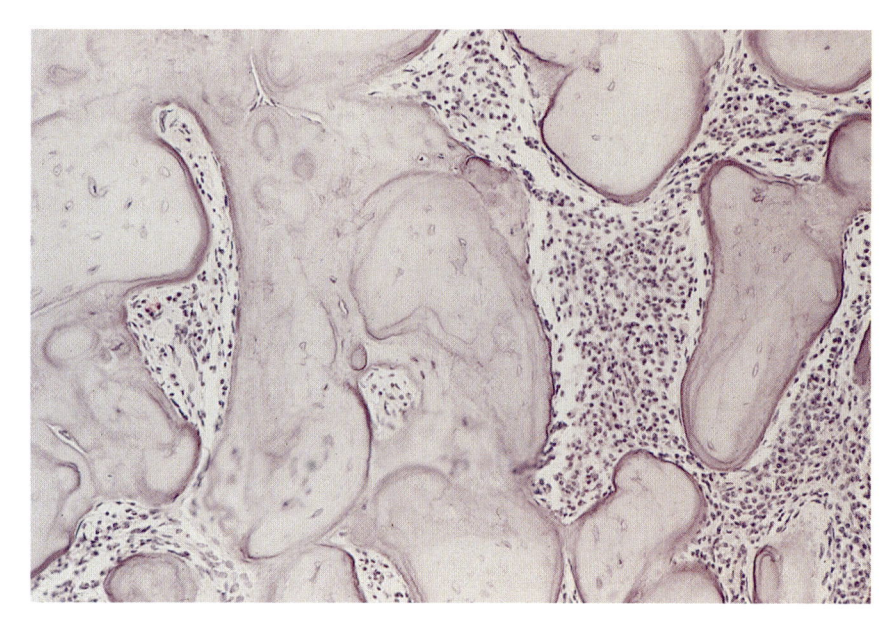

stages and, with maturation, will contain increasing amounts of cementumlike tissue, occasionally interspersed with trabeculae of woven bone[437]. Some authors observed that the cemental masses tend to exhibit striations vertical to their outer surfaces[104]. In case of the presence of an intraoral sinus, varying amounts of inflammatory cells may be present (Fig. 10-36).

222 • Odontogenic tumors

Fig. 10-37a. Because of vague complaints, 47 has been extracted, most likely based on the assumption of a periapical inflammatory lesion.

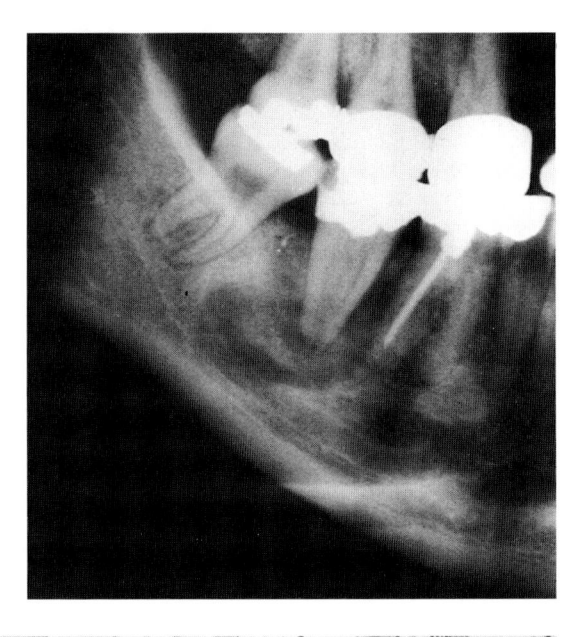

Fig. 10-37b. The apical area was curetted. Histologic examination showed a fibro-osseous cemental lesion.

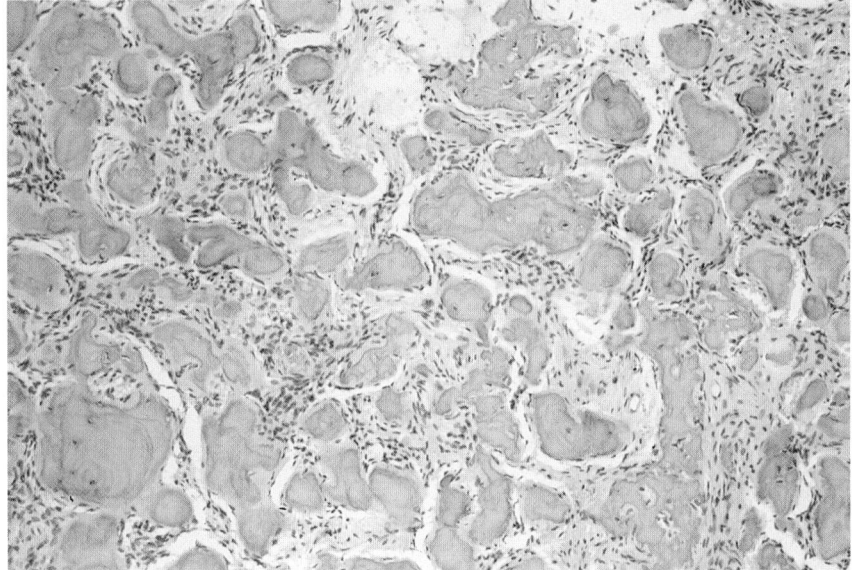

The histologic differential diagnosis includes an ossifying and cementifying fibroma, if such an entity exists (see p. 225). Cementumlike masses may also be encountered in bone lesions in patients suffering from Paget's disease, and in some cases of osteomyelitis. In "bona fide" cases of fibrous dysplasia the occurrence of cementumlike masses is rare. On the other hand, cementumlike changes may be observed in osteosarcomas.

Fig. 10-37c.
The patient was lost to follow-up but returned four years later because of a swelling at the site of extraction. There is expansion of the inferior border

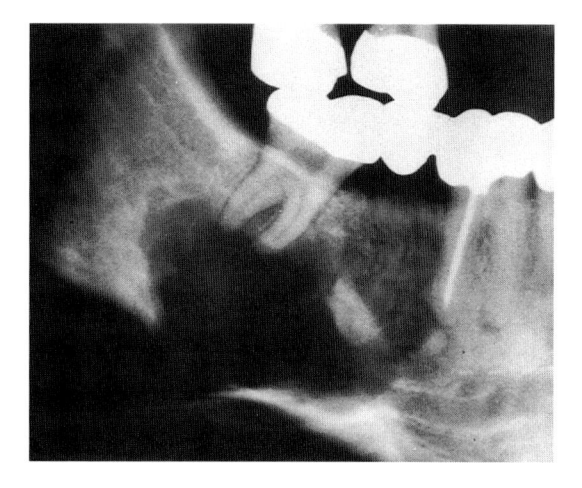

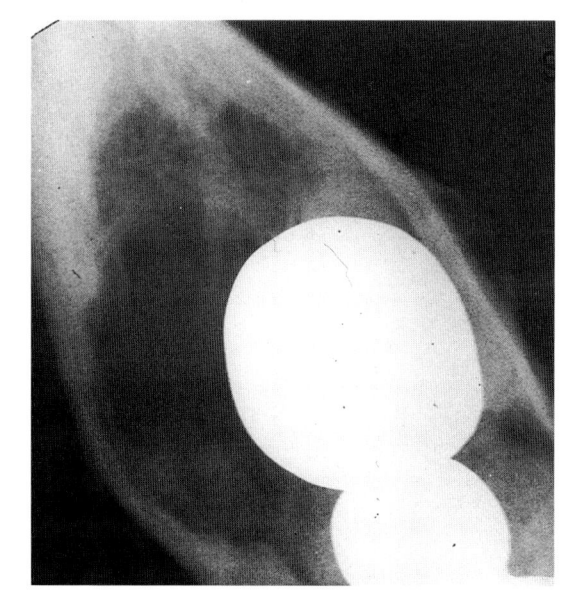

Fig. 10-37d.
and also of the buccal and lingual plates.
The histology was more or less similar. The lesion has been enucleated.

Grading

Neville and Albenesius have proposed a grading system for benign fibro-osseous lesions of periodontal ligament origin[401]. Grade 1 has been defined as the presence of one or more lesions confined to one quadrant or periapical cemental dysplasia confined to the six mandibular anterior teeth. Grade 2 refers to lesions that involve two quadrants, including periapical cemental dysplasia extending beyond the six mandibular anterior teeth. Grades 3 and 4 refer to involvement of three and four jaw quadrants, respectively. It is evident that this grading system can only be used with the availability of full mouth radiographs.

Treatment The majority of the FOCL's probably remain more or less inactive. In a number of cases, which can not be predicted on the basis of patient's data nor on clinical-radiographic criteria (and nor on histologic grounds if a biopsy has been performed), active growth may take place resulting in swelling of the involved part of the jaw (Fig. 10-37). The percentage of cases in which such active growth will take place is not known.

Excochleation of an early lesion with the purpose of preventing a possible active growth, seems not to be justified. Instead, radiographic follow-up may be considered, with radiographs being taken, for instance, every five years. Even that policy may be regarded as "overtreatment".

Although in some cases active and progressive lesions may develop, malignant transformation has not been reported. Therefore, if possible, a conservative surgical approach is recommended as the choice of treatment in case of actively growing lesions, followed by long-term observation[209]. In the presence of secondary infection the supportive administration of antibiotics may be helpful.

Ossifying and cementifying fibroma

Definition and terminology

The term ossifying fibroma has not been used in the WHO monograph on histologic typing of bone tumors[500]. It is stated there that the term is used only for certain fibro-osseous lesions of the jaws, as discussed in the WHO monograph on histological typing of odontogenic tumors, jaw cysts, and allied lesions[437]. In the latter text the cementifying fibroma has been defined as a lesion that consists of cellular fibroblastic tissue, containing rounded or lobulated, heavily calcified, strongly basophilic masses of cementum-like tissue. The ossifying fibroma has been defined as an encapsulated neoplasm that consists of fibrous tissue containing varying amounts of metaplastic bone and mineralized masses that have rounded outlines and few entrapped cells[437].

As a consequence of the discussion in the introductory paragraph on the cementum-containing lesions, with regard to the difficulty of distinguishing between bone and cementum, the term ossifying and cementifying fibroma (OCF) will be used in this text. Nevertheless, there remains some doubt as to whether OCF is an entity on its own, and whether it should be classified as a neoplasm. Some of the OCF's may actually be part of, or represent a form of, fibrous dysplasia. Others may be part of the spectrum of fibro-osseous cemental lesions.

In Makek's classification[352] the terms cementifying fibroma and ossifying fibroma are not used at all, being replaced by (benign) periodontoma and (aggressive) desmo-osteoblastoma either psammons type or trabecular type. The further text on this subject is therefore presented with much reservation.

Epidemiology

In a series of 64 reported cases of what the authors called ossifying fibroma a marked predilection for female patients was observed, with the majority of cases arising in the molar-premolar region of the mandible[179]. Most lesions were encountered in patients above 40 years of age. There was a preference for Caucasians.

A rare case of multiple familial ossifying fibromas has been reported[648].

Clinical aspects

The most common clinical presentation of OCF is a painless, slowly increasing expansion of the jaw. In some cases an aggressive behavior is observed[315, 363]. Small lesions may be discovered as an incidental finding during radiographic examination.

Fig. 10-38a.
Rather well-circumscribed radiolucency with some spotty central calcifications.

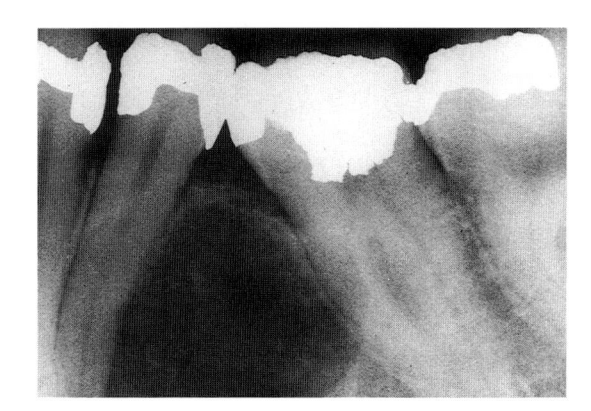

The size may vary from one to several centimeters. In the maxilla, the antrum may become involved[560]. Simultaneous or bilateral occurrence in the mandible and maxilla is not uncommon[259, 564, 665].

Radiographic aspects

Radiographically, the OCF is, by definition, well-circumscribed and is located in the tooth-bearing regions, and not associated with the crown of an impacted tooth. The lesion may be radiolucent with or without central opacities. The pattern may be either unilobular or multilobular. Teeth adjacent to or involved in the lesion may be displaced (Figs. 10-38, 10-39). In a few percent of cases root resorption does occur[179, 181].

Even when it would be possible to make a distinction between an ossifying and a cementifying fibroma histologically, this could not be done on radiographic grounds[257].

Histologic aspects

Although some authors require the histologic presence of a true capsule, the relative ease with which an OCF will shell out of its bony bed is for many other authors the most important factor in differentiating it from (monostotic) fibrous dysplasia.

Eversole observed four hard-tissue configurations, including woven bone trabeculae, lamellar bone trabeculae, ovoid-curvoid deposits, and anastomosing curvilinear trabeculae; with regard to stromal variations a predominant pattern of hypercellularity with moderate vascularity and haphazard collagen orientation was noticed, while a cellular storiform or fasciculated pattern with dystrophic-appearing spheroidal calcification was less common[179]. Based on their large material Eversole et al. stated that there are no spe-

Fig. 10-38b. Histologic examination showed a cellular fibrous lesion that was not really encapsulated.

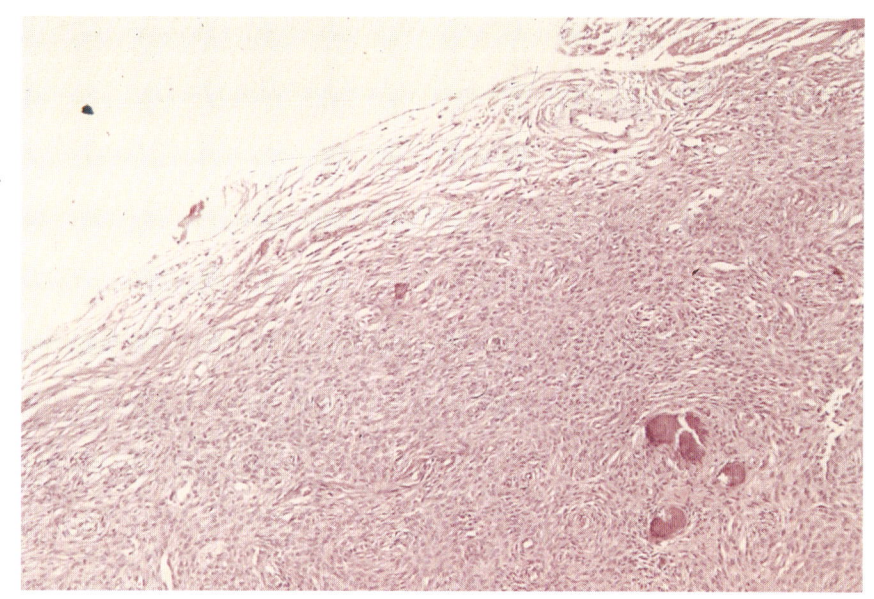

Fig. 10-38c. Scattered cementum-like structures were seen throughout the lesion. Ossifying and cementifying fibroma? (Courtesy Dr. K.G.H. van der Wal, The Netherlands).

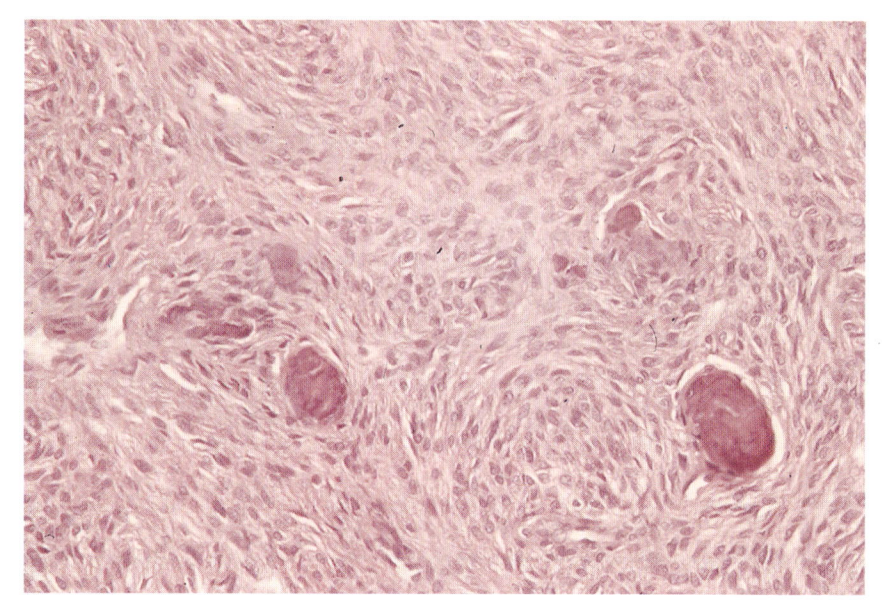

Fig. 10-39a.
Somewhat circumscribed, multilobular and expanding lesion of the mandible. The radiograph is too dark to be able to see a well-circumscribed radiolucency at the extraction site of 25.

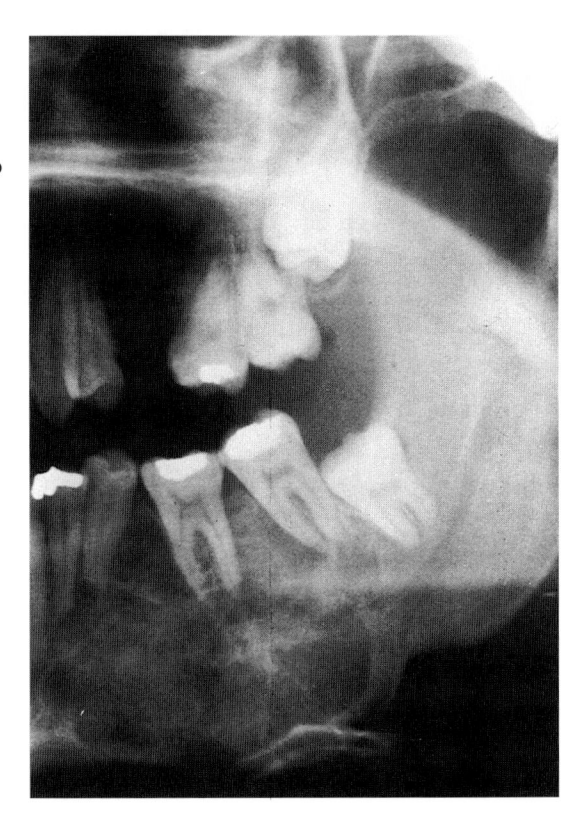

cific clinical, radiologic or microscopic predictor variables that would allow for prognostication. That view has been shared by others[327, 508].

As has been mentioned by Waldron the prefixes "juvenile", "active", "aggressive" etc. are ill-defined both with regard to the terms and the clinical and histologic criteria[597]. Apparently, such terms can only be used with regard to the age of the patient or to the growth rate of the lesion or its tendency to recur[459].

Treatment   In general, complete enucleation has been recommended. Occasionally, a recurrence may be observed[634].

Fig. 10-39b. Both lesions showed the same histologic features.

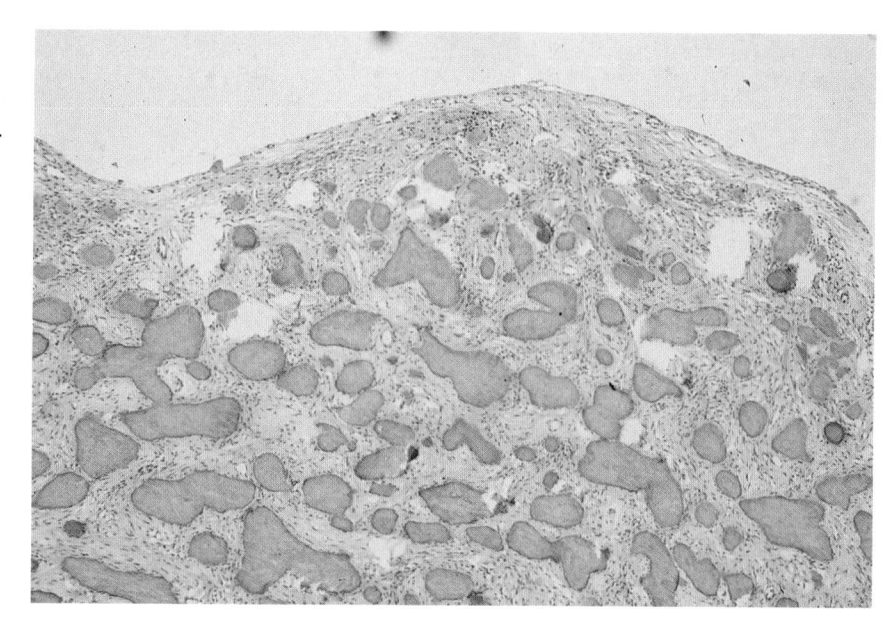

Fig. 10-39c. Ossifying and cementifying fibroma? (Courtesy Dr. G. Beemster, The Netherlands).

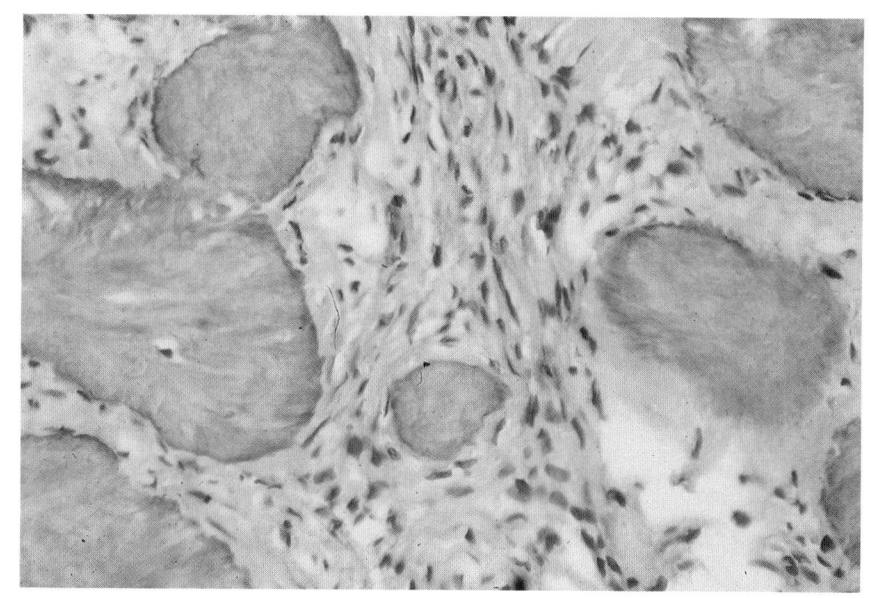

Fig. 10-40a. Destruction of left alveolar ridge by a malignant ameloblastoma. There was anesthesia of the left side of the lower lip.

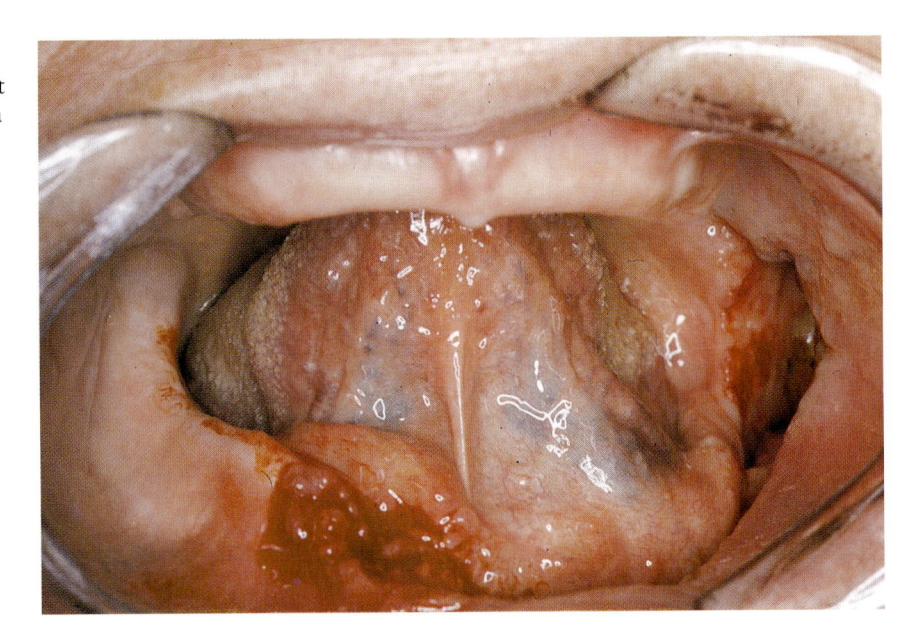

Malignant neoplasms

Odontogenic carcinomas

Malignant ameloblastoma and ameloblastic carcinoma

In the WHO-classification the malignant ameloblastoma is defined as "a neoplasm in which the features of an ameloblastoma are shown by the primary growth in the jaws and by any metastatic growth"[437]. In other words, the biologic behavior of such malignant ameloblastomas could not be predicted on the basis of their morphology. It has been suggested that metastases appear to follow multiple recurrences[328].

Others regard an ameloblastoma as malignant based on such histologic features as polymorphism and mitotic activity, without the requirement of proven metastatic growth (Fig. 10-40). When metastases appear they are usually found in the lungs. In case of lung metastases the occurrence of hypercalcemia has been reported.

The ameloblastic carcinoma is not mentioned separately in the WHO-classification. It is an ameloblastoma in which there is histologic evidence of malignancy in the primary or the recurrent tumor (or metastasis), regardless of whether it has metastasized[127]. It is an extremely rare tumor that will not be discussed here any further[153].

An as yet difficult to classify case of odontogenic carcinoma with sarcomatous proliferation has been reported[650].

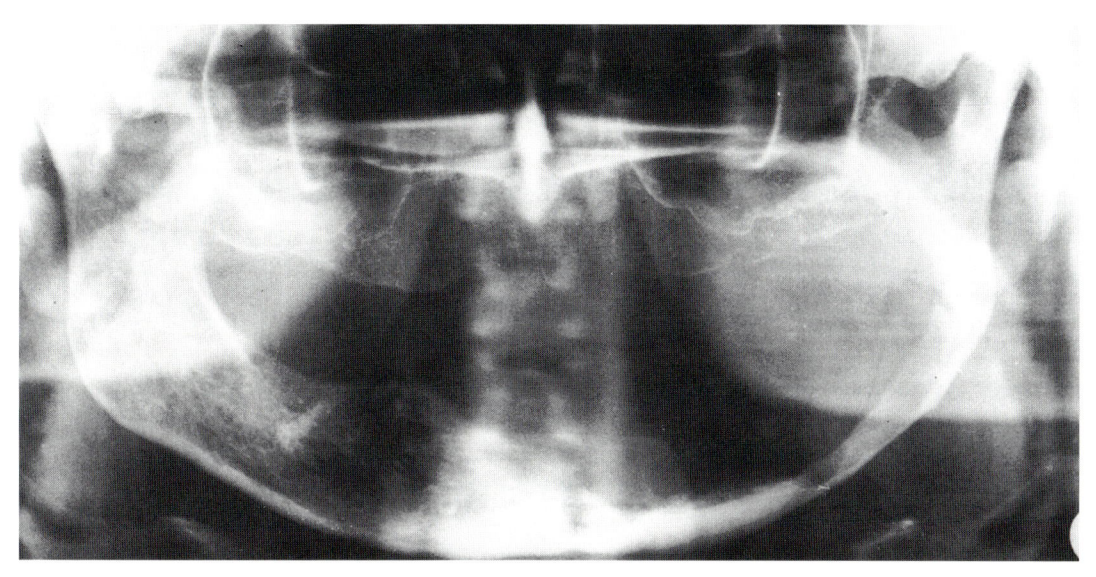

Fig. 10-40b. Destruction of left alveolar ridge by a malignant ameloblastoma.

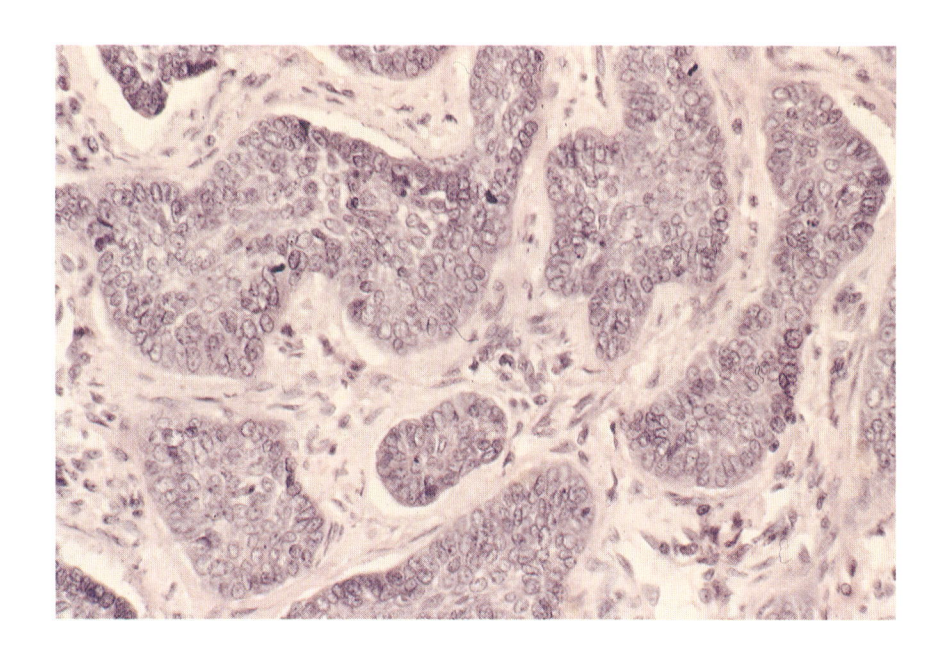

Fig. 10-40c. The biopsy showed the presence of a malignant ameloblastoma.

Primary intraosseous carcinoma

A primary intraosseous carcinoma is a rare neoplasm. The tumor is defined by the WHO as a squamous cell carcinoma arising within the jaws, having no initial connection with the oral mucosa, and presumably developing from residues of the odontogenic epithelium[437]. The malignant transformation that is occasionally found in the lining of a radicular cyst is not regarded as a primary intraosseous carcinoma in the WHO classification, but is classified separately.

The tumor appears more often in the mandible than in the maxilla. Symptoms consist of pain, swelling, and mobility of teeth[482, 635]. Radiographically, there are no special features.

On microscopic examination an alveolar or plexiform pattern of keratinizing or non-keratinizing squamous cells with or without palisading of the peripheral layer can be observed.

Treatment consists of surgical removal. Regional metastatic spread is not uncommon[413].

Other carcinomas arising from odontogenic epithelium

Malignant transformation of the epithelial lining of odontogenic cysts is rare[595]. It may be difficult to really prove that a carcinoma has, indeed, arisen from the epithelial cyst lining rather than developing in close proximity to it (Fig. 10-41).

Clear cell odontogenic tumor/carcinoma

A rather recently described entity is the so-called clear cell odontogenic tumor[249], called by some clear cell odontogenic carcinoma[44].

Malignant neoplasms • 233

Fig. 10-41a.
Radiograph showing an impacted third molar. Notice the irregular outline of the follicle. During removal no abnormalities were observed and no tissue was sent for histologic examination.

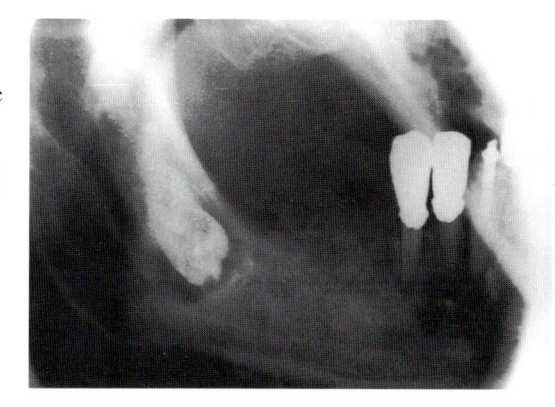

Fig. 10-41b.
Because of disturbed wound healing a new radiograph was taken after two months.

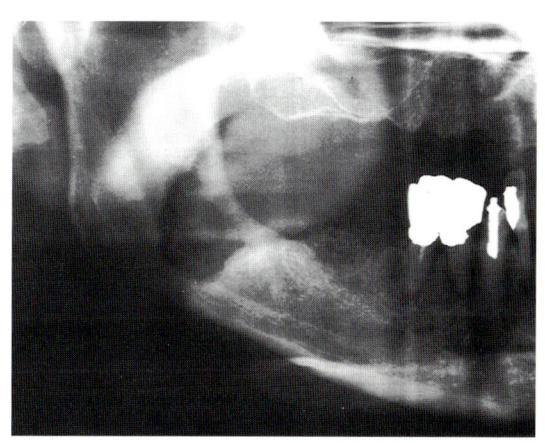

Fig. 10-41c.
A biopsy revealed the presence of a well-differentiated squamous cell carcinoma. Most likely the tumor had originated from the lining of the follicle of the impacted 48.

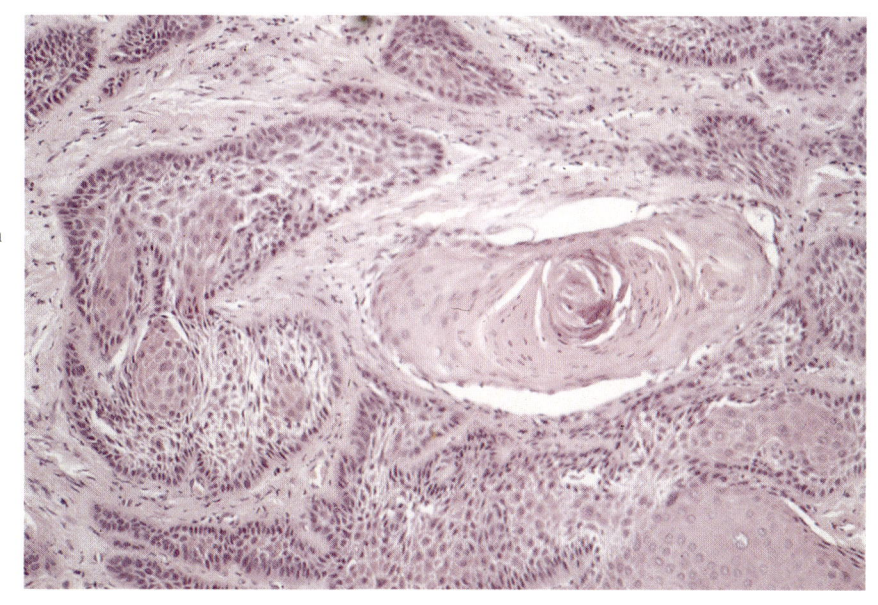

Odontogenic sarcomas

Ameloblastic fibrosarcoma (ameloblastic sarcoma)

As a synonym for ameloblastic fibrosarcoma, the term ameloblastic sarcoma has been used. It is a rare neoplasm of which approximately 50 cases have been reported in the literature[625, 642].

The epithelial component is similar to that of the ameloblastic fibroma, but the mesenchymal tissue is more cellular and shows bizarre fibroblasts with polymorphism and often atypical mitoses. In the presence of dentine the term ameloblastic dentinosarcoma can be used; when both dentine and enamel are present the term ameloblastic odontosarcoma is applied[26].

A radical resection is recommended as the treatment of choice. Also treatment with cytostatic drugs has been reported[223].

Ameloblastic odontosarcoma

The ameloblastic odontosarcoma is an extremely rare tumor that resembles the ameloblastic fibrosarcoma but, in addition, contains small amounts of dysplastic dentine and enamel[434].

Perhaps a distinction should be made between ameloblastic fibro-dentinosarcoma and ameloblastic fibro-odontosarcoma.

Odontogenic carcino-sarcoma

During the 5th meeting of the International Association of Oral Pathologists, held in Tokyo in 1990 a draft has been circulated regarding a revision of the WHO-classification. In that draft the entity of odontogenic carcino-sarcoma has been incorporated in the classification.

CHAPTER 11

Systemic diseases

In this chapter some common and uncommon systemic diseases will be discussed that affect the jaw bones. The lymphoreticular diseases were presented in chapter 9.

Gaucher's disease

Gaucher's disease, a rare disorder of glycosphyngolipid storage, is inherited as an autosomal recessive trait. The disorder is caused by a deficiency of the enzyme glucocerebrosidase, which is responsible for the enzymatic cleavage of glucose from glucosylceramide. The pathologic features of Gaucher's disease are the result of the accumulation of glucosylceramide within the histiocytes of the reticuloendothelial system.

Gaucher's disease is usually classified into three distinct clinical entities, these being the adult, chronic visceral form (type I), the acute, neuropathic form (type II) and the subacute, neuropathic form (type III). In the adult type, radiolucent lesions of the bone are observed in the majority of patients, the femur being the most commonly affected bone. In rare cases the jaws are involved as well[244].

The diagnosis is based on a biopsy, demonstrating the typical Gaucher's cells, and measurement of the serum acid phosphatase and glucocerebrosidase levels.

No treatment is available. In case of splenomegaly a splenectomy may be necessary. With regard to the bone lesions debridement is indicated. Since the replacement of marrow tissue by the Gaucher's cells often results in anemia, leukopenia and thrombocytopenia, the risk of severe hemorrhage should be taken into account.

Histiocytosis X
(Langerhans' cell granulomatosis)

Definition and epidemiology

The etiology and pathogenesis of histiocytosis X are unknown. The disease is characterized by proliferation of tissue macrophages (histiocytes) or of specialized bone marrow-derived cells, called Langerhans' cells[86]. Therefore, the condition could perhaps better be designated "Langerhans' cell disease", "Langerhans cell (eosinophilic) granulomatosis" or Langerhans cell histiocytosis[34, 86, 551].

Three subgroups of histiocytosis X can be distinguished, these being Hand-Schüller-Christian disease, Letterer-Siwe disease and eosinophilic granuloma. Some authors have questioned the aforementioned subclassification and claim that Letterer-Siwe disease is a separate entity.

In 47 nonodontogenic tumors of the jawbones in children, five cases of histiocytosis X were encountered[117]. In a review of 1,120 patients, Hartman reported oral involvement in histiocytosis X in 10% of the cases[256]. Since then, a number of other review articles and case reports have been published[148, 229, 366, 657, 670].

In some cases the oral lesions are the initial manifestation of the disease.

Hand-Schüller-Christian disease

Hand-Schüller-Christian disease is a type of histiocytosis X that appears at a young age, twice as often in boys as in girls. The disease is characterized by extensive lesions in and outside the skeleton and usually has a chronic clinical course. The classical triad consists of one or more punched-out bone lesions of the skull, especially in the temporal bone, unilateral or bilateral exophthalmos, and diabetes insipidus, with or without symptoms of malfunction of the pituitary glands, such as dwarfism.

In the oral cavity there are often nonspecific lesions, e.g. a severe loss of alveolar bone, which may resemble a common periodontal disease[27], or even loss of the entire mandible (Fig. 11-1)[160]. The maxilla is seldom affected. Also the soft tissues may be involved.

The microscopic features can be distinguished in three stages:
1. Proliferation of histiocytes with accumulation of eosinophilic leukocytes; 2. Vascular, granulomatous stage with many histiocytes

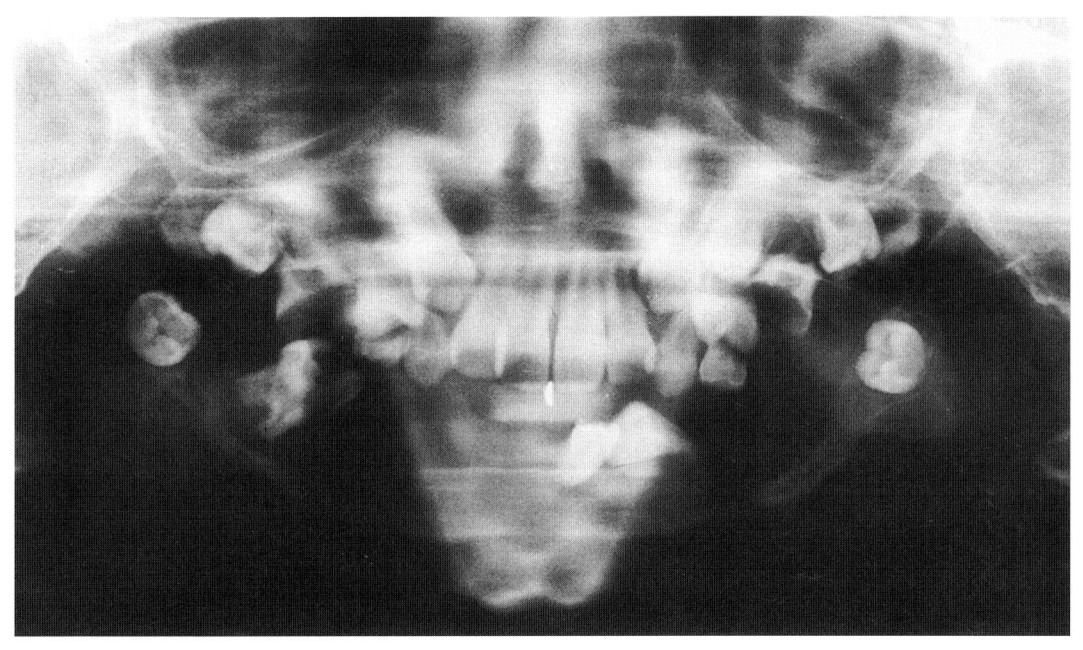

Fig. 11-1. Severe loss of mandibular bone in a nine-year-old girl suffering from Hand-Schüller-Christian disease. (Courtesy Dr. J.A. Tolmeijer, The Netherlands).

and eosinophils; 3. Diffuse, xanthomatous stage with many foam cells.

Treatment consists of curettage or low-dose irradiation. Also chemotherapy can be useful. The prognosis is in general quite favorable. Some patients even undergo spontaneous remission.

Letterer-Siwe disease

Letterer-Siwe disease is the acute type of histiocytosis X, usually seen only in children under the age of three years. According to some authors Letterer-Siwe disease represents an unusual form of malignant lymphoma[86].

The disease often starts with a rash and fever. Splenomegaly, hepatomegaly, and lymphadenopathy are common findings. Later in the process there are deformities of the skeleton. In the oral cavity ulcerations may be present, as well as destruction of the mandible and the maxilla.

The microscopic features resemble those of Hand-Schüller-Christian disease[286].

The prognosis is in general moderate.

238 • Systemic diseases

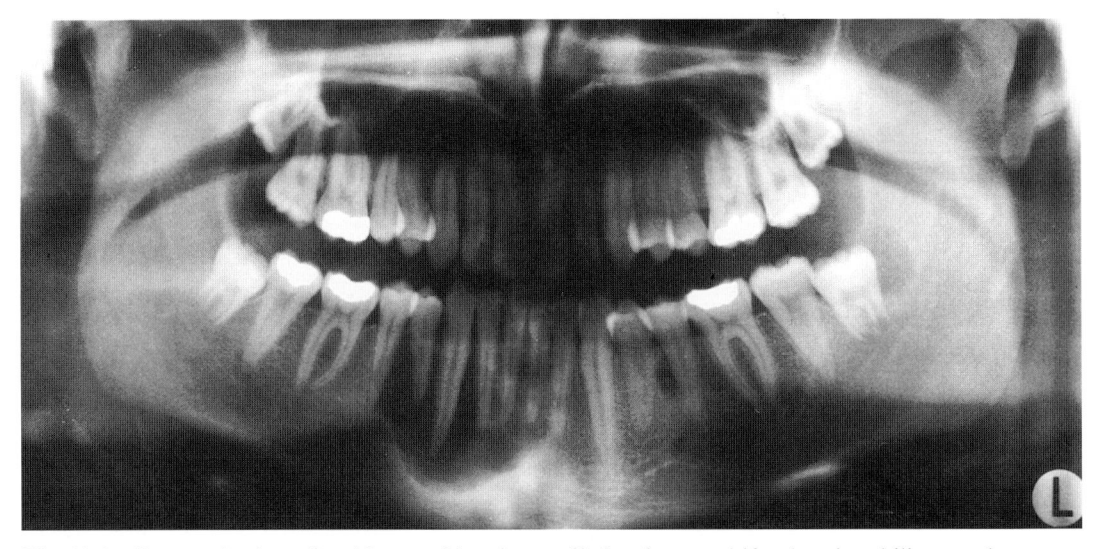

Fig. 11-2a. Panoramic view of an 18-year-old patient suffering from multifocal eosinophilic granuloma (Langerhans' cell granulomatosis). There is a lesion in the right cuspid region of the mandible. The presence of Langerhans' cells was also demonstrated in the lesion distally of 38. Lesions were also present in the right mastoid bone and in one of the ribs.

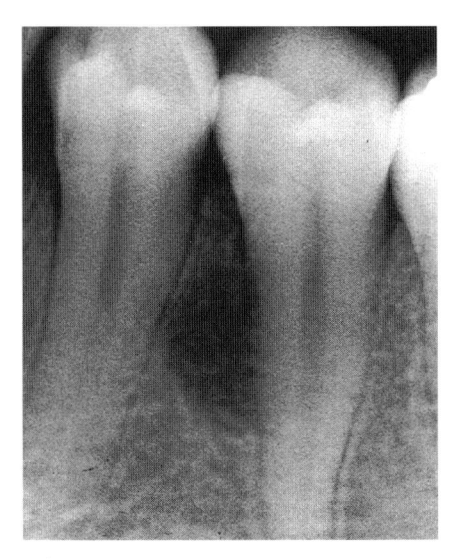

Fig. 11-2b. Detail of the lesion between 34 and 35.

Eosinophilic granuloma

Definition and epidemiology

Eosinophilic granuloma is a disease that in most cases appears in a generalized fashion (multifocal versus unifocal Langerhans' cell granulomatosis) in the bone and is characterized by proliferation of histiocytes and a varying number of eosinophilic leukocytes. The differential diagnosis between unifocal and multifocal presenta-

Fig. 11-2c. High-power view of the biopsy.

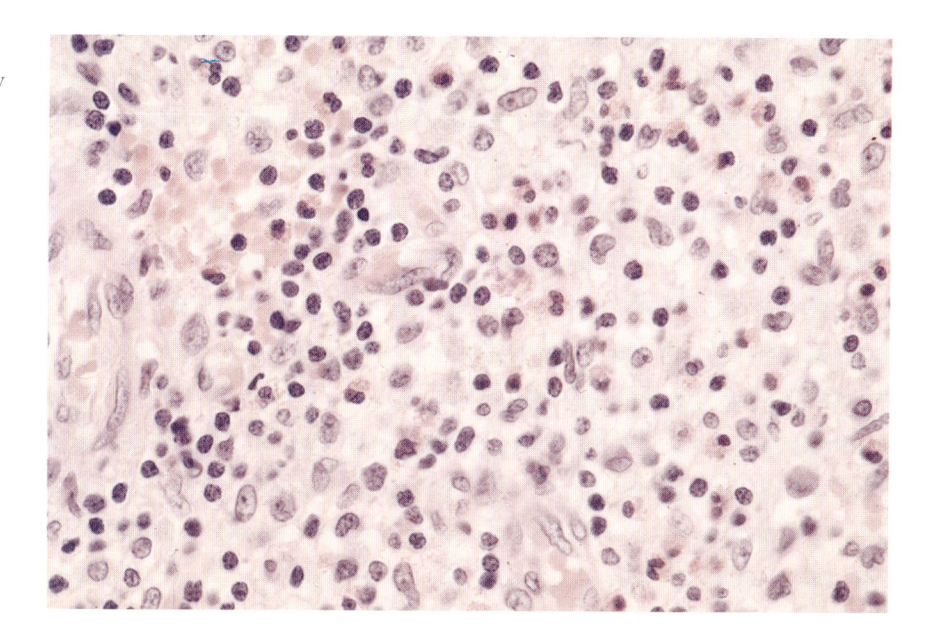

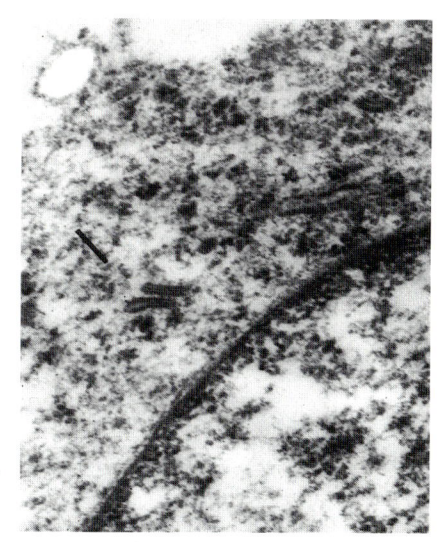

Fig. 11-2d. Ultrastructural examination showed the presence of Birbeck granules in the cytoplasm of the Langerhans' cells. (Orig. magn. x 36,000).

tions is determined by an initial bone scan and by the presence or absence of new lesions over a 12-month period[154]. Common sites of involvement are the skull, mandible, ribs, femur, vertebrae and flat bones.

The disease is mainly seen in older children and young adults, twice as often in males as in females.

Clinical aspects Sometimes it is an incidental finding on the radiograph. On the other hand symptoms such as pain or a slow-growing swelling may be noticed. The disease may first be manifested in the mouth.

Radiographic aspects

The bone lesions are radiolucent and often ill-defined. The lesions in the jaws, more or less limited to the mandible, may also be well-circumscribed and may even mimic the features of a cyst or granuloma and, in some cases, periodontal disease. The lesion may occur in a multifocal fashion (Fig. 11-2)[316].

Histologic aspects

Microscopic examination shows an accumulation of histiocytes in the presence, particularly in the early stage, of many eosinophils. The use of monoclonal antibodies can be of additional help, since the anti-T antibody reacts with the Langerhans' histiocytes[393]. Ultrastructural examination may be helpful as well, since the observation of Langerhans' granules, also referred to as Birbeck granules, in "histiocytic" cells is considered diagnostic.

In a later stage fibrosis takes place and the eosinophils may disappear completely, sometimes giving rise to the features of Hand-Schüller-Christian disease. In the presence of secondary infection, which is not a rare event in the jaws, the histopathologic examination may not at first result in the correct diagnosis.

Treatment

In general, the prognosis of solitary eosinophilic granuloma is favorable. Curettage will usually be sufficient. Clinically the tissue strongly resembles granulation tissue and is very friable. Occasionally, irradiation in a limited dosage of 300-600 rads has been applied successfully. Also the successful intralesional injection of methylprednisolone sodium succinate has been reported, especially in solitary lesions[122, 299]. However, in its disseminated form eosinophilic granuloma is an unpredictable disease for which treatment is not always effective[186]. Recurrences have been observed up to 10 years after first treatment[670].

Osteopetrosis

Definition and epidemiology

Osteopetrosis, also called Albers-Schönberg disease or marble bone disease, is a disease of the skeleton of unknown etiology that affects the growth and remodelling of bone. In most cases heredity seems to play a role. Possibly, the osteoclasts are defective. It is beyond the scope of this text to discuss the regulation of bone cell mechanism in health and disease[243].

Three subtypes are recognized: (1) malignant (recessive) osteopetrosis, (2) benign (dominant) osteopetrosis, and (3) an intermediate (recessive) form with associated carbonic anhydrase II deficiency, renal tubular acidosis, and cerebral calcification[539].

Malignant osteopetrosis is already present at birth or shortly thereafter. Sometimes these children are stillborn. Most bones of the skeleton are involved in this diffuse sclerotic process. In the severe type the foramina of the skull may become obliterated, resulting, among other things, in atrophy of the optical nerve. Hepatosplenomegaly, growth disturbance, deafness, and facial paralysis are common findings. The patients usually die as a result of anemia or secondary infections.

Benign osteopetrosis becomes manifest later in life and is a much less aggressive disease. Quite often multiple fractures or generalized pain in the bones lead to the diagnosis.

For discussion on so-called focal periapical osteopetrosis see chapter 2 p. 36.

Clinical aspects

In the jaws osteomyelitis may develop rather easily in the massive, compact bone after a simple extraction[133]. A simple extraction may also cause a fracture of the bone. The teeth often show hypoplasia of the enamel, dentinal defects, incomplete roots, and increased susceptibility to caries. The eruption of teeth may be delayed, probably due to sclerotic changes of the bone. Ankylosis of cementum to bone is another possible explanation for the delayed or impaired eruption of teeth[653]. An excellent review of the oral and dental findings of osteopetrosis is presented by Ruprecht and coworkers[481].

Radiographic aspects

The radiographs show a diffuse, homogeneous, symmetrically sclerosing aspect of all bones (Fig. 11-3). The marrow spaces are replaced by dense bone, while the cortical plates may be somewhat expanded. Van Buchem et al. have written about a disease that,

242 • Systemic diseases

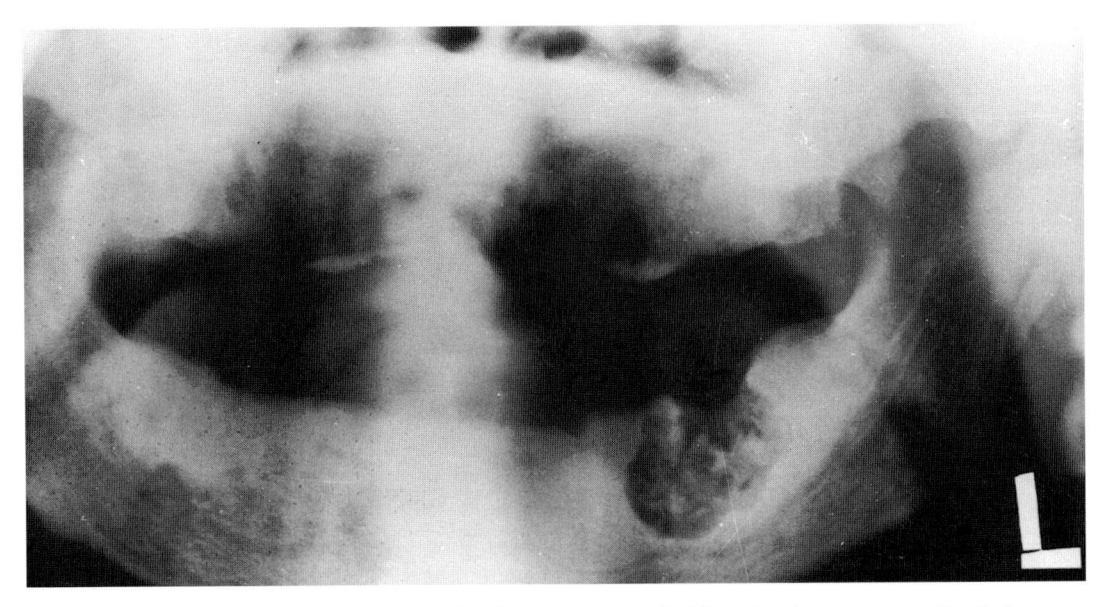

Fig. 11-3a. Panoramic view of patient suffering from osteopetrosis. Note the dense aspect of both the mandible and maxilla. In the left part of the mandible osteomyelitis had developed.

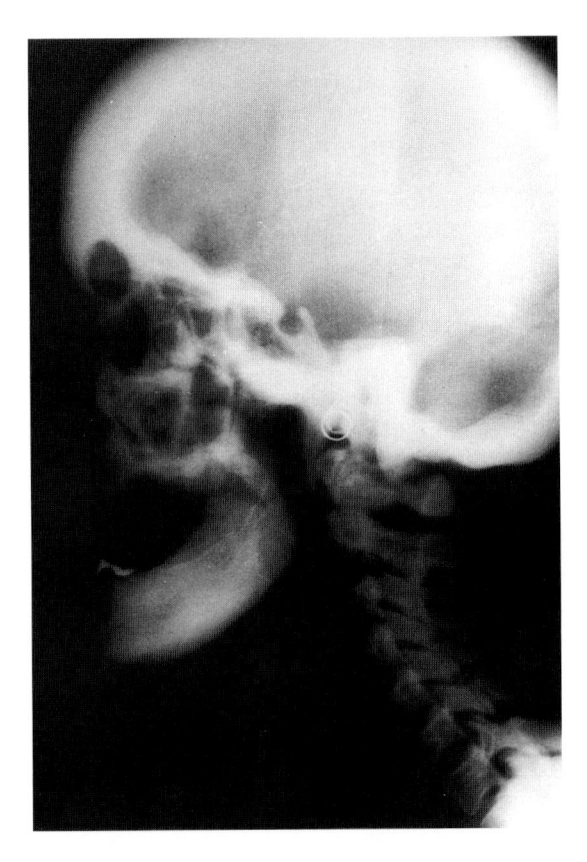

Fig. 11-3b.
Note the thickness and density of the skull bones.

radiographically, shows some similarity to osteopetrosis (See chapter 1 p. 25). Other diseases that should be included in the differential diagnosis are polyostotic fibrous dysplasia (See chapter 4 p. 70), pycnodysostosis (See chapter 1 p. 28), and Engelmann's disease. In the latter entity, also referred to as Camurati-Engelmann's disease or progressive diaphyseal dysplasia, only the diaphyses are involved[144].

Laboratory findings

The laboratory values of the blood may indicate a type of anemia. The values of calcium and phosphate of the serum are usually normal, as is the alkaline phosphatase.

Histologic aspects

On microscopic examination endostal bone formation is seen as well as reduced physiological resorption. In the long bones remnants of cartilage may persist. When polarized light is used, the shortage of collagen fibers is obvious.

Treatment

No effective measures exist to prevent or treat the disease.

Osteoporosis

Osteoporosis may appear in the skeleton, usually later in life, but is seldom seen in the jaws as a generalized disorder. Osteoporosis and mandibular resorption has been studied in rats. A significant difference in mandibular bone resorption was associated with an osteoporotic-inducing diet high in protein and low in calcium[545].

A disorder that may occur in the jaws and whose name, wrongly, suggests a relationship with osteoporosis, is the osteoporotic bone marrow defect. The latter lesion will be discussed in chapter 12 p. 255.

244 • Systemic diseases

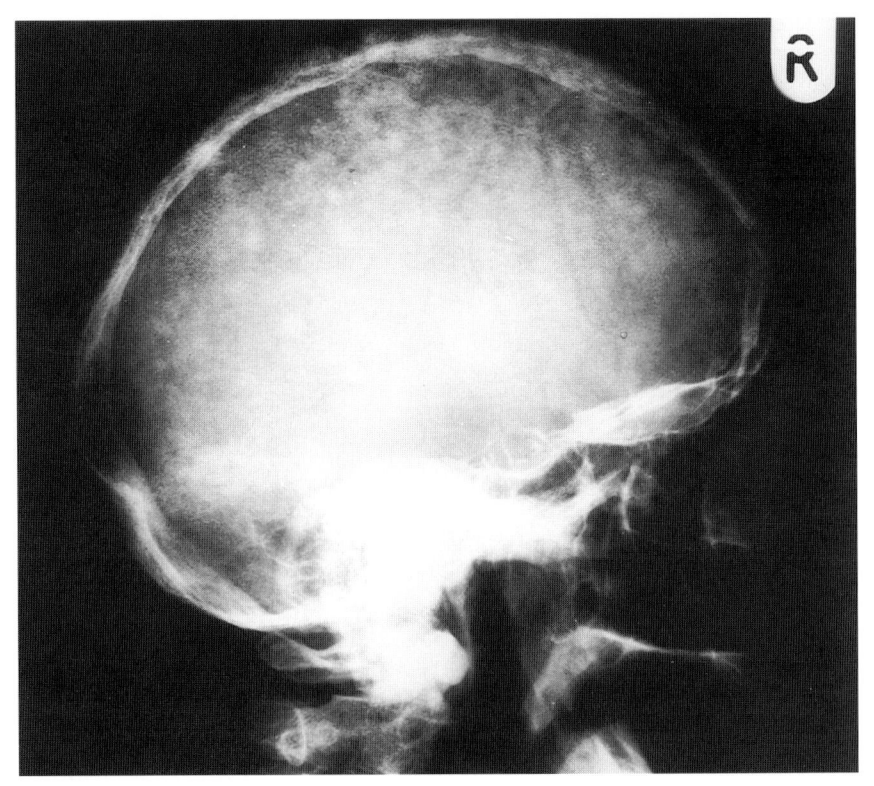

Fig. 11-4a. Lateral skull film of patient with Paget's disease. Notice the "cotton wool" appearance.

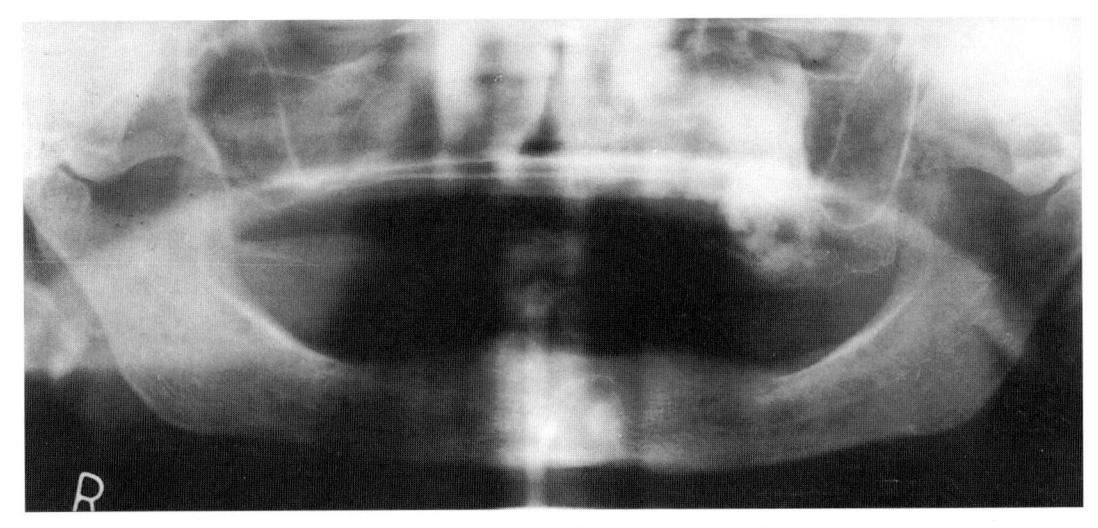

Fig. 11-4b. The panoramic view shows opaque changes in the left part of the maxilla.

Paget's disease

Definition and epidemiology

Paget's disease, also called osteitis deformans, is a disease of unknown etiology, characterized by simultaneous destruction and repair of osseous tissues. The disease may be monostotic or polyostotic.

It has been suggested that osteoclasts of patients having Paget's disease contain antigen substances. These are expected to prove similar to the virus that causes measles[460].

The disorder, first described by Paget in 1899, is most likely to appear in those over 40 years of age and is seen somewhat more often in men than in women. Reliable figures on the prevalence of the disease are not available. The percentages range from 0.1% to 5.0%. Geographical differences are seen, as was reported in a review article of 152 reported cases of Paget's disease of the jaws[540].

Clinical aspects

Paget's disease is a chronic disease, the symptoms of which develop gradually. These consist of bone pain, severe headache, deafness, loss of sight, dizziness, and mental disturbance. A progressive enlargement of the cranium may appear. The vertebral column, the femur, and the tibia may also be expanded. The affected bones feel warm due to increased vascularity and appear to carry an increased risk of fractures.

As opposed to the exuberant facial changes in fibrous dysplasia, extensive alterations in the facial bones with Paget's disease are infrequent[562]. When the jaws are involved, the maxilla is more frequently affected than the mandible, the ratio being approximately 3:1. In some instances both jaws are involved. Expansion of the bone takes place and a flattening of the palate as well. Diastemata may develop and the teeth tend to migrate palatally. On extraction of teeth in an affected part of the bone there is often disturbed wound healing, even to the extent of the development of osteomyelitis[77]. A rare case of Paget's disease with involvement of the dental pulp has been reported[21].

Radiographic aspects

The radiograph shows osteolytic foci in the skeleton and in the cranium, interspersed by areas of somewhat more radiopaque structure, resulting in a "cotton wool" appearance (Fig. 11-4). In case of jaw involvement the radiographic aspect may mimic chronic diffuse sclerosing osteomyelitis. The teeth may show hypercementosis (Fig. 11-5). Resorption of teeth has also been reported[542] as

Fig. 11-5.
Hypercementosis of upper incisors in a patient with Paget's disease.

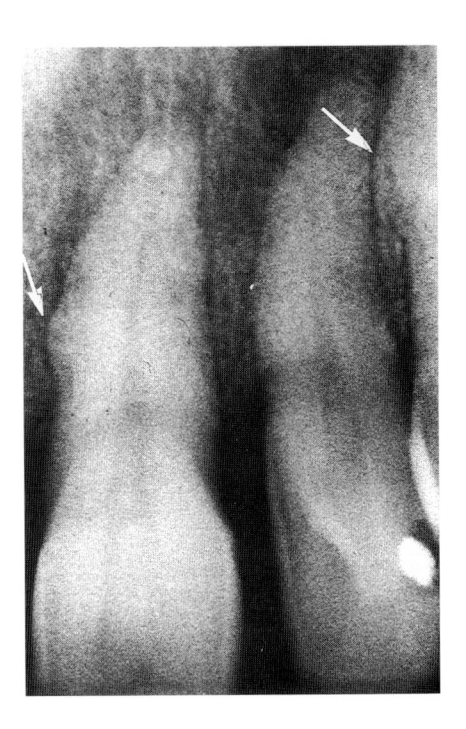

well as loss of the lamina dura and calcifications of the pulp chamber[421].

Laboratory findings   The serum calcium and phosphorus values are usually normal. The alkaline phosphatase may be considerably raised. The disease often proceeds with exacerbations and remissions. During remissions the value of alkaline phosphatase is usually normal.

Histologic aspects   The microscopic aspect usually shows considerable osteoblastic and osteoclastic activity, all in a disorderly pattern. At the same time there is increased vascularity. The formation of mosaic bone is classic. This is bone that has been partly resorbed and rebuilt in an alternating fashion, resulting in numerous reversal lines. Occasionally, cementumlike masses can be observed. The stroma is of a fibrous nature. Often lymphocytic infiltrates can be observed in edematous areas (Fig. 11-6).

Treatment   At present no effective therapy exists for Paget's disease, although rather recently the successful use of a single infusion of the biphosphanate AHPrBP (APD) has been reported[572]. Malignant transformation into an osteogenic sarcoma occurs in less than 1% of patients with Paget's disease.

Fig. 11-6. Low-power view of maxillary lesion in Paget's disease. Notice the disorderly pattern of the bone trabeculae, the osteoblastic rimming and the vascularity of the marrow.

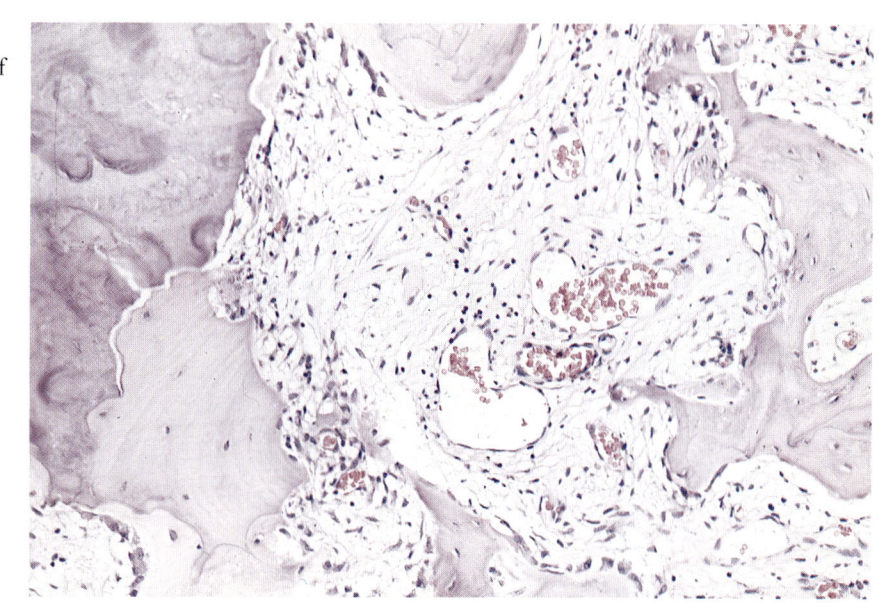

Fig. 11-7.
Part of panoramic view of patient suffering from renal osteodystrophy. Thinning and almost absent cortical bone at the angle of the mandible and delicate trabecular pattern of the bone of the ascending ramus.

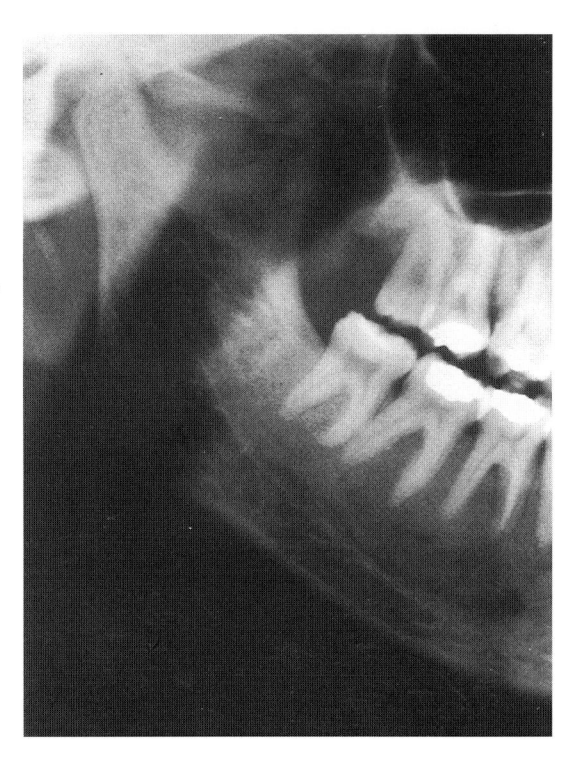

Renal osteodystrophy

Renal osteodystrophy refers to the bone changes that occur secondary to chronic renal failure and chronic hemodialysis. These bone changes include osteitis fibrosa cystica, focal osteosclerosis, osteoclastoma ("brown tumors") and osteomalacia. The pathophysiologic mechanisms involved in renal dystrophy have been reviewed by Brenner and Rector[89].

The radiographic changes in the jaws of 38 patients with severe renal disease have been described by Kelly et al.[309]. Partial or total loss of the lamina dura, delicate or absent trabecular pattern, and an overall granular or chalky-white appearance associated with an increase in radiographic density were the most common findings. Others have noticed a significant decrease in the thickness of the mandibular angular cortex (Fig. 11-7)[83]. A paper has been published favoring maxillomandibular above hands roentgenographs in the evaluation of renal osteodystrophy[362]. In reply to the latter paper it has been stated that radiography of the hands remains the method of choice for evaluating the onset and the follow-up of renal osteodystrophy[288].

Sarcoidosis

Sarcoidosis is a systemic disease of unknown etiology characterized by the presence of non-caseating giant cell granulomas in several organs. The disease may appear as an acute disease accompanied by fever or as a more chronic respiratory disease.

Sarcoid lesions may occur in the lungs, the skin, the eyes and also in the oral mucosa. Involvement of the jaw bones is exceptional[587].

Scleroderma

In patients with scleroderma (progressive systemic sclerosis) osteolysis in the region of the coronoid process, condylar process, and angle of the mandible has been reported (Fig. 11-8). The osteolysis, either bilateral or unilateral[438], is possibly due to excessive pressure from the skin or to muscle atrophy[510]. Another explanation is the involvement of small arterial branches of the internal maxillary artery by the progressive systemic sclerosis[453].

Thalassemia

The thalassemias are a group of inherited pathologic hemoglobin conditions resulting from a quantitative reduction of a specific globin chain. Normal adult hemoglobin consists of two alpha (α) and two beta (β) chains. The thalassemias exhibit an imbalance in the production of either α or β chains. The imbalance is due to disturbances in the control mechanism of protein synthesis and results in altered function of the hemoglobin molecule and altered structure of erythrocytes. Hemolysis is the most important consequence. The thalassemias are classified according to the chain that is produced at the reduced rate. A homozygous, heterozygous, or double heterozygous form may be distinguished.

In the heterozygous α- or β-thalassemia, also called thalassemia minor, the disease tends to be mild, with minimal clinical expression. Homozygous and double heterozygous forms may become severe and are called thalassemia major, also referred to as Cooley's anemia or Mediterranean anemia. Within the thalassemia major group there are many genetic defects that produce various clinical and hematologic findings.

Fig. 11-8a. Patient suffering from scleroderma.

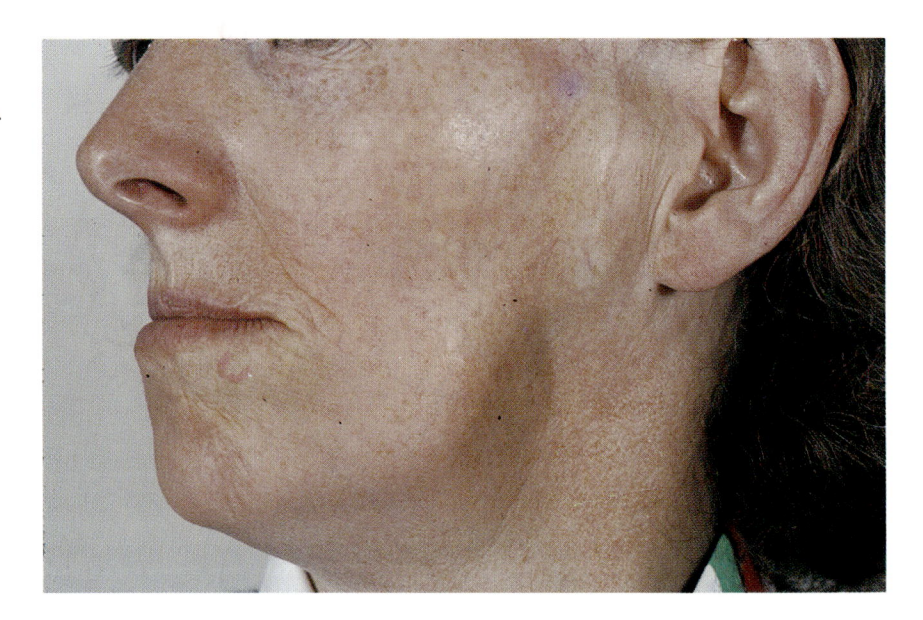

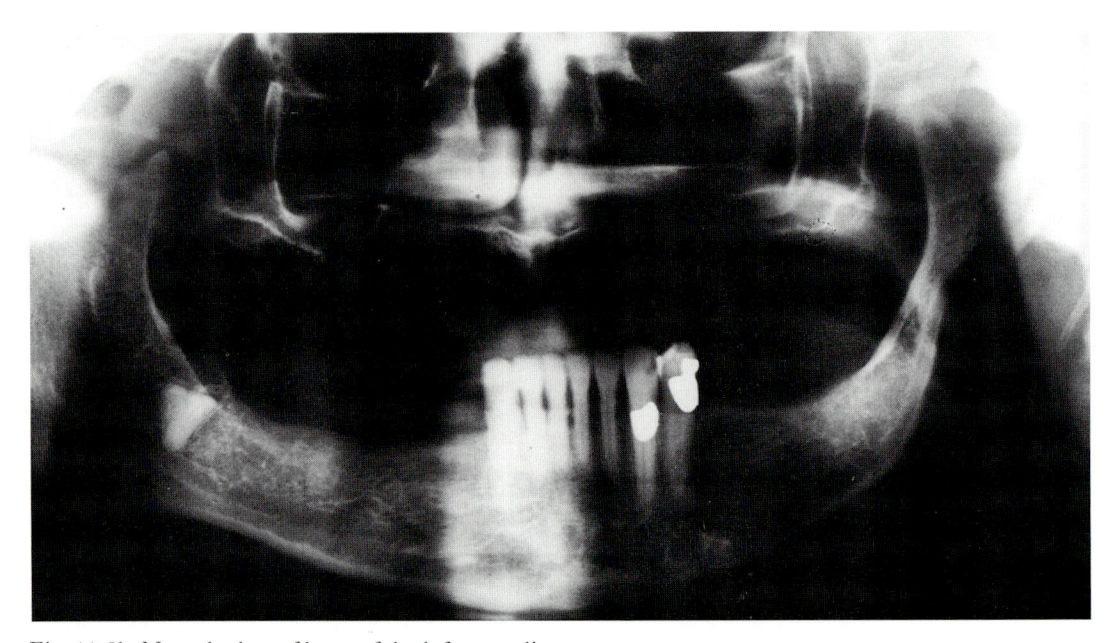

Fig. 11-8b. Note the loss of bone of the left ascending ramus.

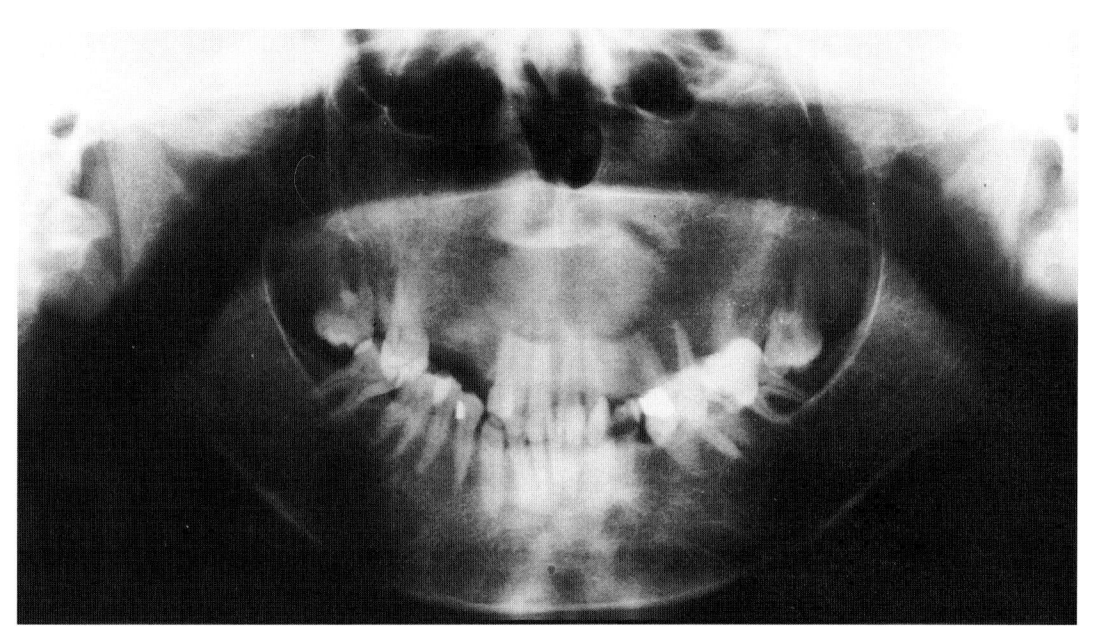

Fig. 11-9a. Panoramic view of patient suffering from thalassemia. The changes are more marked in the maxilla than in the mandible.

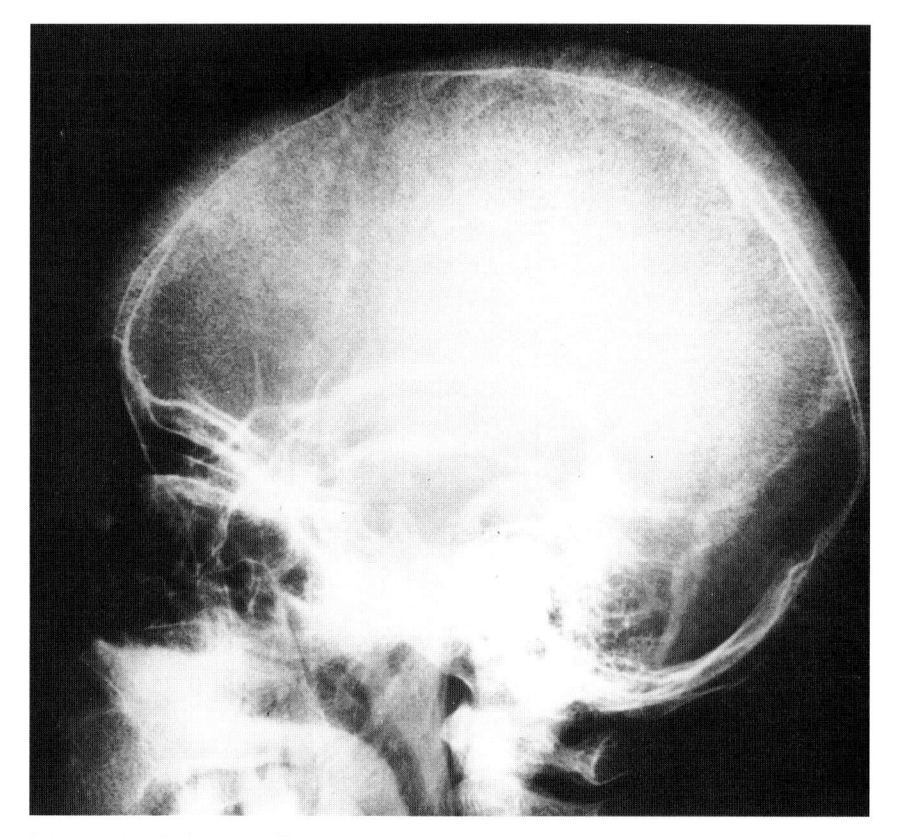

Fig. 11-9b. "Hair-on-end" appearance.

Fig. 11-9c. Low-power view of biopsy of the maxilla. (Courtesy Drs. J. Hes and K. de Man, The Netherlands).

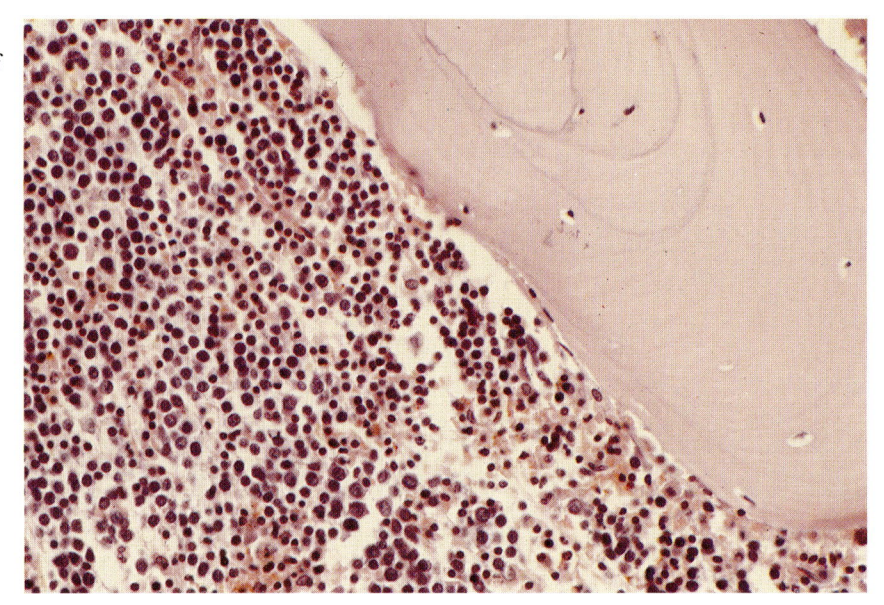

Extreme hypertrophy of the erythroid marrow in medullary and sometimes extramedullary sites is a well-recognized feature of thalassemia major. Involvement of the facial skeleton resulting in severe disfigurement has been described in several reports (Fig. 11-9).

Under the impact of this disorder, a typical facial appearance develops: high and bulging cheek bones, retraction of the upper lip, protrusion of the anterior teeth and spacing of other teeth, overbite or open bite, and varying degrees of malocclusion.

The skeletal changes are the result of proliferation of the bone marrow in the facial skeleton. This proliferated marrow is extensively used as an ancillary hematopoietic organ to compensate for the chronic hemolysis.

Usually the mandible becomes less enlarged than the maxilla. The dense cortical plates of the mandible apparently prevent the expansion. The bony changes may occur early in life and tend to persist, particularly in the skull.

Persons suffering from thalassemia major are significantly retarded in all aspects of their growth.

A separate paper is devoted to the changes visible in radiographs used in dentistry[442]. Another paper deals with the oral manifestations and complications[149]. Furthermore, a patient has been described suffering from homozygous β-thalassemia in whom a surgical correction had been performed of a bimaxillary hyperplasia[266a].

CHAPTER 12

Miscellaneous lesions and disorders of bone

Atrophy of the alveolar ridges

When a tooth has been removed, the alveolar bone will resorb in time. In some patients this resorption proceeds very slowly, while in others a more rapid resorption may be observed. The atrophy is usually much more distinct in the mandible than in the maxilla (Fig. 12-1).

The factors playing a role in the process of the resorption are not fully understood. The age of the patient at the time of the removal of a tooth seems to play a role, as does the condition of the periodontium at the time of the extraction[570]. In a study of 14 patients with advanced mandibular atrophy, four of them exhibited gener-

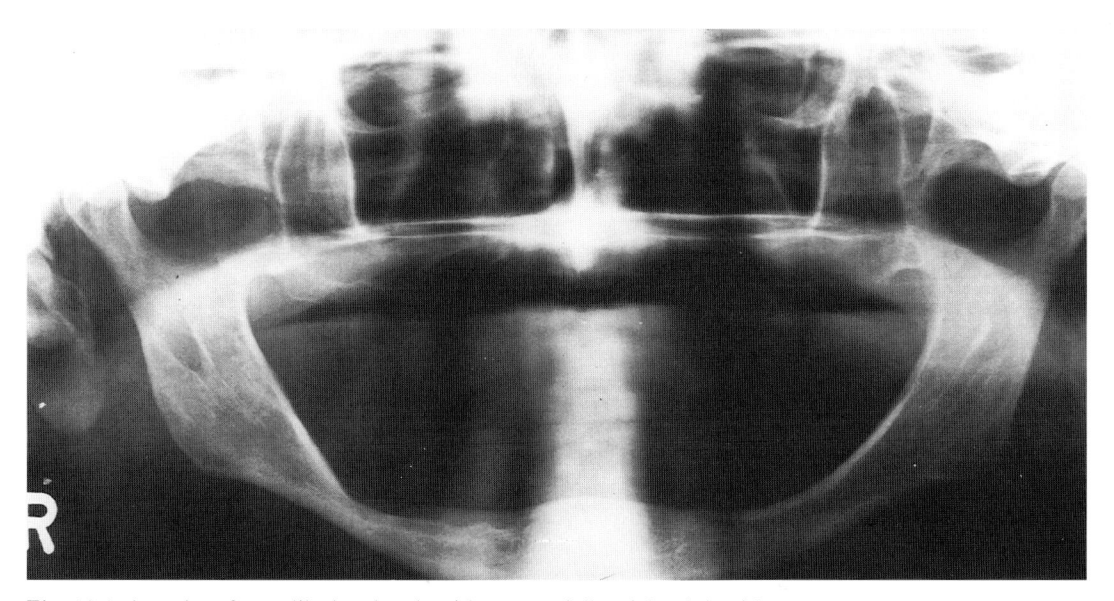

Fig. 12-1. Atrophy of mandibular alveolar ridge, especially of the right side.

alized bone disease[50, 51]. Other authors have confirmed the possible relation between mandibular atrophy and metabolic bone loss[85, 241, 242]. A thickness of the mandibular angular cortex at gonion of less than 1 mm has been shown to be indicative of metabolic bone loss[84].

A study has been carried out to analyze the pattern of the age-related bone loss in the mandibular cortex[631]. The analysis showed that cortical porosity and the percentage of Haversian canals showing resorption are unrelated to sex and increased after the age of 50 years. In an animal experiment a significant difference in mandibular bone resorption was associated with an osteoporotic-inducing diet[545].

It is beyond the scope of this book to discuss the various treatment modalities, such as vestibuloplasty, ridge augmentation, insertion of implants, etc. This also holds true for the possible influence of nutritional regimens[68].

Fibrous or sclerotic healing of extraction wounds

In case of loss of both the buccal and lingual, or palatal, cortical bone plates the alveolus of an extracted tooth may fail to ossify. Instead, fibrous tissue is formed, resulting in a permanent asymptomatic radiolucency at the site of extraction. On the other hand, sclerotic healing may occur.

Both conditions are usually encountered as an incidental finding on the radiograph (Fig. 12-2).

In case of doubt the taking of a biopsy is indicated to rule out any other disease. No further treatment is required.

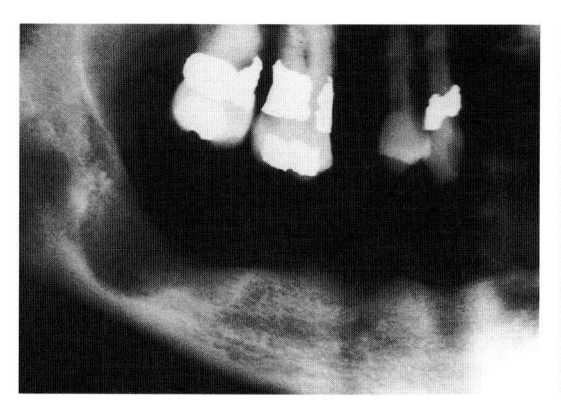

Fig. 12-2a.
Rather well-defined, non-characteristic radiolucency in lower third molar region. The last extraction had taken place at least 10 years previously. On exploration, fibrous tissue was encountered. Histopathologic examination further supported a final diagnosis of "fibrous healing".

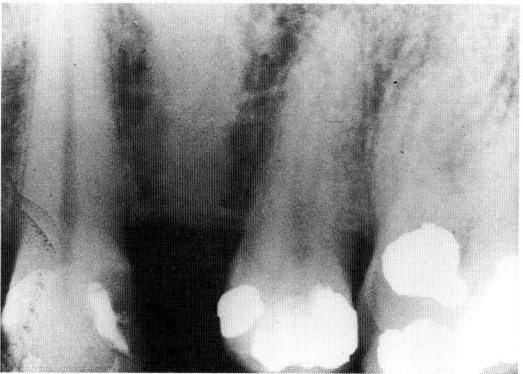

Fig. 12-2b.
Incidental finding of sclerotic alveolus on a radiograph. No signs or symptoms. The 24 had been extracted many years previously. No biopsy has been taken. Therefore, apart from the diagnosis "sclerotic healing", also the possibility of a fibro-osseous cemental lesion and focal chronic osteomyelitis should be taken into account.

Focal osteoporotic bone marrow defect

Definition and epidemiology

The focal osteoporotic bone marrow defect, exclusively occurring in the jaws, is usually described as a harmless, solitary lesion in the jaws - mainly in the mandible - in which the presence of normal hematopoietic marrow is observed. Also the term hematopoietic marrow defect has been used[335].

No data are available concerning the occurrence in the various races. Focal osteoporotic bone marrow defect is seen particularly in women[485]. The average age at the time of diagnosis is about 40 years[618].

Pathogenesis

At birth, bone marrow is of the red, blood-forming type. In adults, however, red bone marrow has largely been replaced by the yellow, fatty type, except in the condyles and the angles of the mandible. The presence of red bone marrow in other sites in the mandible can be explained in various ways: 1. Persistent embryologic red bone marrow remnants; 2. Hyperplasia of red bone marrow due to an increased need for red blood cells in the body, such as in sickle-cell anemia[493]; 3. Abnormal healing of bone tissue after extraction of a tooth or as the result of an inflammatory process.

Clinical aspects

Focal osteoporotic bone marrow defect is usually located in the molar region of the mandible, quite often in a place where a tooth was extracted in the past. It is often detected as an incidental finding on a radiograph. However, pain and swelling may occur[354].

Radiographic aspects

The radiograph may show a circumscribed lucency, but may also show an ill-defined area with a honeycombed structure. Opacities in the center of the lesion have also been described[502]. The size may vary from a few millimeters to some centimeters (Fig. 12-3). The radiographic aspect is not at all pathognomonic and may mimic, among other lesions, a residual cyst, a solitary bone cyst, or a central giant cell granuloma.

Makek and Lello distinguished five groups: 1) those associated with soft or hard tissue third molar impactions; 2) those resembling solitary and aneurysmal bone cysts; 3) those with diffuse, irregular serpiginous borders; 4) square lesions with intraluminal trabeculation; and 5) those related to adjacent dentally treated teeth[354].

Histologic aspects

Histologic examination shows normal hematopoietic tissue.

Treatment

The only way to establish the diagnosis is by histologic examination. This implies the treatment as well.

Focal osteoporotic bone marrow defect • 257

Fig. 12-3a.
Incidental finding. Somewhat scalloped outline of radiolucency below apices of vital 35-37.

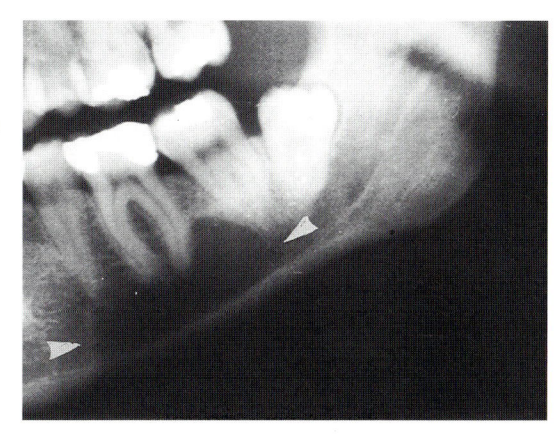

Fig. 12-3b.
The biopsy showed normal hematopoietic tissue, compatible with the diagnosis of focal osteoporotic bone marrow defect.

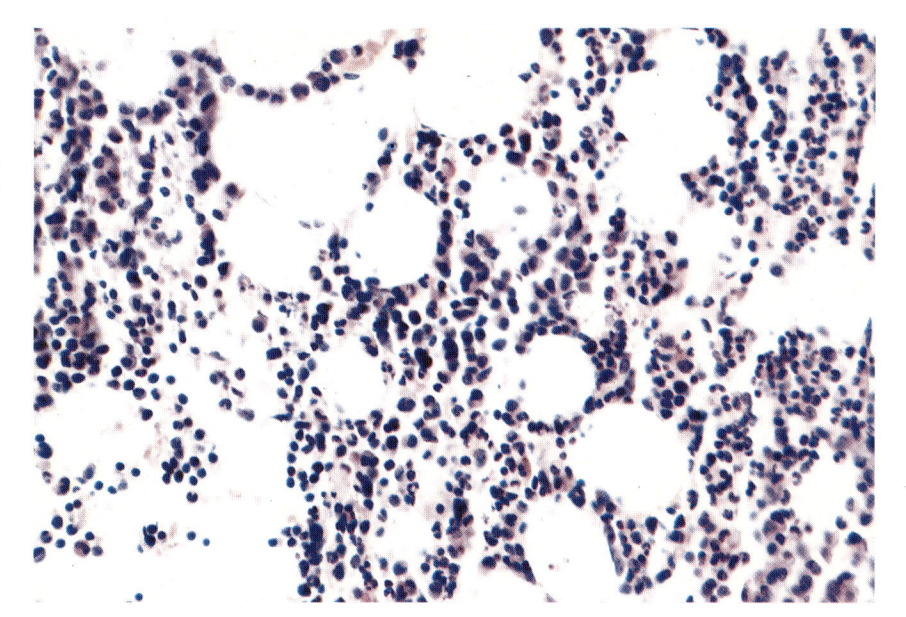

Hemophilic pseudotumor of bone

Bleeding in hemophilic patients, caused for instance by trauma, may result in osteolytic lesions of the bones. Only a very few cases have been reported of such cases involving the jaws. The lesion manifests itself as a painless swelling of several months' duration.

In a review of the English language literature eight patients, all boys, ranging from one to 16 years, were disclosed[91]. In all cases the mandible was involved, occasionally bilaterally.

Radiographically, both bone destruction and new bone formation may be observed.

It has been suggested that surgical removal be undertaken only when a conservative approach, e.g. by Factor-VIII replacement, has failed.

Massive osteolysis

Definition and epidemiology

Massive osteolysis, also known as phantom bone disease or progressive resorption of bone, is a chronic disorder of unknown etiology characterized by spontaneous, progressive resorption of one or more bones. The disorder is possibly related to hemangiomatosis[500].

The involved bones may eventually disappear completely. No evidence has been found of genetic transmission of the disease.

There is no preference for race, sex or age, although in most patients the disease develops before the third decade. A few, rather recent cases have been reported of involvement of the mandible/or maxilla[203, 264]. Also parietal bone involvement has been mentioned in the literature[75].

Clinical aspects

The disorder is not characterized by pain. Even slight trauma may lead to a fracture.

Laboratory findings

Laboratory studies are generally unrevealing.

Radiographic aspects

Radiographically, intramedullary and subcortical radiolucent foci can be seen in the first stage of the disease. Finally, complete resorption takes place unless spontaneous arrest occurs. Progression to adjacent bones, denying joint bounderies, is not uncommon.

Scintigraphic aspects

Bone scans may reveal either decreased or increased isotope uptake.

Histologic aspects	Histologically, a proliferative vascular fibrous connective tissue stroma can be seen, replacing normal bone trabeculae. Osteoblastic and osteoclastic activity is relatively rare[203].
Treatment	Treatment is actually not available. Attempts with bone grafts have resulted in only a limited success. After spontaneous arrest of the disease, reossification does not occur. The disease may result in severe disability, especially in patients with rib and vertebral involvement.

Overprojection of radiopaque structures

Especially with the use of panoramic radiographs various calcified structures of the oral and perioral structures may be projected on the radiographs. Examples are sialoliths from the submandibular glands, calcified lymphnodes, phleboliths in patients with congenital hemangiomas, so-called antroliths, pilomatrixomas or osteomas of the skin, and amalgam fragments in the oral mucosa or, occasionally, in the bone itself. Such radiopacities can be misleading,

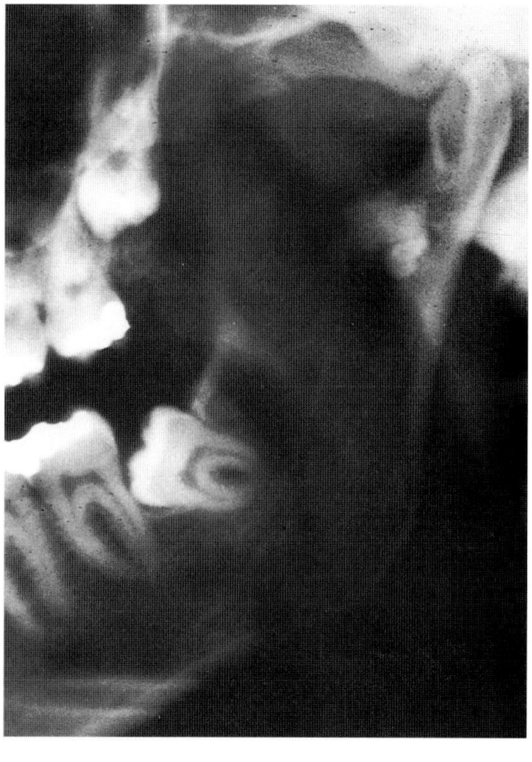

Fig. 12-4.
Opacity "in" ascending ramus caused by overprojection of a pilomatrixoma of the skin.

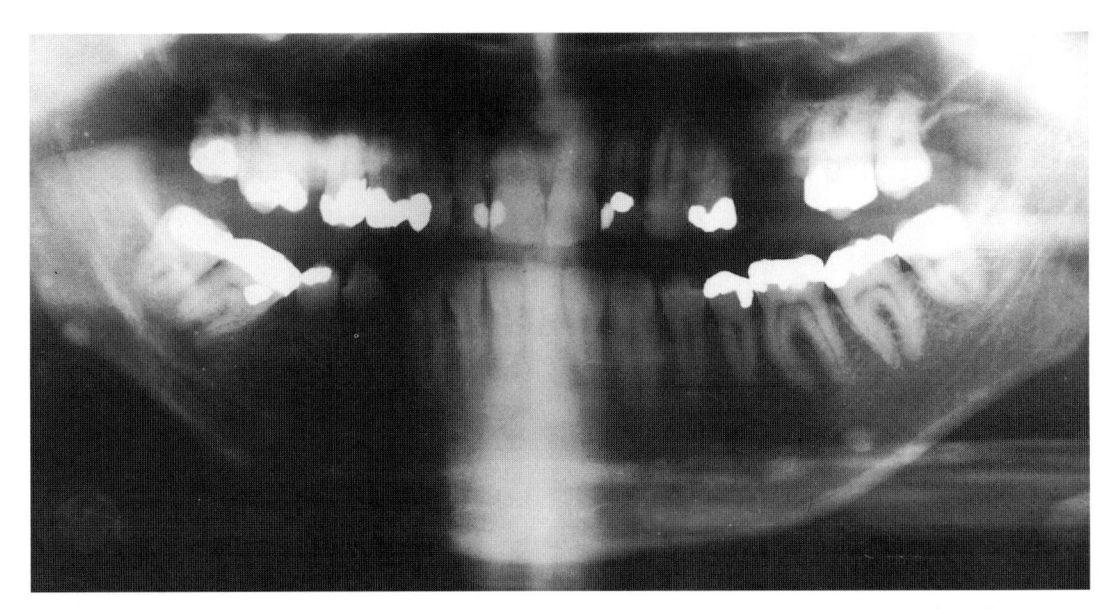

Fig. 12-5. Multiple opacities scattered "throughout" the mandible as a result of overprojection of phleboliths in patient with multiple congenital soft tissue hemangiomas in the orofacial region.

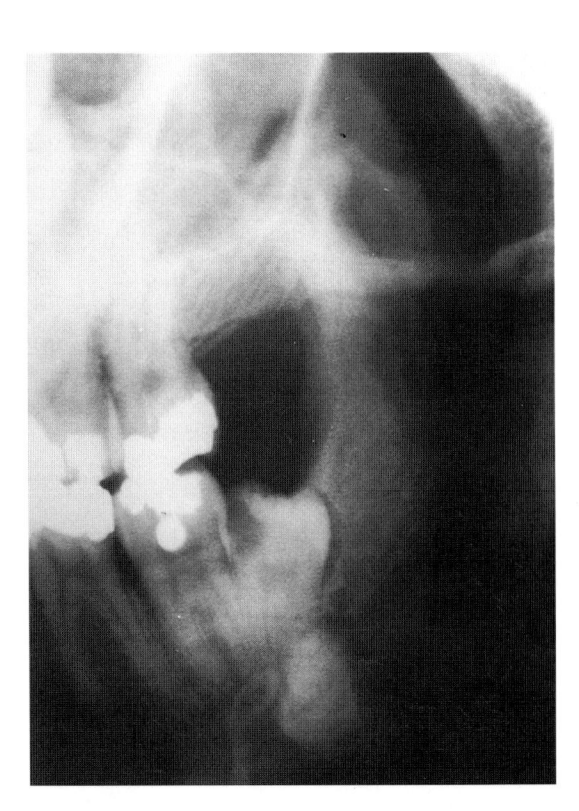

Fig. 12-6. Overprojection of a sialolith at the apex of the partially erupted 38.

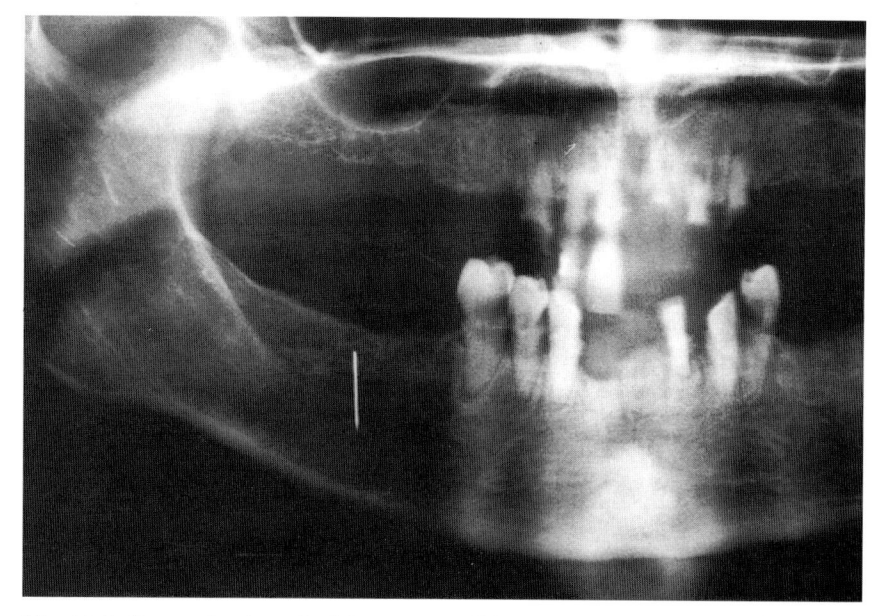

Fig. 12-7. Overprojection of a "charm needle" in the cheek of a 60-year-old woman. Incidental finding.

indeed, as is shown in Figs. 12.4-12.6. Even talismans, also referred to as "charm needles", introduced under the skin, may be observed as an incidental finding on a radiograph (Fig. 12-7)[339].

Careful examination of the soft tissues is in most cases sufficient to arrive at a correct diagnosis. Furthermore, there is the option of taking an additional radiograph in a direction perpendicular to the first one.

262 • Miscellaneous lesions and disorders of bone

Fig. 12-8a. Squamous cell carcinoma of the mucosa of the alveolar ridge,

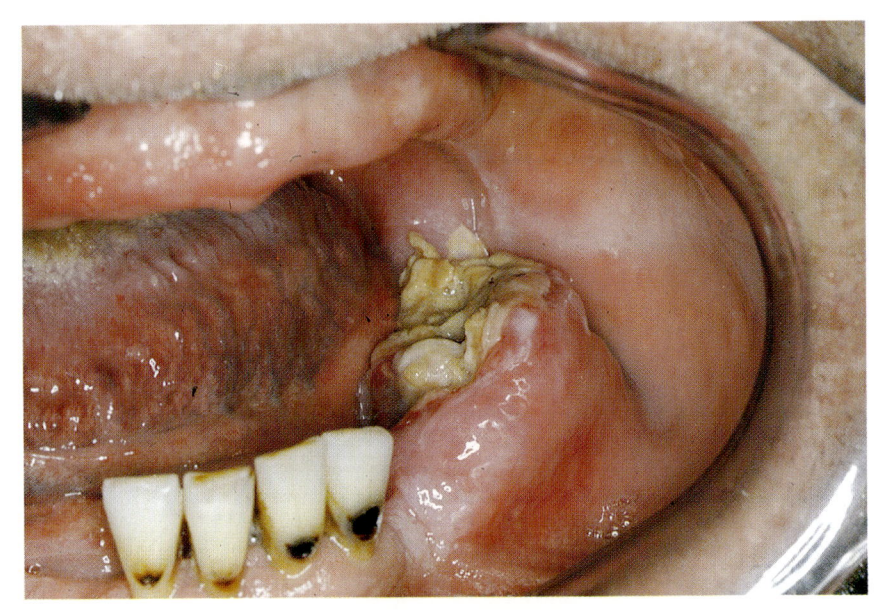

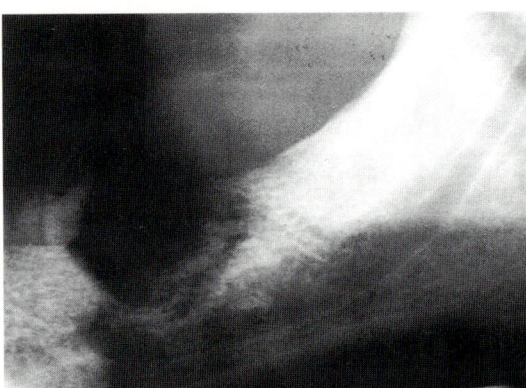

Fig. 12-8b. causing severe bone destruction.

Squamous cell carcinoma

A few reports deal with the mode of invasion of squamous cell carcinoma of the oral mucosa into the underlying bone[410, 536]. In general, an ill-defined, destructive, radiolucent change can be observed. In a number of cases diffuse growth in the dental canal and, if teeth are present, in the periodontal ligament can be seen. In some instances a periosteal reaction is present[368]. Occasionally, the tumor has actually spread well around the mandible without demonstrable radiographic changes.

Apart from conventional radiographs, CT-scans can be helpful in detecting bone invasion[121].

Uncontrolled growth of alveolar processes

A rare case of uncontrolled growth of the alveolar processes of the mandible and maxilla in a 20-month-old child has been reported. The postmortem histologic examination showed a soft and hard tissue mass, consisting of fibrous connective tissue with foci of calcification. No mitoses were present. A diagnosis of embryonic connective tissue was made[343].

CHAPTER 13

Disorders of the temporomandibular joint

Introduction

As in all diseases, the history as presented by the patient with a possible disorder of the temporomandibular joint (TMJ) should be fully scrutinized. The clinical examination of the TMJ comprises palpation of the condyles. Attention is given to possible pain on palpation and the presence of clicking sounds during opening or closing of the mandible. Such clicking may be either unilateral or bilateral. The mobility of the mandible and the exact pattern during opening and closing are also noted. There may be deviations or irregularities in the sagittal or vertical direction, or both. Furthermore, attention should be given to possible spasms of the masticatory and non-masticatory muscles in the head and neck region.

The dentition must be carefully examined as well, especially with regard to the occlusion, the possible presence of abrasion, and the possible presence of a midline deviation.

For the radiographic examination the panoramic view is often used. An advantage of that view is that both condyles are presented in the same view, enabling comparison. However, the image of the condyles is not always clear. Special radiographic view for evaluation of the TMJ are Parma's view and Schüller's views. Schüller's view is well-suited to evaluating the articular space. Both views require a separate image of each condyle. A disadvantage of Parma's view is the high skin dosage. Tomography can also be used to examine the TMJ[475]. Other techniques include CAT-scanning, magnetic resonance imaging (MRI)[250], arthrography[103] and arthrotomography. Double-contrast arthrotomography and MRI have been shown to be very valuable in making the diagnosis of internal derangement[265, 608]. It has been stressed, indeed, that often various radiographic exposures are required to obtain the minimum amount of information necessary for assessment of condyle morphology[471].

Sonography can be helpful for computerized recordings of joint sounds[263]. At present, arthroscopy is gaining in popularity for the diagnosis and also for the treatment of several of the TMJ-disorders[67, 321].

Ankylosis

One of the most common fractures of the jaws is the fracture through or just under the condyle of the mandible, sometimes bilaterally. In this event a hematoma may arise inside the capsule of the joint. Bone formation may then take place in the hematoma, resulting in a bony ankylosis. Ankylosis may also be of a fibrous nature.

In a series of 76 patients in Nigeria cancrum oris was the cause of ankylosis in almost 50% of the cases, trauma accounting for 30% and the remaining cases being due to osteomyelitis[8]. In that paper a distinction was made between extra-articular ankylosis and intracapsular ankylosis. The majority of the cases of infective origin were extra-articular and of a fibrous nature; most of the cases due to trauma were intracapsular. An ankylosis of the TMJ may also be the result of birth delivery with the aid of a forceps.

If ankylosis develops in the TMJ at an early age, it will often lead to permanent functional and esthetic problems. It is now possible - with a fair chance of permanent success - to operate on an ankylotic TMJ and to restore the mobility of the mandible. Recurrent ankylosis has been described in a patient with chronic psoriasis[552].

Arthrogryposis

Arthrogryposis multiple congenita (AMC) is a rare disorder, characterized by multiple fixed joint deformities. It is defined as a congenital, nonprogressive limitation of movement in two or more joints in different body areas. Often all limbs are involved. However, asymmetrical involvement may also occur. Maxillofacial manifestations of AMC include micrognathia and limited jaw opening[176].

Neuromuscular disorders are probably the most frequent causes.

Chondromatosis

Chondromatosis is a benign proliferation of cartilage-like structures from the synovial membrane. The cartilage-like structures may become detached and enter the joint space as loose bodies.

The knee and elbow are the most commonly involved sites. Chondromatosis or osteochondromatosis of the TMJ is a rather rare phenomenon[73, 145, 198, 350, 406, 503, 592]. The condition is usually mono-articular and occurs mainly in middle-aged women.

Swelling, complaints of pain and also trismus may occur. Clinically, the condition may be confused with an anomaly of the parotid gland[574].

Radiologically, the joint space is widened. Cartilagenous bodies, which may undergo partial calcification and ossification, are not always visible on the radiograph and may be encountered as an incidental finding during a surgical procedure on a painful joint.

A good clinical result can be obtained by removal of all particles and by synovectomy. Condylectomy is seldom required.

Condylar changes in systemic disease

The complete resorption of the mandibular condyle in progressive systemic sclerosis has been reported (See also p. 249).

Cysts and neoplasms

The occurrence of cysts or neoplasms in the TMJ is rare. The literature describes a synovial cyst of the TMJ that appeared clinically as a tumor of the parotid gland[294]. We have had a similar experience with an odontogenic keratocyst in the ascending ramus of the mandible, extending into the condyle.

There have been reports of an osteosarcoma[6], an osteochondroma[64, 195, 338], an osteoblastoma[607], a chondroblastoma[546], a chondrosarcoma[407], a non-osteogenic fibroma[22], and an eosinophilic granuloma[426, 569]. Although even more rare than the occurrence of primary tumors, a metastatic process occurring in the condyle has been mentioned in a number of reports[143, 261, 425].

Hyperplasia of the condyles
(Bifid mandibular condyle)

Unilateral hyperplasia of the mandibular condyles is quite uncommon. It is a benign enlargement that sometimes results in a doubling of the condyles, giving the impression of a bifid condyle[42, 236, 340]. A few cases of bilateral bifid condyles have been reported[364].

A preceding trauma or an inflammatory process is possibly the cause. The lesion is occasionally accompanied by pain. Serious occlusal disturbance may arise. Hearing loss has been described due to obstruction of the external auditory meatus[519].

Treatment may consist of resection of the involved condyle. Also various types of osteotomies have been performed to correct jaw deformities[285].

Hypoplasia of the condyles

Hypoplasia of the mandibular condyles may be either congenital or acquired[55]. Causes that may lead to the acquired type are, e.g. delivery by forceps at birth, trauma, or irradiation in the TMJ region. Odontogenic infections may also play a role in the etiology of hypoplasia of the condyles. Depending on the extent of hypoplasia, the growth disturbance of the homolateral part of the mandible will lead to a more or less serious deformity of the face. The older the patient is at the time of the growth disturbance, the smaller the deformity of the face will be.

The growth center in the condyle cannot be stimulated. In some cases a cosmetically acceptable result may be obtained by means of an osteotomy. An unusual case of spontaneous regeneration of an unilaterally absent mandibular condyle has been reported[308].

Hyperplasia of the coronoid process

Enlargement of the coronoid process is uncommon, and may be unilateral or bilateral[219, 246].

The etiology is not clear. Trauma may play a role, as it does with disorders of the condyles. Two cases of bilateral symmetrical hyperplasia of the coronoid processes in sisters have been described, suggesting a hereditary etiology[649]. The abnormality occurs predominantly in males, and is characterized by progressive, asymptomatic limitation of mandibular movements[525].

An osteoma of the coronoid process has also been described as a cause of enlargement[419].

Treatment consists of surgical correction. This can usually be carried out intraorally.

Pain dysfunction syndrome
(arthrosis deformans; osteoarthrosis)

Terminology — Disorders in the TMJ may cause symptoms such as tenderness, pain, clicking sounds (crepitus) on moving the mandible, trismus, and even complete immobility of the mandible. In the past various terms have been used for this condition, such as arthrosis deformans and osteoarthrosis. At present, much attention is being paid to a possible incorrect position of the disc, also referred to as internal derangement. Three groups are currently recognized: normal disc position, anterior displacement with reduction, and anterior displacement without reduction. In anterior displacement with reduction there is normalization of the disc position during opening. In anterior displacement without reduction, also referred to as closed lock, the disc lies in the displaced position during all mandibular movements.

Epidemiology — The pain dysfunction syndrome is more common in women than in men, which probably indicates that women pay more attention to oral health than men. In a group of 367 patients, joint dysfunction was observed mostly in the 20-30 years age group[416].

Etiology — The cause of the symptoms may be a neuromuscular dysfunction as a result of occlusal disturbances of the dentition, trauma, prolonged dental treatment, or such habits as continual grinding of the teeth at night, also referred to as bruxism. Stress also seems to play a role in the pain dysfunction syndrome. Some cases have been reported of the simultaneous occurrence of arthritis of the TMJ and psoriasis[455]. Uncommon causes of TMJ-symptoms are calcium pyrophosphate dihydrate (CPPD) arthropathy[594], tuberculous osteoarthritis[571], sarcoid arthritis[505], gonococcal arthritis[116] and rheumatoid arthritis[16].

Fig. 13-1.
Radiographic aspect of arthrosis deformans.

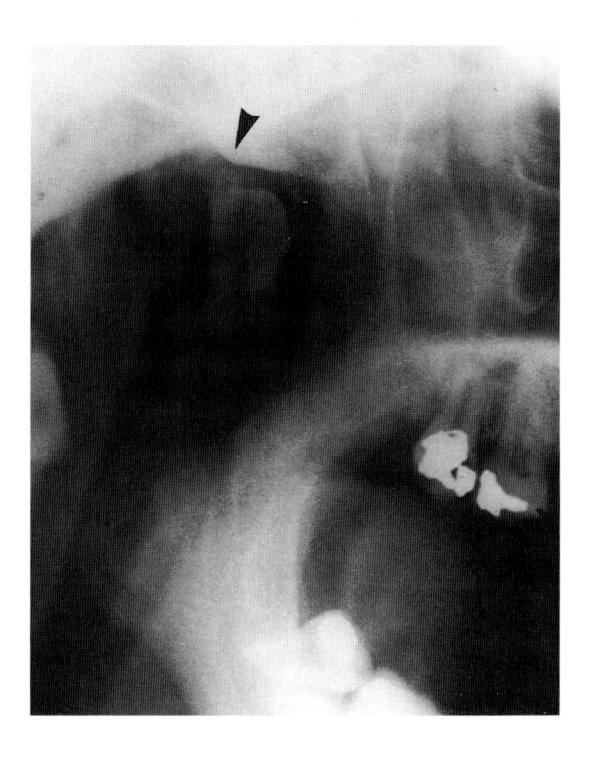

Clinical aspects   Patients sometimes complain of the jaws being locked, especially on waking up in the morning. When pain appears - often experienced by the patient as an earache - it may be local pain, but the pain may also radiate to the forehead, the temporal bone, the occipital area, or the neck. The pain is usually most intense at the end of the day. Some patients complain of a "tired" or dull feeling in the TMJ, while others refer to a sharp pain. In many cases there is also tenderness of the masticatory muscles. Furthermore, the pain can be experienced in other regions, even in the suprahyoid region.

Radiographic aspects   On radiographic examination changes of the TMJ can be observed only in long-existing and severe cases of osteoarthrosis of the condyle (Fig. 13-1). A radiologic grading system has been proposed by Rohlin and Petersson, based on lateral and anteroposterior tomography, and panoramic radiographs[476]. Although that system was designed for patients with rheumatoid arthritis, it seems a useful one for other causes of temporomandibular joint conditions, including osteoarthrosis.

Staging   Based on clinical, radiologic and surgical findings of 740 joints, Wil-

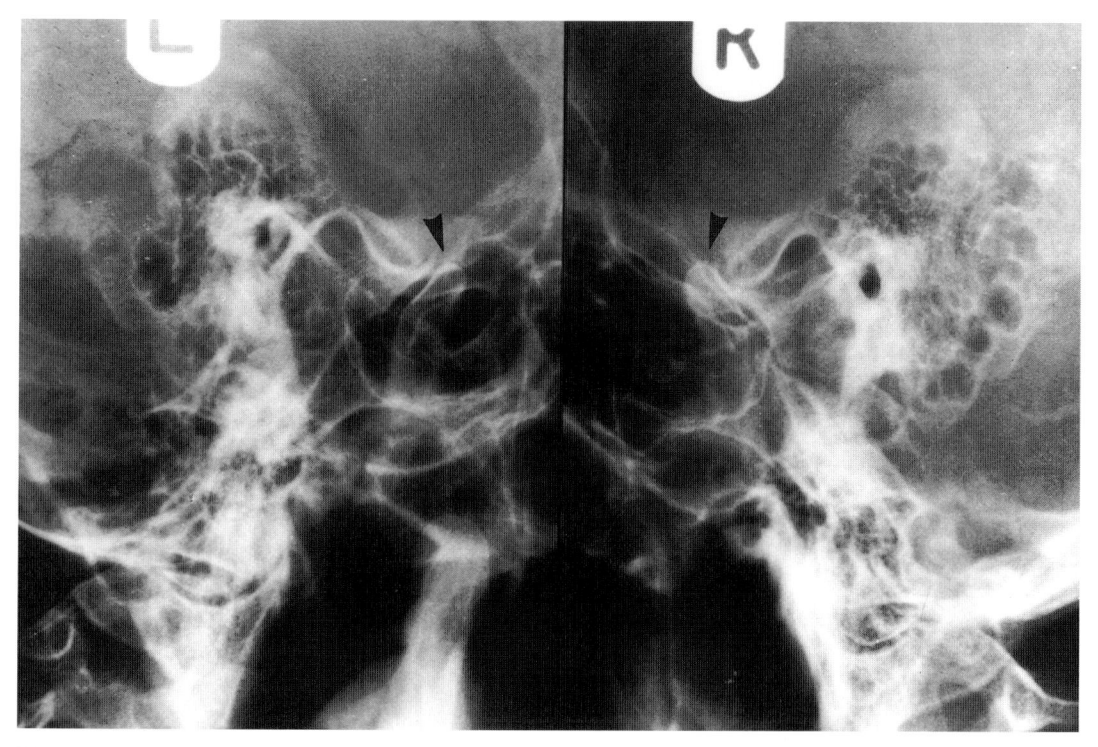

Fig. 13-2. Bilateral (sub)luxation of the condyles. This patient was in fact able to close the mandible normally.

kes[613] has proposed staging criteria for internal derangements. A distinction was made between five stages: early, early/intermediate, intermediate, intermediate/late and late stage.

Histologic aspects

Histological examination of 52 surgically removed condyles in patients who failed to respond to conservative management of their temporomandibular joint problem showed inflammatory changes only in rare instances[472]. Furthermore, the proliferative, intermediate and cartilage zones were frequently absent either partly or completely in older subjects. A semi-quantitative study of the condyles in jaw dysfunction has been reported by Slootweg and de Wilde[538]. The literature also contains a report of the macroscopic and microscopic appearance of radiologic findings in temporomandibular joints from elderly individuals[17].

In a study of 17 surgically removed discs chondrocytes, a surface layer of proliferative connective tissue, vessels, and splitting were seen, all being features that were not observed in normal specimens[322].

Treatment   Treatment is primarily aimed at improving the occlusion of the dentition. Various registration methods can be applied to determine the ideal position of the mandible in relation to the maxilla. Several types of soft and hard splints can be used. Physiotherapy and muscle relaxants may be of additional help. Some clinicians administer local anesthetics in the joint space, followed by muscle exercises. In the past, the successful use of intermaxillary fixation for some weeks has also been reported[416]. Surgical treatment is only indicated in severe and persistent cases. In the past the articular disc was removed, but in spite of some reported good long-term results[579] this is rarely done now. At present, much attention is being given to the surgical repositioning of the articular disc and the repair of possible perforations in the disc or the posterior attachment. Probably, internal derangement is a frequent cause of such perforations[79]. Eminectomy may be part of the surgical procedure.

Also the condylar head or only its surface can be removed, the latter procedure being referred to as a condylar shave. Some practitioners have tried to relieve TMJ pain by intersecting the auriculotemporal nerve. In the past, corticosteroids were injected into the articular spaces. Although at first the symptoms appear to be relieved, over time the results usually are disappointing. Likewise, meniscal and glenoid fossa implants are rarely used nowadays.

(Sub)luxation

Luxations of the TMJ are in many cases simply subluxations. The patient is able to return the mandible to the normal position (Fig. 13-2). A true luxation exists if the patient is not able to return the mandible to its correct position and requires help from a doctor or dentist.

To manually reposition the mandible one should first exert a downward pressure on the mandible and then a dorsal one. This dorsal movement usually takes place spontaneously. Administering a sedative may reduce muscle spasms and thereby facilitate the repositioning procedure or even bring about a spontaneous repositioning. If a patient has recurrent, true luxations of the TMJ, surgical intervention is indicated. Techniques vary from increasing the articular eminence of the temporal bone in order to reduce the mobility of the condyle, to techniques that remove the articular eminence, thus allowing the condyle to easily move forward and backward.

Trismus

Limited ability to open the mouth is called trismus. Unfortunately, no strict criteria can be given for the normal mouth opening, due to individual differences. The maximum can be scored by measuring the distance between the central incisors of the mandible and the maxilla or, in case of an edentulous patient, the distance in the midline between the alveolar ridges of the mandible and the maxilla.

Trismus may be caused by various disorders, e.g., by neuromuscular disturbances as part of the pain dysfunction syndrome, by ankylosis of the joint, by an enlargement of the coronoid process, or by arthritis. A rare cause of trismus is myositis ossificans of the masseter muscle. After the removal of a third molar from the mandible, transient trismus is rather common, usually lasting only a couple of days or a week but in exceptional cases for up to a few months. Occasionally, a benign or malignant disease in or in the vicinity of the TMJ appears to be the cause[581].

Treatment consists of elimination of the cause and includes physiotherapy to improve the condition. Forceful opening of the mouth under general anesthesia seldom if ever leads to a good result. Further discussion of treatment is beyond the scope of this book.

References

1. Abbas F, Bras J. Intra-osseous salivary gland inclusion of the mandible. *Int J Oral Maxillofac Surg* 1985; 14: 560-3.
2. Abdin HA, Prabhu SR. Leiomyosarcoma of mandible in a Sudanese female. *Int J Oral Maxillofac Surg* 1985; 14: 85-8.
3. Abdul-Karim FW, Ayala AG, Chawla SP, et al. Malignant fibrous histiocytoma of Jaws. *Cancer* 1985; 56: 1590-6.
4. Abiose BO, Ajagbe HA, Thomas O. Fibromyxomas of the jawbones - a study of ten cases. *Br J Oral Maxillofac Surg* 1987; 25: 415-21.
5. Abrams AM, Kirby JW, Melrose RJ. Cementoblastoma; a clinical-pathologic study of seven new cases. *Oral Surg, Oral Med, Oral Pathol* 1974; 38: 394-403.
6. Abubaker AO, Braun TW, Sotereanos GC, et al. Osteosarcoma of the mandibular condyle. *J Oral Maxillofac Surg* 1986; 44: 126-31.
7. Ackermann G, Cohen MA, Altini M. The paradental cyst: A clinicopathologic study of 50 cases. *Oral Surg, Oral Med, Oral Pathol* 1987; 64: 308-12.
8. Adekeye EO. Ankylosis of the mandible: analysis of 76 cases. *J Oral Maxillofac Surg* 1983; 41: 442-9.
9. Adekeye EO, Cornah J. Osteomyelitis of the jaws: a review of 141 cases. *Br J Oral Maxillofac Surg* 1985; 23: 24-35.
10. Adekeye EO, Edwards MB, Goubran GF. Fibro-osseous lesions of the skull, face and jaws in Kaduna, Nigeria. *Br J Oral Maxillofac Surg* 1980; 18: 57-72.
11. Aderhold L. Die lokale Behandlung von Knocheninfektionen mit der Gentamicin-PMMA-Minikette in der Kiefer- und Gesichtschirurgie. Eine klinische und pharmakokinetische Studie. *Dtsch Z Mund-Kiefer-Gesichts Chir* 1985; 9: 94-101.
12. Adler CP. Tumour-like lesions in the femur with cementum-like material. Does a 'cementoma' of long bone exist? *Skeletal Radiol* 1985; 14: 26-37.
13. Ahlfors E, Larsson A, Sjögren S. The odontogenic keratocyst: a benign cystic tumor? *J Oral Maxillofac Surg* 1984; 42: 10-9.
14. Aitasalo K, Neva M. Morphometry of orthopantomographic mandibular bone changes during radiotherapy. *Acta Radiologica Diagnosis* 1985; 26: 551-6.
15. Ajagbe HA, Daramola JO, Junaid TA. Chondrosarcoma of the jaw; review of fourteen cases. *J Oral Maxillofac Surg* 1985; 43: 763-6.
16. Akerman S, Kopp S, Nilner M, et al. Relationship between clinical and radiologic findings of the temporomandibular joint in rheumatoid arthritis. *Oral Surg, Oral Med, Oral Pathol* 1988; 66: 639-43.
17. Akerman S, Kopp S, Rohlin M. Macroscopic and microscopic appearance of radiologic findings in temporomandibular joints from elderly individuals. An autopsy study. *Int J Oral Maxillofac Surg* 1988; 17: 58-63.
18. Akinwande J, Odukoya O, Nwoku AL, et al. Burkitt's lymphoma of the jaws in Lagos. Ten-year review. *J Maxillofac Surg* 1986; 14: 323-8.
19. Akker van den HP, Kuiper L, Peeters FLM. Embolization of an arteriovenous malformation of the mandible. *J Oral Maxillofac Surg* 1987; 45: 255-60.
20. Alattar MM, Baughman RA, Collet WK. A survey of panoramic radiographs for evaluation of normal and pathologic findings. *Oral Surg, Oral Med, Oral Pathol* 1980; 50: 472-8.
21. Aldred MJ, Cooke BED. Paget's disease of bone with involvement of the dental pulp. *J Oral Pathol Med* 1989; 18: 184-5.
22. Aldred MJ, Breckon JJW, Holland CS. Non-osteogenic fibroma of the mandibular condyle. *Br J Oral Maxillofac Surg* 1989; 27: 412-7.
23. Ali A, Campbell HD. Central cavernous haemangioma of an edentulous maxilla. *Br J Oral Maxillofac Surg* 1983; 21: 63-8.
24. Allard RHB. Nasolabial cyst. Review of the literature and report of 7 cases. *Int J Oral Maxillofac Surg* 1982; 11: 351-9.

25. Altini M, Peters E, White B, et al. Botryomycosis of the oral regions. *J Oral Pathol* 1986; 15: 297-9.

26. Altini M, Thompson SH, Lownie JF, et al. Ameloblastic sarcoma of the mandible. *J Oral Maxillofac Surg* 1985; 43: 789-94.

27. Altshuler L, Sclaroff A, Eppley B. Total mandibular replacement in a patient with Hand-Schüller-Christian Disease. *J Oral Maxillofac Surg* 1985; 43: 966-71.

28. Amarjit S, Bhardwaj DN, Nagpal BL. Intraosseous liposarcoma of the maxilla and mandible: report of two cases. *J Oral Maxillofac Surg* 1979; 37: 593-6.

29. Anavi Y, Herman GE, Graybill S, et al. Malignant fibrous histiocytoma of the mandible. *Oral Surg, Oral Med, Oral Pathol* 1989; 68: 436-43.

30. Anderson JH, Grisius RJ, McKean TW. Arteriovenous malformation of the mandible. *Oral Surg, Oral Med, Oral Pathol* 1981; 52: 118-25.

31. Anker AH, Radden BG. Dentinoma of the mandible. *Oral Surg, Oral Med, Oral Pathol* 1989; 67: 731-3.

32. Anneroth G, Hall G, Stuge U. Nasopalatine duct cyst. *Int J Oral Maxillofac Surg* 1986; 15: 572-80.

33. Anneroth G, Johansson B. Peripheral ameloblastoma. *Int J Oral Maxillofac Surg* 1985; 14: 295-9.

34. Anonsen CK, Donaldson SS. Langerhans' cell histiocytosis of the head and neck. *Laryngoscope* 1987; 97: 537-42.

35. Antalovska Z, Bartakova V, Chylkova V, et al. Ergebnisse der unspezifischen Immunotherapie bei den sklerotisierenden Kieferosteomyelitiden. *Dtsch Z Zahn-Mund-Kieferheilkd* 1983; 71: 810-9.

36. Antoine P, Raphael B, Bachelot H, et al. Neuroblastome primitif de la mandibule. A propos d'un cas. *Rev Stomatol Chir maxillofac* 1984; 85: 314-9.

37. Antoniades K, Eleftheriades I, Karakasis D. The Gardner syndrome. *Int J Oral Maxillofac Surg* 1987; 16: 480-3.

38. Atkinson CH, Harwood AR, Cummings BJ. Ameloblastoma of the jaw. A reappraisal of the role of megavoltage irradiation. *Cancer* 1984; 53: 869-73.

39. Auclair PL, Cuenin P, Kratochvil FJ, et al. A clinical and histomorphologic comparison of the central giant cell granuloma and the central giant cell tumor. *Oral Surg, Oral Med, Oral Pathol* 1988; 66: 197-208.

40. Awang MN. The aetiology of dry socket: a review. *Int Dent J* 1989; 39: 236-40.

41. Bacchini P, Marchetti C, Mancini L, et al. Ewing's sarcoma of the mandible and maxilla. *Oral Surg, Oral Med, Oral Pathol* 1986; 61: 278-83.

42. Balciunas BA. Bifid mandibular condyle. *J Oral Maxillofac Surg* 1986; 44: 324-5.

43. Bang G, Baardsen R, Gilhuus-Moe O. Infantile fibrosarcoma in the mandible: case report. *J Oral Pathol, Med* 1989; 18: 339-43.

44. Bang G, Koppang HS, Hansen LS, et al. Clear cell odontogenic carcinoma: report of three cases with pulmonary and lymphnode metastases. *J Oral Pathol, Med* 1989; 18: 113-8.

45. Barrett AP, Waters BE, Griffiths CJ. A critical evaluation of panoramic radiography as a screening procedure in dental practice. *Oral Surg, Oral Med, Oral Pathol* 1984; 57: 673-7.

46. Barsekow F, Kameke von A. Zur Differentialdiagnose und Therapie der aneurysmatischen Knochenzysten. *Dtsch Z Mund-Kiefer-Gesichts Chir* 1984; 8: 211-3.

47. Batsakis JG. *Tumors of the Head and Neck*, 2nd edn. The Williams and Wilkins Company, Baltimore. 1979.

48. Batsakis JG, Raymond AK. Chondromyxoid fibroma. *Ann Otol Rhinol Laryngol* 1989; 98: 571-2.

49. Bauer HCF, Kreicsbergs A, Silfersward C, et al. DNA analysis in the differential diagnosis of osteosarcoma. *Cancer* 1988; 61: 1430-6.

50. Bays RA. The influence of systemic bone disease on bone resorption following mandibular augmentation. *Oral Surg, Oral Med, Oral Pathol* 1983; 55: 223-31.

51. Bays RA, Weinstein RS. Systemic bone disease in patients with mandibular atrophy. *J Oral Maxillofac Surg* 1982; 40: 270-2.

52. Becker S und Härle F. Die latente Knochenhöhle, ein Fall seltener Lokalisation. *Dtsch Z Mund-Kiefer-Gesichts Chir* 1986; 10: 60-1.

53. Belfiglio EJ, Wonderlich ST, Fox LJ. Myospherulosis of the alveolus secondary to the use of Terra-cortril and Gelfoam. *Oral Surg, Oral Med, Oral Pathol* 1986; 61: 12-4.

54. Benca PG, Mostofi R, Kuo PC. Proliferative periostitis (Garré's osteomyelitis). *Oral Surg, Oral Med, Oral Pathol* 1987; 63: 258-60.

55. Berger SS, Stewart RE. Mandibular hypoplasia secondary to perinatal trauma: report of case. *J Oral Maxillofac Surg* 1977; 35: 578-82.

56. Bergh van den JPA, Waal van der I. Ewing's sarcoma of the mandible: Report of a case. *J Oral Maxillofac Surg* 1988; 46: 798-800.

57. Bernstein ML, Miller RL, Steiner M. The differentiation of malignant lymphoma from anaplastic seminoma in a patient presenting with testicular and jaw swelling. *Oral Surg, Oral Med, Oral Pathol* 1983; 56: 378-87.

58. Bersch W, Foitzik Ch, Neuner M. Zur Differentialdiagnose myxoid-fibromatöser Gewebe der Kieferknochen bei Kindern und Jugendlichen. *Dtsch Z Mund-Kiefer-Gesichts Chir* 1988; 12: 110-2.

59. Bersch W, Scheunemann H, Müntefering H, et al. Desmoplastisches Fibrom im Bereich der Mandibula. Ein kasuistischer Beitrag. *Dtsch Z Mund-Kiefer-Gesichts Chir* 1986; 10: 257-63.

60. Berthold H, Burkhardt A, Läng H. Einfache (solitäre) Knochenzysten im Kieferbereich. *Dtsch Z Mund-Kiefer-Gesichts Chir* 1987; 11: 278-87.

61. Bertoni F, Present D, Marchetti C, et al. Desmoplastic fibroma of the jaw: the experience of the Istituto Beretta. *Oral Surg, Oral Med, Oral Pathol* 1986; 61: 179-84.

62. Bertoni F, Unni KK, Beabout JW, et al. Chondroblastoma of the skull and facial bones. *Am J Clin Pathol* 1987; 88: 1-9.

63. Bertoni F, Unni KK, McLeod RA. Xanthoma of bone. *Am J Clin Pathol* 1988; 90: 377-84.

64. Bessho K, Murakami K-I, Iizuka T, et al. Osteoma in mandibular condyle. *Int J Oral Maxillofac Surg* 1987; 16: 372-5.

65. Beumer J, Harrison R, Sanders B, et al. Osteoradionecrosis: predisposing factors and outcomes of therapy. *Head & Neck Surgery* 1984; 6: 819-27.

66. Beyer D, Herzog M, Zanella FE, et al. *Röntgendiagnostik von Zahn- und Kiefererkrankungen.* Springer Verlag, Berlin. 1987.

67. Bibb CA, Pullinger AG, Baldioceda F, et al. Temporomandibular joint comparative imaging: Diagnostic efficacy of arthroscopy compared to tomography and arthrography. *Oral Surg, Oral Med, Oral Pathol* 1989; 68: 352-9.

68. Blank RP, Diehl HA, Ballard GT, et al. Calcium metabolism and osteoporotic ridge resorption: a protein connection. *J Prosthet Dent* 1987; 58: 590-5.

69. Blankestijn J, Panders AK, Wymenga JPH. Ameloblastic fibroma of the mandible. *Br J Oral Maxillofac Surg* 1986; 24: 417-21.

70. Blarcom van CW, Masson JK, Dahlin DC. Fibrosarcoma of the mandible. A clinicopathologic study. *Oral Surg, Oral Med, Oral Pathol* 1971; 32: 428-39.

71. Block MS, Cade JE, Rodriguez FH. Malignant fibrous histiocytoma in the maxilla: review of the literature and report of a case. *J Oral Maxillofac Surg* 1986; 44: 402-12.

72. Block MS, Zide MF, Kent JW. Excision of sclerosing osteomyelitis and reconstruction with particulate hydroxylapatite. *J Oral Maxillofac Surg* 1986; 44: 244-6.

73. Bont de LGM, Liem RSB, Boering G. Synovial chondromatosis of the temporomandibular joint: a light and electron microscopic study. *Oral Surg, Oral Med, Oral Pathol* 1988; 66: 593-8.

74. Bosshardt LL, Wash Y, Gordon RC, et al. Recurrent peripheral osteoma of the mandible. *J Oral Maxillofac Surg* 1971; 29: 446-50.

75. Bouwsma C, Go G, Panders AK, et al. Massive osteolysis of the skull and its therapeutic implications; a case report. *J Neurol, Neurosurg, and Psychiatry* 1989; 52: 279-81.

76. Bradley N, Thomas DM, Antoniades K, et al. Squamous cell carcinoma arising in an odontogenic cyst. *Int J Oral Maxillofac Surg* 1985; 17: 260-3.

77. Brady FA, Roser SM, Sapp JPh. Osteomyelitis of the mandible as a complicating factor in Paget's disease of bone. *Br J Oral Maxillofac Surg* 1979; 17: 33-42.

78. Brady FA, Sapp JPh, Christensen RE. Extracondylar osteochondromas of the jaws. *Oral Surg, Oral Med, Oral Pathol* 1978; 46: 658-68.

79. Brand JW, Whinery JG, Anderson QN, et al. The effects of temporomandibular joint internal derangement and degenerative joint disease on tomographic and arthrotomographic images. *Oral Surg, Oral Med, Oral Pathol* 1989; 67: 220-3.

80. Brannon RB. The odontogenic keratocyst. A clinicopathologic study of 312 cases. Part I. Clinical features. *Oral Surg, Oral Med, Oral Pathol* 1976; 42: 54-72.

81. Brannon RB. The odontogenic keratocyst. A clinicopathologic study of 312 cases. Part II. Histologic features. *Oral Surg, Oral Med, Oral Pathol* 1977; 43: 233-55.

82. Bras J, Donner R, van der Kwast WAM, et al. Juxtacortical osteogenic sarcoma of the jaws. Review of the literature and report of a case. *Oral Surg, Oral Med, Oral Pathol* 1980; 50: 535-44.

83. Bras J, van Ooy CP, Abraham-Inpijn L, et al. Radiographic interpretation of the mandibular angular cortex: a diagnostic tool in metabolic bone loss. Part II. Renal osteodystrophy. *Oral Surg, Oral Med, Oral Pathol* 1982; 53: 647-50.

84. Bras J, van Ooy CP, van den Akker HP. Mandibular atrophy and metabolic bone loss. *Int J Oral Maxillofac Surg* 1985; 14: 16-21.

85. Bras J, van Ooy CP, Duns JY, et al. Mandibular atrophy and metabolic bone loss. A radiologic analysis of 126 edentulous patients. *Int J Oral Maxillofac Surg* 1983; 12: 309-13.

86. Braunwald E, Isselbacher KJ, Petersdorf RG, et al. (eds.): *Harrison's principles of internal medicine*, 11th edn, vol.I. McGraw Hill Book Company, New York-Toronto. 1987.

87. Brecht K, Johnson CM. Complete mandibular agenesis. Report of a case. *Arch Otolaryngol* 1985; 111: 132-4.

88. Bredenkamp JK, Zimmerman MC, Mickel RA. Maxillary ameloblastoma. A potentially lethal neoplasm. *Arch Otolaryngol Head Neck Surg* 1989; 115: 99-104.

89. Brenner BM, Rector RC. *The Kidney*, vol. II, pp. 2213-69. W.B. Saunders, Philadelphia. 1981.

90. Brocheriou C, Payen J. Tumeurs cartilagineuses des maxillaires. A propos de 11 observations. *Ann Anat Pathol (Paris)* 1975; 20: 23-4.

91. Brook AH, Bedi R, Chan Lui WY, et al. Haemophilic pseudotumours of the mandible: report of a case in a one-year-old child. *Br J Oral Maxillofac Surg* 1985; 23: 47-52.

92. Brown AMS, Bell RAF. Osteomyelitis of the mandible in metastatic staphylococcal infection. *Br J Oral Maxillofac Surg* 1987; 25: 334-40.

93. Brown OE, Finn R. Mucormycosis of the mandible. *J Oral Maxillofac Surg* 1986; 44: 132-6.

94. Burg J, Landat F, Ducours JL. Chémodectome; a propos d'un cas situé sur le trajet du nerf dentaire inferieur. *Rev Stomatol Chir maxillofac* 1985; 86: 46-8.

95. Buchner A, Hansen LS. The histomorphologic spectrum of the gingival cyst in the adult. *Oral Surg, Oral Med, Oral Pathol* 1979; 48: 532-9.

96. Burkes EJ, Kelly DE. Primary mandibular neuroblastoma. *J Oral Maxillofac Surg* 1980; 38: 128-31.

97. Burkhardt A. Klassifizierung von fibromatösen Kieferläsionen mit Hartgewebsbildung - Neue Aspekte. *Dtsch Z Mund-Kiefer-Gesichts Chir* 1986; 10: 225-30.

98. Burkhardt A. Dentin formation in so-called "fibro-osteo-cemental" lesions of the jaw: Histologic, electron microscopic, and immunohistochemical investigations. *Oral Surg, Oral Med, Oral Pathol* 1989; 68: 729-38.

99. Burkhardt A, Berthold H. Cherubismus. Klinische und morphologische Beobachtungen. *Dtsch Z Mund-Kiefer-Gesichts Chir* 1986; 10: 257-63.

100. Cale AE, Freedman PD, Kerpel SM, et al. Benign fibrous histiocytoma of the maxilla. *Oral Surg, Oral Med, Oral Pathol* 1989; 68: 444-50.

101. Camarda AJ, Pham J, Forest D. Mandibular infected buccal cyst: report of two cases. *J Oral Maxillofac Surg* 1989; 47: 528-34.

102. Campbell AM, Rennie JS, Moos KF, et al. Neuroblastoma presenting as mandibular swelling in a two-year-old girl. A short case report. *Br J Oral Maxillofac Surg* 1987; 25: 422-6.

103. Campbell RL, Alexander JM. Temporomandibular joint arthrography: negative pressure, nontomographic techniques. *Oral Surg, Oral Med, Oral Pathol* 1983; 55: 121-6.

104. Cannon JS, Keller EE, Dahlin DC. Gigantiform cementoma: report of two cases (mother and son). *J Oral Maxillofac Surg* 1980; 38: 65-70.

105. Cannon ML, Cooley RO, Gonzalez-Crussi F, et al. Oral manifestations of malignant histiocytosis (histiocytic medullary reticulosis). *Oral Surg, Oral Med, Oral Pathol* 1982; 54: 180-6.

106. Chan CW, Kung TM, Ma L. Teleangiectatic osteosarcoma of the mandible. *Cancer* 1986; 58: 2110-5.

107. Chapman PJ, Romaniuk K. Traumatic bone cyst of the mandible; regression following aspiration. *Int J Oral Maxillofac Surg* 1985; 14: 290-4.

108. Chen CY, Ohba T. An analysis of radiological findings of Stafne's idiopathic bone cavity. *Dentomaxillofac Radiol* 1981; 10: 18-23.

109. Chin DC. Treatment of maxillary hemangioma with a sclerosing agent. *Oral Surg, Oral Med, Oral Pathol* 1983; 55: 247-9.

110. Chomette G, Auriol M, Guilbert F. Cherubism; histo-enzymological and ultrastructural study. *Int J Oral Maxillofac Surg* 1988; 17: 219-23.

111. Chomette G, Auriol M, Princ G, et al. Le leiomyosarcome osseux; étude ultrastructurale et histoenzymologique. A propos d'un cas de siège mandibulaire. *Sem Hop Paris* 1984; 60: 2379-84.

112. Chou L, Hansen LS. Ganglioneuroma of the mandible. *Oral Surg, Oral Med, Oral Pathol* 1989; 68: 201-5.

113. Christensen RE. Mesenchymal chondrosarcoma of the jaws. *Oral Surg, Oral Med, Oral Pathol* 1982; 54: 197-206.

114. Christensen RE, Propper RH. Intraosseous mandibular cyst with sebaceous differentiation. *Oral Surg, Oral Med, Oral Pathol* 1982; 53: 591-5.

115. Christensen RE, Sanders B, Mudd B. Local recurrence of solitary plasmacytoma of the mandible. *J Oral Maxillofac Surg* 1978; 36: 311-3.

116. Chue PWY. Gonococcal arthritis of the temporomandibular joint. *Oral Surg, Oral Med, Oral Pathol* 1975; 39: 572-7.

117. Chuong R, Kaban LB. Diagnosis and treatment of jaw tumors in children. *J Oral Maxillofac Surg* 43: 1985; 323-32.

118. Chuong R, Kaban LB, Kozakewich H, et al. Central giant cell lesions of the jaws: a clinicopathologic study. *J Oral Maxillofac Surg* 1986; 44: 708-13.

119. Clark JL, Unni KK, Dahlin DC, et al. Osteosarcoma of the jaw. *Cancer* 1983; 51: 2311-6.

120. Clausen F, Poulsen H. Metastatic carcinoma to the jaws. *Acta Pathol Microbiol Scand* 1963; 57: 361-74.

121. Close LG, Merkel M, Burns DK, et al. Computed tomography in the assessment of mandibular invasion by intraoral carcinoma. *Ann Otol Rhinol Laryngol* 1986; 95: 383-8.

122. Cohen M, Zornoza J, Cangir A, et al. Direct injection of methylprednisolone sodium succinate in the treatment of solitary eosinophilic granuloma of bone. A report of 9 cases. *Radiology* 1980; 136: 289-93.

123. Cohen MA, Grossman ES, Thompson SH. Features of central giant cell granuloma of the jaws xenografted in nude mice. *Oral Surg, Oral Med, Oral Pathol* 1988; 66: 209-17.

124. Colm SJ, Abrams MB, Waldron CA. Recurrent osteoblastoma of the mandible: report of a case. *J Oral Maxillofac Surg* 1988; 46: 881-5.

125. Corio RJ, Crawford BE, Schaberg SJ. Benign cementoblastoma. *Oral Surg, Oral Med, Oral Pathol* 1976; 41: 524-30.

126. Corio RL, Goldblatt LI, Edwards PA. Paraoral cartilage analogue of fibromatosis. *Oral Surg, Oral Med, Oral Pathol* 1981; 52: 56-60.

127. Corio RL, Goldblatt LI, Edwards PA, et al. Ameloblastic carcinoma: a clinicopathologic study and assessment of eight cases. *Oral Surg, Oral Med, Oral Pathol* 1987; 64: 570-6.

128. Correl RW, Jensen JL, Rhyne RR. Lingual cortical mandibular defects. *Oral Surg, Oral Med, Oral Pathol* 1980; 50: 287-91.

129. Coulon JP, Lechien P, Reychler H. Revue de la littérature recente à propos d'un cas de lymphome de Burkitt a localisation maxillo-faciale. *Rev Stomatol Chir Maxillofac* 1986; 87: 201-11.

130. Courtney RM, Kerr DA. The odontogenic adenomatoid tumor; a comprehensive study of twenty new cases. *Oral Surg, Oral Med, Oral Pathol* 1975; 39: 424-35.

131. Craig GT. The paradental cyst. *A specific inflammatory cyst. Br Dent J* 1976; 141: 9-14.

132. Craig GT, Holland CS, Hindle MO. Dermoid cyst of the mandible. *Br J Oral Maxillofac Surg* 1980; 18: 230-7.

133. Crockett DM, Stanley RB, Lubba R. Osteomyelitis of the maxilla in a patient with osteopetrosis. *Otolaryngol Head Neck Surg* 1986; 95: 117-21.

134. Curtis AB. Childhood leukemias; osseous changes in jaws on panoramic dental radiographs. *J Am Dent Assoc* 1971; 83: 844-7.

135. Cutler LS, Chaudry AP, Topazian R. Melanotic neuroectodermal tumor of infancy: an ultrastructural study, literature review and reevaluation. *Cancer* 1981; 48: 257-70.

136. Dabska M, Huvos AG. Mesenchymal chondrosarcoma in the young. A clinicopathologic study of 19 patients with explanation of histogenesis. *Virchows Arch (Pathol Anat)* 1983; 399: 89-104.

137. Dahl I, Akerman M, Angervall L. Ewing's sarcoma of bone. A correlative cytological and histological study of 14 cases. *Acta Path Microbiol Immunol Scand Sect A* 1986; 94: 363-9.

138. Dahlin DC. *Bone tumors: general aspects and data on 6221 cases*, 3rd edn., pp. 274-87. Charles C. Thomas, Springfield, Ill. 1978.

139. Dahlin DC, Unni KK, Matsuno T. Malignant (fibrous) histocytoma of bone; fact or fancy? *Cancer* 1977; 39: 1508-16.

140. D'Ambrosio JA, Langlais RP, Young RS. Jaw and skull changes in neurofibromatosis. *Oral Surg, Oral Med, Oral Pathol* 1988; 66: 391-6.

141. Daramola JO. Massive osteomyelitis of the mandible complicating sickle cell disease: report of case. *J Oral Maxillofac Surg* 1981; 39: 144-6.

142. Davies HT, Bradley N, Bowerman JE. Oral nodular fasciitis. *Br J Oral Maxillofac Surg* 1989; 27: 147-51.

143. DeBoom GW, Jensen JL, Siegel W, et al. Metastatic tumors of the mandibular condyle. Review of the literature and report of a case. *Oral Surg, Oral Med, Oral Pathol* 1985; 60: 512-6.

144. Demas PN, Sotereanos GC. Facial-skeletal manifestations of Engelmann's disease. *Oral Surg, Oral Med, Oral Pathol* 1989; 68: 686-90.

145. Demeulemeester LJ-MJ, Bossuyt M, Casselman J, et al. Synovial chondromatosis of the temporomandibular joint. *Int J Oral Maxillofac Surg* 1988; 17: 181-2.

146. DePablos PL, Ramos I, De La Calle H. Brown tumor in the palate associated with primary hyperparathyrodism. *J Oral Maxillofac Surg* 1987; 45: 719-20.

147. Difiore PM, Hartwell GR. Median mandibular lateral periodontal cyst. *Oral Surg, Oral Med, Oral Pathol* 1987; 63: 545-50.

148. Diner PA, Brocheriou C, Crépy C, et al. Histiocytose mandibulaire. *Rev Stomatol Chir maxillofac* 1982; 83: 355-9.

149. Dis ML van, Langlais RP. The thalassemias: oral manifestations and complications. *Oral Surg, Oral Med, Oral Pathol* 1986; 62: 229-33.

150. Domarus Von H, Ziegner E, Froster-Iskenius U, et al. Spontane Neumutation als Ursache eines Gardner-Syndroms. *Dtsch Z Mund-Kiefer-Gesichts Chir* 1983; 7: 471-7.

151. Dominguez FV, Keszler A. Comparative study of keratocysts, associated and non-associated with nevoid basal cell carcinoma syndrome. *J Oral Pathol* 1988; 17: 39-42.

152. Donath K. The diagnostic value of the new method for the study of undecalcified bones and teeth with attached soft tissue (Sawing and Grinding Technique). *Path Res Pract* 1985; 179: 631-3.

153. Dorner L, Sear AJ, Smith GT. A case of ameloblastic carcinoma with pulmonary metastases. *Br J Oral Maxillofac Surg* 1988; 26: 503-10.

154. Duncan WK, Post CA, McCoy BP. Eosinophilic granuloma. *Oral Surg, Oral Med, Oral Pathol* 1988; 65: 736-41.

155. Dunlap CL, Barker BF. Giant-cell hyalin angiopathy. *Oral Surg, Oral Med, Oral Pathol* 1977; 44: 587-91.

156. Dunlap CL, Barker BF. Central odontogenic fibroma of the WHO type. *Oral Surg, Oral Med, Oral Pathol* 1987; 57: 390-4.

157. Dunlap CL, Neville B, Vickers RA, et al. The Noonan syndrome/cherubism association. *Oral Surg, Oral Med, Oral Pathol* 1989; 67: 698-705.

158. Dyson DP. Van Buchem's disease (hyperostosis corticalis generalisata familiaris). A case report. *Br J Oral Maxillofac Surg* 1972; 9: 237-45.

159. Eggert JH. Diagnostik und Therapie des multiplen Myeloms -Fallbetreibung mit fünfjähriger Verlaufskontrolle. *Dtsch Zahnärztl Z* 1982; 37: 1007-14.

160. Eggert JH. Vollstandige Unterkieferresorption beim Morbus Schüller-Christian (Histiocytosis-X). *Dtsch Z Mund-Kiefer-Gesichts Chir* 1982; 6: 324-31.

161. Eisenbud L, Attie J, Garlick J, et al. Aneurysmal bone cyst of the mandible. *Oral Surg, Oral Med, Oral Pathol* 1987; 64: 202-6.

162. Eisenbud L, Kahn LB, Friedman E. Benign osteoblastoma of the mandible: fifteen years follow-up showing spontaneous regression after biopsy. *J Oral Maxillofac Surg* 1987; 45: 53-7.

163. Eisenbud L, Sciubba J, Mir R, et al. Oral presentations in non-Hodgkin's lymphoma: a review of thirty-one cases. Part II. Fourteen cases arising in bone. *Oral Surg, Oral Med, Oral Pathol* 1984; 57: 272-80.

164. Eisenbud L, Stern M, Rothberg M, et al. Central giant cell granuloma of the jaws: experiences in the management of thirty-seven cases. *J Oral Maxillofac Surg* 1988; 46: 376-84.

165. Eliasson S, Isacsson G, Köndell PA. Lateral periodontal cysts. Clinical, radiographical and histopathological findings. *Int J Oral Maxillofac Surg* 1989; 18: 191-3.

166. El-Labban NG, Kramer IRH. The nature of the hyaline rings in chronic periostitis and other conditions: an ultrastructural study. *Oral Surg, Oral Med, Oral Pathol* 1981; 51: 509-15.

167. El-Laban NG, Lee KW. Myofibroblasts in central giant cell granuloma of the jaws: an ultrastructural study. *Histopathology* 1983; 7: 907-18.

168. El-Laban NG, Lee KW. Vascular degeneration in adenomatoid odontogenic tumour: an ultrastructural study. *J Oral Pathol* 1988; 17: 298-305.

169. Ellis GL, Abrams AM, Melrose RJ. Intraosseous benign neural sheath neoplasms of the jaws. Report of seven new cases and review of the literature. *Oral Surg, Oral Med, Oral Pathol* 1977; 44: 731-43.

170. Ellis GL, Brannon RB. Intraosseous lymphangioma of the mandible. *Skeletal Radiol* 1980; 5: 253-6.

171. Ellis GL, Kratochvil FJ. Epithelioid hemangioendothelioma of the head and neck: a clinicopathologic report of twelve cases. *Oral Surg, Oral Med, Oral Pathol* 1986; 61: 61-8.

172. El-Mofty S, Refai H. Benign osteoblastoma of the maxilla. *J Oral Maxillofac Surg* 1989; 47: 60-4.

173. Elzay RP, Mills S, Kay S. Fibrous defect (nonossifying fibroma) of the mandible. *Oral Surg, Oral Med, Oral Pathol* 1984; 58: 402-7.

174. Epstein JB, Hatcher DC, Graham M. Bone scintigraphy of fibro-osseous lesions of the jaw. *Oral Surg, Oral Med, Oral Pathol* 1981; 51: 346-50.

175. Epstein JB, Voss NJS, Stevenson-Moore P. Maxillofacial manifestations of multiple myeloma. An unusual case and review of the literature. *Oral Surg, Oral Med, Oral Pathol* 1984; 57: 267-71.

176. Epstein JB, Wittenberg GJ. Maxillofacial manifestations and management of arthrogryposis: literature review and case report. *J Oral Maxillofac Surg* 1987; 45: 274-9.

177. Epstein JB, Wong FLW, Stevenson-Moore P. Osteoradionecrosis: clinical experience and a proposal for classification. *J Oral Maxillofac Surg* 1987; 45: 104-10.

178. Eversole LR, Leider AS, Corwin JO, et al. Proliferative periostitis of Garré: its differentiation from other neoperiostoses. *J Oral Maxillofac Surg* 1979; 37: 725-31.

179. Eversole LR, Leider AS, Nelson K. Ossifying fibroma: a clinicopathologic study of sixty-four cases. *Oral Surg, Oral Med, Oral Pathol* 1985; 60: 505-11.

180. Eversole LR, Leider AS, Strub D. Radiographic characteristics of cystogenic ameloblastoma. *Oral Surg, Oral Med, Oral Pathol* 1984; 57: 572-7.

181. Eversole LR, Merrel PW, Strub D. Radiographic characteristics of central ossifying fibroma. *Oral Surg, Oral Med, Oral Pathol* 1985; 59: 522-7.

182. Eversole LR, Sabes WR, Brandebura J, et al. Medulloblastoma: extradural metastasis to the jaw. *Oral Surg, Oral Med, Oral Pathol* 1972; 34: 634-40.

183. Eversole LR, Stone CE, Strub D. Focal sclerosing osteomyelitis/focal periapical osteopetrosis: Radiographic patterns. *Oral Surg, Oral Med, Oral Pathol* 1984; 58: 456-60.

184. Fantasia JE. Lateral periodontal cyst. An analysis of forty-six cases. *Oral Surg, Oral Med, Oral Pathol* 1979; 48: 237-43.

185. Farman AG, Kay S. Oral leiomyosarcoma. Report of a case and review of the literature pertaining to smooth-muscle tumors of the oral cavity. *Oral Surg, Oral Med, Oral Pathol* 1977; 43: 402-9.

186. Favara BE, McCarthy RC, Mierau GW. Histiocytosis X. *Human Pathol* 1983; 14: 663-76.

187. Feinberg SE, Finkelstein MW, Page HL, et al. Recurrent "traumatic" bone cysts of the mandible. *Oral Surg, Oral Med, Oral Pathol* 1984; 57: 418-22.

188. Ficarra G, Kaban LB, Hansen LS. Central giant cell lesions of the mandible and maxilla: a clinicopathologic and cytometric study. *Oral Surg, Oral Med, Oral Pathol* 1987; 64: 44-9.

189. Ficarra G, Silverman S, Quivey JM, et al. Granulocytic sarcoma (chloroma) of the oral cavity: a case with a leukemic presentation. *Oral Surg, Oral Med, Oral Pathol 1987; 63: 709-14.*

190. Field EA, Nind D. Varga E, et al. The effect of chlorhexidine irrigation on the incidence of dry socket: a pilot study. *Br J Oral Maxillofac Surg* 1988; 26: 395-401.

191. Field EA, Speechley JA, Rotter E, et al. Dry socket incidence compared after a 12 year interval. *Br J Oral Maxillofac Surg* 1985; 23: 419-27.

192. Finn DG, Goepfert H, Batsakis JG. Chondrosarcoma of the head and neck. *Laryngoscope* 1984; 94: 1539-44.

193. Fleiner B, Schluter E. Das maligne fibröse Histiozytom der Kiefer-Gesichtsregion. *Dtsch Z Mund-Kiefer-Gesichts Chir* 1988; 12: 83-96.

194. Florine BL, Simonton SC, Sane SM, et al. Clear cell sarcoma of the kidney; report of a case with mandibular metastasis simulating a benign myxomatous tumor. *Oral Surg, Oral Med, Oral Pathol* 1988; 65: 567-74.

195. Forssell H, Happonen R-P, Forssell K, et al. Osteochondroma of the mandibular condyle. Report of a case and review of the literature. *Br J Oral Maxillofac Surg* 1985; 23: 183-9.

196. Forssell K, Forssell H, Happonen R-P, et al. Simple bone cyst - Review of the literature and analysis of 23 cases. *Int J Oral Maxillofac Surg* 1988; 17: 21-4.

197. Forssell K, Forssell H, Kahnberg K-E. Recurrence of a keratocyst - a long term follow-up study. *Int J Oral Maxillofac Surg* 1988; 17: 25-8.

198. Forssell K, Happonen R-P, Forssell H. Synovial chondromatosis of the temporomandibular joint. Report of a case and review of the literature. *Int J Oral Maxillofac Surg* 1988; 17: 237-41.

199. Forteza G, Colmenero B, Lopez-Barea F. Osteogenic sarcoma of the maxilla and mandible. *Oral Surg, Oral Med, Oral Pathol* 1986; 62: 179-84.

200. Frame JW, Putnam G, Wake MJC, et al. Therapeutic arterial embolisation of vascular lesions in the maxillofacial region. *Br J Oral Maxillofac Surg* 1987; 25: 181-94.

201. Franklin CD, Craig GT, Smith CJ. Quantitative analysis of histologic parameters in giant cell lesions of the jaws and long bones. *Histopathology* 1979; 3: 511-22.

202. Franklin CD, Pindborg JJ. The calcifying epithelial odontogenic tumor. A review and analysis of 113 cases. *Oral Surg, Oral Med, Oral Pathol* 1976; 42: 753-65.

203. Frederiksen NL, Wesley RK, Sciubba JJ, et al. Massive osteolysis of the maxillofacial skeleton: a clinical, radiographic, histologic, and ultrastructural study. *Oral Surg, Oral Med, Oral Pathol* 1983; 55: 470-80.

204. Freedman PD, Cardo VA, Kerpel SM, et al. Desmoplastic fibroma (fibromatosis) of the jaw bones. Report of a case and review of the literature. *Oral Surg, Oral Med, Oral Pathol* 1978; 46: 386-95.

205. Freilich RE. Adenocarcinoma of the pancreas metastatic to the mandible. *J Oral Maxillofac Surg* 1986; 44: 735-7.

206. Fujii N, Eliseo ML. Chondromyxoid fibroma of the maxilla. *J Oral Maxillofac Surg* 1988; 46: 235-8.

207. Fujita S, Takahashi H, Okabe H, et al. A case of benign cementoblastoma. *Oral Surg, Oral Med, Oral Pathol* 1989; 68: 64-8.

208. Fukuda Y, Ishida T, Fujimoto M, et al. Malignant lymphoma of the oral cavity: clinicopathologic analysis of 20 cases. *J Oral Pathol* 1987; 16: 8-12.

209. Fun-Chee L, Jinn-Fei Y. Florid osseous dysplasia in Orientals. *Oral Surg, Oral Med, Oral Pathol* 1989; 68: 748-53.

210. Gardner DG. The central odontogenic fibroma: an attempt at clarification. *Oral Surg, Oral Med, Oral Pathol* 1980; 50: 425-32.

211. Gardner DG. Radiotherapy in the treatment of ameloblastoma. *Int J Oral Maxillofacial Surg* 1988; 17: 201-5.

212. Gardner DG. An evaluation of reported cases of median mandibular cysts. *Oral Surg, Oral Med, Oral Pathol* 1988; 65: 208-13.

213. Gardner DG, Kessler HP, Morency R, et al. The glandular odontogenic cyst: an apparent entity. *J Oral Pathol* 1988; 17: 359-66.

214. Gardner DG, Mills DM. The widened periodontal ligament of osteosarcoma of the jaws. *Oral Surg, Oral Med, Oral Pathol* 1976; 41: 652-6.

215. Gardner DG, Yaacob HB, Hamid JA. Teratoma of the maxilla. *Oral Surg, Oral Med, Oral Pathol* 1987; 64: 68-71.

216. Garrington GE, Collett WK. Chondrosarcoma. I. A selected literature review. *J Oral Pathol* 1988; 17: 1-11.

217. Garrington GE, Collett WK. Chondrosarcoma. II. Chondrosarcoma of the jaws: analysis of 37 cases. *J Oral Pathol* 1988; 17: 12-20.

218. George DI, Gould AR, Miller RL, et al. Desmoplastic fibroma of the maxilla. *J Oral Maxillofac Surg* 1985; 43: 718-25.

219. Giacomuzzi D. Bilateral enlargement of mandibular coronoid processes: review of the literature and report of case. *J Oral Maxillofac Surg* 1986; 44: 728-31.

220. Giansanti JS. The pattern and width of the collagen bundles in bone and cementum. *Oral Surg, Oral Med, Oral Pathol* 1970; 30: 508-14.

221. Giles DL, McDonald PJ. Pathologic fracture of mandibular condyle due to carcinoma of the rectum. *Oral Surg, Oral Med, Oral Pathol* 1982; 53: 247-9.

222. Gingell JC, Beckerman T, Levy BA, et al. Central mucoepidermoid carcinoma. Review of the literature and report of a case associated with an apical periodontal cyst. *Oral Surg, Oral Med, Oral Pathol* 1984; 57: 436-40.

223. Goldstein G, Parker FP, Hugh GSF. Ameloblastic sarcoma: pathogenesis and treatment with chemotherapy. *Cancer* 1976; 37: 1673-8.

224. Goldstein H, McNeil BJ, Zufall E, et al. Is there still a place for bone scanning in Ewing's sarcoma? *J Nucl Med* 1980; 21: 10-2.

225. Goodpasture HC, Carlson T, Ellis B, et al. Alternaria osteomyelitis. Evidence of specific immunologic tolerance. *Arch Pathol Lab Med* 1983; 107: 528-30.

226. Gorab GN, Brahney Chr, Aria AA. Unusual presentation of a Stafne bone cyst. *Oral Surg, Oral Med, Oral Pathol* 1986; 61: 213-5.

227. Gorlin RJ, Pindborg JJ, Cohen MM. *Syndromes of the head and neck*, 2nd edn. McGraw Hill, New York. 1976.

228. Gorsky M, Silverman S, Greenspan D, et al. Metastatic chordoma to the mandible. *Oral Surg, Oral Med, Oral Pathol* 1983; 55: 601-4.

229. Gorsky M, Silverman S, Lozada F, et al. Histiocytosis X: Occurrence and oral involvement in six adolescent and adult patients. *Oral Surg, Oral Med, Oral Pathol* 1983; 55: 24-8.

230. Götzfried HF, Paulus GW, Feistal H. Diagnostik und Verlaufskontrolle der Kieferosteomyelitis durch 4-Phasen-und markierte Leukozytenszintigraphie. *Fortschr Kiefer Gesichts Chir* 1987; 32: 172-5.

231. Gould AR, Mascaro JJ. Intraosseous lipogranuloma presenting with mental nerve paresthesia. *J Oral Maxillofac Surg* 1984; 42: 124-7.

232. Greer RO, Johnson M. Botryoid odontogenic cyst: clinicopathologic analysis of ten cases with three recurrences. *J Oral Maxillofac Surg* 1988; 46: 574-9.

233. Griffin ThJ, Hurst PS, Swanson J. Non-Hodgkin's lymphoma: a case involving four third molar extraction sites. *Oral Surg, Oral Med, Oral Pathol* 1988; 65: 671-4.

234. Grünebaum M. Nonfamilial cherubism: report of two cases. *J Oral Maxillofac Surg* 1973; 31: 632-5.

235. Gundlach KKH, Buurman R. Dysplasia cleidocranialis - histologische Befunde am Zahnzement. *Dtsch Zahnärztl Z* 1978; 33: 574-8.

236. Gundlach KKH, Fuhrmann A, Beckmann-van der Ven G. The double-headed mandibular condyle. *Oral Surg, Oral Med, Oral Pathol* 1987; 64: 249-53.

237. Gupta DS, Gupta MK. Odontoblastoma. *J Oral Maxillofac Surg* 1986; 44: 146-8.

238. Gupta DS, Gupta MK, Borle RM. Osteomyelitis of the mandible in marble bone disease. *Int J Oral Maxillofac Surg* 1986; 15: 201-5.

239. Gupta DS, Gupta MK, Naider G. Mandibular osteomyelitis caused by Actinomyces Israelii. Report of a case. *J Maxillofac Surg* 1986; 14: 291-3.

240. Gutierrez MM, Mora RG. Nevoid basal cell carcinoma syndrome. *J Am Acad Dermatol* 1986; 15: 1023-30.

241. Habets LLMH, Bras J, van den Akker HP, et al. Mandibular atrophy and metabolic bone less. A 5-year follow-up. *Int J Oral Maxillofac Surg* 1987; 16: 131-8.

242. Habets LLMH, Bras J, Borgmeyer-Hoelen AMMJ. Mandibular atrophy and metabolic bone loss. Endocrinology, radiology and histomorphometry. *Int J Oral Maxillofac Surg* 1988; 17: 208-11.

243. Hagel-Bradway S, Dziak R. Regulation of bone cell metabolism. *J Oral Pathol Med* 1989; 18: 344-51.

244. Hall MB, Brown RW, Baughman RA. Gaucher's disease affecting the mandible. *J Oral Maxillofac Surg* 1985; 43: 210-3.

245. Hall MB, Sclar AG, Gardner DF. Albright's syndrome with reactivation of fibrous dysplasia secondary to pituitary adenoma and further complicated by osteogenic sarcoma. Report of a case. *Oral Surg, Oral Med, Oral Pathol* 1984; 57: 616-9.

246. Hall RE, Orbach S, Landesberg R. Bilateral hyperplasia of the mandibular coronoid processes: a report of two cases. *Oral Surg, Oral Med, Oral Pathol* 1989; 67: 141-5.

247. Hamner JE, Scofield HH, Cornyn J. Benign fibro-osseous lesions of periodontal membrane origin. *Cancer* 1968; 22: 861-78.

248. Handlers JP, Abrams AM, Melrose RJ, et al. Fibrosarcoma of the mandible presenting as a periodontal problem. *J Oral Pathol* 1985; 14: 351-6.

249. Hansen LS, Eversole LR, Green TL, et al. Clear cell odontogenic tumor - a new histologic variant with aggressive potential. *Head & Neck Surg* 1985; 8: 115-23.

250. Hansson L-G, Westesson P-L, Katzberg RW, et al. MR Imaging of the temporomandibular joint: comparison of images of autopsy specimens made at 0.3 T and 1.5 T with anatomic cryosections. *AJR* 1989; 152: 1241-4.

251. Happonen R-P, Aho HJ, Ekfors TO, et al. Chondromyxoid fibroma of the mandible. Ultrastructural comparison with a typical chondromyxoid fibroma of the femur. *Proc Finn Dent Soc* 1984; 80: 230-7.

252. Happonen R-P, Ekfors T, Suonpää J, et al. Malignant fibrous histiocytoma of the jaws: Report of two cases. *J Oral Maxillofac Surg* 1988; 46: 690-3.

253. Hardt N, Hofer B. *Szintigraphie der Kiefer- und Gesichtsschädel-Erkrankungen.* Quintessenz, Berlin. 1988.

254. Harrison JD, Martin IC. Oral vegetable granuloma: ultrastructural and histological study. *J Oral Pathol* 1986; 15: 322-6.

255. Harsanyi BB, Larsson A. Xanthomatous lesions of the mandible: osseous expression of non-X histiocytosis and benign fibrous histiocytoma. *Oral Surg, Oral Med, Oral Pathol* 1988; 65: 551-66.

256. Hartman KS. Histiocytosis X: a review of 114 cases with oral involvement. *Oral Surg, Oral Med, Oral Pathol* 1980; 49: 38-54.

257. Hartmann N, Gundlach KKH. Ossifizierendes und zementbildendes Fibrom im klinischen und röntgenologischen Vergleich. *Dtsch Z Mund-Kiefer-Gesichts Chir* 1986; 10: 245-8.

258. Hashimoto N, Kurihara K, Yamasaki H, et al. Pathological characteristics of metastatic carcinoma in the human mandible. *J Oral Pathol* 1987; 16: 362-7.

259. Hauser MS, Freije S, Payne RW, et al. Bilateral ossifying fibroma of the maxillary sinus. *Oral Surg, Oral Med, Oral Pathol* 1989; 68: 759-63.

260. Hawkins PL, Sadeghi EM. Ameloblastic fibro-odontoma: report of case. *J Oral Maxillofac Surg* 1986; 44: 1014-9.

261. Hecker R, Noon W, Elliott M. Adenocarcinoma metastatic to the temporomandibular joint. *J Oral Maxillofac Surg* 1985; 43: 629-31.

262. Heeten den GJ, Schraffordt Koops H, Kamps WA, et al. Treatment of malignant fibrous histiocytoma of bone; a plea for primary chemotherapy. *Cancer* 1985; 56: 37-40.

263. Heffez L, Blaustein D. Advances in sonography of the temporo-mandibular joint. *Oral Surg, Oral Med, Oral Pathol* 1986; 62: 486-95.

264. Heffez L, Doku HChr, Carter BL, et al. Perspectives on massive osteolysis. *Oral Surg, Oral Med, Oral Pathol* 1983; 5: 331-43.

265. Heffez L, Mafee MF, Langer B. Double-contrast arthrography of the temporomandibular joint: Role of direct sagittal CT imaging. *Oral Surg, Oral Med, Oral Pathol* 1988; 65: 511-4.

266. Heffez L, Mafee MF, Vaiana J. The role of magnetic resonance imaging in the diagnosis and management of ameloblastoma. *Oral Surg, Oral Med, Oral Pathol* 1988; 65: 2-12.

266a. Hes J, van der Waal I, de Man K. Bimaxillary hyperplasia: The facial expression of homozygous β-thalassemia. *Oral Surg, Oral Pathol, Oral Med* 1990; 69: 185-90.

267. Hesseling P, Wood RE, Nortjé CJ, et al. African Burkitt's lymphoma in the Cape province of South Africa and Namibia. *Oral Surg, Oral Med, Oral Pathol* 1989; 68: 162-6.

268. Heydt D, Thompson SH, Shakenovsky BN. Transition of apical periodontal cysts to intramedullary osteomyelitis: a clinicopathological analysis. *J Endod* 1985; 11: 67-70.

269. Heymer B, Kreidler J, Adler C-P. Strahleninduziertes Osteosarkom des Unterkiefers. *Dtsch Z Mund-Kiefer-Gesichts Chir* 1988; 12: 113-9.

270. Hietanen J, Lukinmaa P-L, Calonius P-EB, et al. Desmoplastic fibroma involving the mandible. *Br J Oral Maxillofac Surg* 1986; 24: 442-7.

271. Hietanen J, Matilla K, Calonius P-EB, et al. Central neurilemmomas of the mandible. Report of two cases. *Int J Oral Maxillofac Surg* 1984; 13: 166-71.

272. High AS, Hirschmann PN. Age changes in residual radicular cysts. *J Oral Pathol* 1986; 15: 524-8.

273. Higuchi Y, Nakamura N, Tashiro N. Clinicopathologic study of cemento-osseous dysplasia producing cysts of the mandible. Report of four cases. *Oral Surg, Oral Med, Oral Pathol* 1988; 65: 339-42.

274. Hirschberg A, Dayan D, Buchner A, et al. Cholesterol granuloma of the jaws. *Int J Oral Maxillofac Surg* 1988; 17: 230-1.

275. Hirota J, Osaki T. Primary central adenoid cystic carcinoma of the mandible. *J Oral Maxillofac Surg* 1989; 47: 176-9.

276. Hoen MM, Downs RH, LaBounty GL, et al. Osteomyelitis of the maxilla with associated vertical root fracture and Pseudomonas infection. *Oral Surg, Oral Med, Oral Pathol* 1988; 66: 494-8.

277. Hoffman S, Jacoway JR, Krolls SO. *Intraosseous and parosteal tumors of the jaws*. Armed Forces Institute of Pathology, Washington D.C. 1987.

278. Hollins RR, Lydiatt DD, Markin RS, et al. Mesenchymal chondrosarcoma: a case report. *J Oral Maxillofac Surg* 1987; 45: 72-5.

279. Horch H-H, Schaefer HE, Féaux de Lacroix W. Zum sogenannten "kongenitalen melanotischen neuroektodermalen" Tumor des Kiefer-Gesichtsbereichs. *Dtsch Z Mund-Kiefer-Gesichts Chir* 1982; 6: 207-16.

280. Hudson JW, Jaffrey B, Chase DC, et al. Malignant teratoma of the mandible. *J Oral Maxillofac Surg* 1983; 41: 540-3.

281. Hupp JR, Collins FJV, Ross A, et al. A review of Burkitt's lymphoma. Importance of radiographic diagnosis. *J Maxillofac Surg* 1982; 10: 240-5.

282. Hupp JR, Topazian RG, Krutchkoff DJ. The melanotic neuroectodermal tumor of infancy; report of two cases and review of the literature. *Int J Oral Maxillofac Surg* 1981; 10: 432-46.

283. Huvos AG, Heilweil M, Bretsky SS. The pathology of malignant fibrous histiocytoma. A study of 130 patients. *Am J Surg Pathol* 1985; 9: 853-71.

284. Hyman J, Bakker V. Xeroradiographic detection of tooth and bone pathology. *Oral Surg, Oral Med, Oral Pathol* 1979; 47: 482-4.

285. Iannetti G, Cascone P, Belli E, et al. Condylar hyperplasia: Cephalometric study, treatment planning, and surgical correction (our experience). *Oral Surg, Oral Med, Oral Pathol* 1989; 68: 673-81.

286. Ide F, Sano R, Shimura H, et al. An ultrastructural and immunohistochemical study on mandibular lesion of Letterer-Siwe disease. *J Oral Pathol* 1981; 10: 386-97.

287. Ikemura K, Horie A, Tashiro H, et al. Simultaneous occurrence of a calcifying odontogenic cyst and its malignant transformation. *Cancer* 1985; 56: 2861-5.

288. Innocenti M, Bonucchi D, Zaltron D, et al. Maxillomandibular versus hands roentgenographs in the evaluation of renal osteodystrophy. *Nephron* 1987; 46: 208-9.

289. Iwu CO. Osteomyelitis of the mandible in sickle cell homozygous patients in Nigeria. *Br J Oral Maxillofac Surg* 1989; 27: 429-34.

290. Jacobsson S. Diffuse sclerosing osteomyelitis of the mandible. *Int J Oral Maxillofac Surg* 1984; 13: 363-85.

291. Jacobsson S, Heyden G. Chronic sclerosing osteomyelitis of the mandible. Histologic and histochemical findings. *Oral Surg, Oral Med, Oral Pathol* 1977; 43: 357-64.

292. Jacobsson S, Hollender L. Treatment and prognosis of diffuse sclerosing osteomyelitis of the mandible. *Oral Surg, Oral Med, Oral Pathol* 1980; 49: 7-14.

293. Jacobsson S, Hollender L, Lindberg S, et al. Chronic sclerosing osteomyelitis of the mandible. Scintigraphic and radiographic findings. *Oral Surg, Oral Med, Oral Pathol* 1978; 45: 167-74.

294. Janecka IP, Conley JJ. Synovial cyst of temporo-mandibular joint imitating a parotid tumour (a case report). *J Maxillofac Surg* 1978; 6: 154-6.

295. Jensen J, Sindet-Pedersen S, Simonsen EK. A comparative study of treatment of keratocysts by enucleation or enucleation combined with cryotherapy. *J Cranio-Max-Fac Surg* 1988; 16: 362-5.

296. Johnson RE, Scheithauer BW, Dahlin DC. Melanotic neuro-ectodermal tumor of infancy. A review of seven cases. *Cancer* 1983; 52: 661-6.

297. Jones DC. Adenocarcinoma of the esophagus presenting as a mandibular metastasis. *J Oral Maxillofac Surg* 1989; 47: 504-7.

298. Jones GM, Eveson JW, Sheperd JP. Central odontogenic fibroma. A report of two controversial cases illustrating diagnostic dilemmas. *Br J Oral Maxillofac Surg* 1989; 27: 406-11.

299. Jones LR, Toth BB, Cangir A. Treatment for solitary eosinophilic granuloma of the mandible by steroid injection: report of a case. *J Oral Maxillofac Surg* 1989; 47: 306-9.

300. Juniper RP. Caffey's disease. *Br J Oral Maxillofac Surg* 1982; 20: 281-7.

301. Kameyama Y, Maeda H, Nakane S, et al. Malignant Schwannoma of the maxilla in a patient without neurofibromatosis. *Histopathology* 1987; 11: 1205-10.

302. Kameyama Y, Takehana, S, Mizohata, M, et al. A clinicopathological study of ameloblastomas. *Int J Oral Maxillofac Surg* 1987; 16: 706-12.

303. Katou F, Motegi K, Baba S. Mandibular lesions in patients with adenomatosis coli. *J Cranio-Max-Fac Surg* 1989; 17: 354-8.

304. Kaugars GE. Botryoid odontogenic cyst. *Oral Surg, Oral Med, Oral Pathol* 1986; 62: 555-9.

305. Kaugars GE, Cale AE. Traumatic bone cysts. *Oral Surg, Oral Med, Oral Pathol* 1987; 63: 318-24.

306. Kayavis JG, Papanayotou PH, Antoniadis DZ. Reticulum cell sarcoma of the mandible: report of case. *J Oral Maxillofac Surg* 1980; 38: 210-1.

307. Keeney GL, Unni KK, Beabout JW, et al. Adamantinoma of long bones. A clinicopathologic study of 85 cases. *Cancer* 1989; 64: 730-7.

308. Keizer S, Tuinzing DB. Spontaneous regeneration of a unilaterally absent mandibular condyle. *J Oral Maxillofac Surg* 1985; 43: 130-2.

309. Kelly WH, Mirahmadi MK, Simon JHS, et al. Radiographic changes of the jaw bones in end stage renal disease. *Oral Surg, Oral Med, Oral Pathol* 1980; 50: 372-81.

310. Khanna S, Khanna NN. Primary tumors of the jaws in children. *J Oral Maxillofac Surg* 1979; 37: 800-4.

311. Kluin PM, Slootweg PJ, Schuurman HJ, et al. Primary B-cell malignant lymphoma of the maxilla with a sarcomatous pattern and multilobulated nuclei. *Cancer* 1984; 54: 1598-605.

312. Koch PhE, Hammer WB. Cleidocranial dysostosis: review of the literature and report of case. *J Oral Maxillofac Surg* 1978; 36: 39-42.

313. Komisar A, Silver C, Kalnicki S. Osteoradionecrosis of the maxilla and skull base. *Laryngoscope* 1985; 95: 24-8.

314. Köndell PA, Grantström M, Heimdahl A, et al. Experimental mandibular Staphylococcus aureus osteomyelitis; antibody response and treatment with dicloxacillin. *Int J Oral Maxillofac Surg* 1986; 15: 620-8.

315. Kristensen S, Tveteras K. Aggressive cementifying fibroma of the maxilla. *Arch Otorhinolaryngol* 1986; 243: 102-5.

316. Krutchkoff DJ, Jones CR. Multifocal eosinophilic granuloma: a clinical pathologic conference. *J Oral Pathol* 1984; 13: 472-88.

317. Krutchkoff DJ, Runstad L. Unusually aggressive osteomyelitis of the jaws; a report of two cases. *Oral Surg, Oral Med, Oral Pathol* 1989; 67: 499-507.

318. Kubo K, Miyatani H, Takenoshita Y, et al. Widespread radiopacity of jaw bones in familial adenomatosis coli. *J Cranio-Max-Fac Surg* 1989; 17: 350-3.

319. Kuepper RC, Harrigan WF. Treatment of mandibular cherubism. *J Oral Maxillofac Surg* 1978; 36: 638-41.

320. Kummoona R, Al-Hetie T. Skeletal bone scanning in "Middle East" jaw lymphoma. *Oral Surg, Oral Med, Oral Pathol* 1982; 54: 473-6.

321. Kurita K, Bronstein SL, Westesson P-L, et al. Arthroscopic diagnosis of perforation and adhesions of the temporomandibular joint: Correlation with postmortem morphology. *Oral Surg, Oral Med, Oral Pathol* 1989; 68: 130-4.

322. Kurita K, Westesson P-L, Sternby NH, et al. Histologic features of the temporomandibular joint disk and posterior disk attachment: Comparison of symptom-free persons with normally positioned disks and patients with internal derangement. *Oral Surg, Oral Med, Oral Pathol* 1989; 67: 635-43.

323. Kuroi M. Simple bone cyst of the jaw: review of the literature and report of case. *J Oral Maxillofac Surg* 1980; 38: 456-9.

324. Kwon PH, Horswell BB, Gatto DJ. Desmoplastic fibroma of the jaws: surgical management and review of the literature. *Head & Neck Surg* 1989; 11: 67-75.

325. Lainson PA, Khowassah MA, Tewfik HH. Seminoma metastatic to the jaws. *Oral Surg, Oral Med, Oral Pathol* 1975; 40: 404-8.

326. Lambertenghi-Deliliers G, Bruno E, Cortelezzi A, et al. Incidence of jaw lesions in 193 patients with multiple myeloma. *Oral Surg, Oral Med, Oral Pathol* 1988; 65: 533-7.

327. Langdon JD, Rapidis AD, Patel MF. Ossifying fibroma - one disease or six? An analysis of 39 fibro-osseous lesions of the jaws. *Br J Oral Maxillofac Surg* 1976; 14: 1-11.

328. Laughlin EH. Metastasizing ameloblastoma. *Cancer* 1989; 64: 776-80.

329. Leider AS, Eversole LR, Barkin ME. Cystic ameloblastoma; a clinicopathologic analysis. *Oral Surg, Oral Med, Oral Pathol* 1985; 60: 624-30.

330. Leider AS, Jonker LA, Cook HE. Multicentric familial squamous odontogenic tumor. *Oral Surg, Oral Med, Oral Pathol* 1989; 68: 175-81.

331. Lello GE, Makek M. Calcifying odontogenic cyst. *Int J Oral Maxillofac Surg* 1986; 15: 637-44.

332. Lello GE, Raubenheimer E. Hodgkin's disease presenting in the maxilla. A case report. *Int J Oral Maxillofac Surg* 1989; 18: 7-9.

333. Lewars PHD. Chronic periostitis in the mandible underneath artificial dentures. *Br J Oral Maxillofac Surg* 1971; 8: 264-9.

334. Lindquist C, Teppo L, Sane J, et al. Osteosarcoma of the mandible: analysis of nine cases. *J Oral Maxillofac Surg* 1986; 44: 759-64.

335. Lipani CS, Natiella JR, Greene GW. The hematopoietic defect of the jaws: a report of sixteen cases. *J Oral Pathol* 1982; 11: 411-6.

336. Llewelyn J, Sugar AW. Neurillemmoma of the mandible. Report of a case. *Br J Oral Maxillofac Surg* 1989; 27: 512-6.

337. Llombart-Bosch A, Blache R, Peydro-Olaya A. Ultrastructural study of 28 cases of Ewing's sarcoma: typical and atypical forms. *Cancer* 1978; 41: 1362-73.

338. Loftus MJ, Bennett JA, Fantasia JE. Osteochondroma of the mandibular condyles. *Oral Surg, Oral Med, Oral Pathol* 1986; 61: 221-6.

339. Loh FC, Yeo JF. Talisman in the orofacial region. *Oral Surg, Oral Med, Oral Pathol* 1989; 68: 252-5.

340. Loh FC, Yeo JF. Bifid mandibular condyle. *Oral Surg, Oral Med, Oral Pathol* 1990; 69: 24-7.

341. Loh HS. A retrospective evaluation of 23 reported cases of solitary plasmacytoma of the mandible, with an additional case report. *Br J Oral Maxillofac Surg* 1984; 22: 216-24.

342. Lombardi T, Kuffer R, Bernard J-P, et al. Immunohistochemical staining for vimentin filaments and S-100 proteins in myxoma of the jaws. *J Oral Pathol* 1988; 17: 175-7.

343. Looby JP. Uncontrolled growth of the alveolar processes of the maxilla and mandible in a 20-month-old child. *Oral Surg, Oral Med, Oral Pathol* 1977; 43: 855-8.

344. Lovely FW. Recurrent aneurysmal bone cyst of the mandible. *J Oral Maxillofac Surg* 1983; 41: 192-5.

345. Löwicke G, Teuber S. Fernmetastasen im Unterkiefer. *Dtsch Z Mund-Kiefer-Gesichts Chir* 1987; 11: 316-8.

346. Lukes RJ. The immunologic approach to the pathology of malignant lymphomas. *Am J Clin Pathol* 1979; 72: 657-69.

347. Lukinmaa P-L, Hietanen J, Laitinen J-M, et al. Mandibular dentinoma. *J Oral Maxillofac Surg* 1987; 45: 60-4.

348. Lukinmaa P-L, Hietanen J, Swan H, et al. Maxillary fibrosarcoma with extracellular immuno-characterization. *Br J Oral Maxillofac Surg* 1988; 26: 36-44.

349. Lustmann J, Gazit D, Ulmansky M, et al. Chondromyxoid fibroma of the jaws: a clinicopathological study. *J Oral Pathol* 1986; 15: 343-6.

350. Lustmann J, Zeltser R. Synovial chondromatosis of the temporomandibular joint. Review of the literature and case report. *Int J Oral Maxillofac Surg* 1989; 18: 90-4.

351. Makek M. Non-ossifying fibroma of the mandible. *Arch Orthop Traum Surg* 1980; 96: 225-7.

352. Makek M. *Clinical Pathology of Fibro-Osteo-Cemental Lesions in the Cranio-Facial and Jaw Bones.* Karger, Basel-New York. 1983.

353. Makek M, Grätz KW, Sailer HF. Das nicht-ossifizierende Fibrom des Unterkiefers. *Dtsch Z Mund Kiefer Gesichs Chir* 1988; 12: 451-5.

354. Makek M, Lello GE. Focal osteoporotic bone marrow defects of the jaws. *J Oral Maxillofac Surg* 1986; 44: 268-73.

355. Malmström M, Fyhrquist F, Kosunen TU, et al. Immunological features of patients with chronic sclerosing osteomyelitis of the mandible. *Int J Oral Maxillofac Surg* 1983; 12: 6-13.

356. Marmary Y, Horne T, Azaz B. Hyperostosis corticalis generalisata: surgical management and long-term follow-up of one patient. *Int J Oral Maxillofac Surg* 1989; 18: 155-7.

357. Martinez V, Sissons HA. Aneurysmal bone cyst. A review of 123 cases including primary lesions and those secondary to other bone pathology. *Cancer* 1988; 61: 2291-304.

358. Marunick MT, Leveque F. Osteoradionecrosis related to mastication and parafunction. *Oral Surg, Oral Med, Oral Pathol* 1989; 68: 582-5.

359. Marx RE. A new concept in the treatment of osteoradionecrosis. *J Oral Maxillofac Surg* 1983; 41: 351-7.

360. Marx RE. Osteoradionecrosis: a new concept of its pathophysiology. *J Oral Maxillofac Surg* 1983; 41: 283-8.

361. Mast HL, Nissenblatt MJ. Metastatic colon carcinoma to the jaw: a case report and review of the literature. *J Surg Oncol* 1987; 34: 202-7.

362. Maxwell DR, Spolnik KJ, Cockerill EM, et al. Roentgenographic manifestations of maxillomandibular renal osteodystrophy. *Nephron* 1985; 41: 223-9.

363. Mayo K, Scott RF. Persistent cemento-ossifying fibroma of the mandible: report of a case and review of the literature. *J Oral Maxillofac Surg* 1988; 46: 58-63.

364. McCormick SU, McCormick SA, Graves RW, et al. Bilateral bifid mandibular condyles. Report of three cases. *Oral Surg, Oral Med, Oral Pathol* 1989; 68: 555-7.

365. McDonald DJ, Sim FH, McLeod RA, et al. Giant-cell tumor of bone. *J Bone Joint Surg* 1986; 68-A: 235-42.

366. McDonald JS, Miller RL, Bernstein ML, et al. Histiocytosis X: a clinical presentation. *J Oral Pathol* 1980; 9: 342-9.

367. McGregor AJ, Lewis DA. Metastasis of carcinoma of the lung by implantation in tooth sockets. *Br J Oral Maxillofac Surg* 1972; 9: 195-9.

368. McGregor IA, MacDonald DG. Spread of squamous cell carcinoma to the nonirradiated edentulous mandible - a preliminary report. *Head & Neck Surg* 1987; 9: 157-61.

369. McMillan MD, Ferguson JW, Kardos TB. Mandibular vascular leiomyoma. *Oral Surg, Oral Med, Oral Pathol* 1986; 62: 427-33.

370. McMillan MD, Kardos TB, Edwards JL, et al. Giant cell hyalin angiopathy or pulse granuloma. *Oral Surg, Oral Med, Oral Pathol* 1981; 52: 178-86.

371. Meechan JG MacGregor IDM, Roger SN, et al. The effect of smoking on immediate post-extraction socket filling with blood and on the incidence of painful socket. *Br J Oral Maxillofac Surg* 1988; 26: 402-9.

372. Melrose RJ, Abrams AM. Juvenile fibromatosis affecting the jaws. Report of three cases. *Oral Surg, Oral Med, Oral Pathol* 1980; 49: 317-24.

373. Melrose RJ, Abrams AA, Mills BG. Florid osseous dysplasia; a clinical-pathologic study of thirty-four cases. *Oral Surg, Oral Med, Oral Pathol* 1976; 41: 62-82.

374. Merkesteijn van JPR, Bakker DJ, van der Waal I, et al. Hyperbaric oxygen treatment of chronic osteomyelitis of the jaws. *Int J Oral Maxillofac Surg* 1984; 13: 386-95.

375. Merkesteijn van JPR, Bras J, Vermeeren JIJF, et al. Osteomyelitis of the jaws in pycnodysostosis. *Int J Oral Maxillofac Surg* 1987; 16: 615-9.

376. Merkesteijn van JPR, Groot RH, Bras J, et al. Diffuse sclerosing osteomyelitis of the mandible: clinical, radiographic and histologic findings in twenty-seven patients. *J Oral Maxillofac Surg* 1988; 46: 825-9.

377. Miles DA, Lovas JL, Cohen MM. Hemimaxillofacial dysplasia: A newly recognized disorder of facial asymmetry, hypertrichosis of the facial skin, unilateral enlargement of the maxilla, and hypoplastic teeth in two patients. *Oral Surg, Oral Med, Oral Pathol* 1987; 64: 445-8.

378. Miller WB, Ausich JE, McDaniel RK. Mandibular intraosseous lipoma. *J Oral Maxillofac Surg* 1982; 40: 594-6.

379. Mills BG. Comparison of the ultrastructure of a malignant tumor of mandible containing giant cells with Paget's disease of bone. *J Oral Pathol* 1981; 10: 203-15.

380. Milobsky SA, Milobsky L, Epstein LI. Metastatic renal adenocarcinoma presenting as periapical pathosis in the maxilla. *Oral Surg, Oral Med, Oral Pathol* 1975; 39: 30-3.

381. Mincer HH, McCoy JM, Turner JE. Pulse granuloma of the alveolar ridge. *Oral Surg, Oral Med, Oral Pathol* 1979; 48: 126-30.

382. Mintz GA, Abrams AM, Carlsen GD, et al. Primary malignant giant cell tumor of the mandible: report of a case and review of the literature. *Oral Surg, Oral Med, Oral Pathol* 1981; 51: 164-71.

383. Mizuno A, Kawabata T, Nakano Y, et al. Lingual mandibular bone defect-idiopathic bone cavity. Report of a case. *Int J Oral Maxillofac Surg* 1983; 12: 64-8.

384. Mock D, Rosen IB. Osteosarcoma in irradiated fibrous dysplasia. *J Oral Pathol* 1986; 15: 1-4.

385. Molla MR, Ijuhin N, Sugata T, et al. Chondrosarcoma of the jaw: report of two cases. *J Oral Maxillofac Surg* 1987; 45: 453-7.

386. Moloy PJ, Kowall KA, Siegel WM. Fibrosarcoma of the mandible following supravoltage irradiation: Report of a case. *Arch Otolaryngol Head Neck Surg* 1989; 115: 1250-2.

387. Monje F, Gil-Diez JL, Campano FJ, et al. Mandibular lesion as the first evidence of multiple myeloma. Case report. *J Cranio-Max-Fac Surg* 1989; 17: 315-7.

388. Moreillon MC, Schroeder HE. Numerical frequency of epithelial abnormalities, particularly microkeratocysts, in the developing human oral mucosa. *Oral Surg, Oral Med, Oral Pathol* 1982; 53: 44-55.

389. Morton ME, Simpson W. The management of osteoradionecrosis of the jaws. *Br J Oral Maxillofac Surg* 1986; 24: 332-41.

390. Mosby EL, Albright JE, Messer EJ, et al. Xanthoma of the mandible. (I and II). *J Oral Maxillofac Surg* 1983; 41: 180-1. 268-70.

391. Mostofi R, Marchmont-Robinson H, Freije S. Spontaneous tooth exfoliation and osteonecrosis following a herpes zoster infection of the fifth cranial nerve. *J Oral Maxillofac Surg* 1987; 45: 264-6.

392. Müller H, Slootweg PJ. The ameloblastoma, the controversial approach to therapy. *J Maxillofac Surg* 1985; 13: 79-84.

393. Murphy GF, Bahn AK, Sato S, et al. Characterization of Langerhans cells by the use of monoclonal antibodies. *Lab Invest* 1981; 45: 465-8.

394. Murray CG, Herson J, Daly TE, et al. Radiation necrosis of the mandible: a 10 year study. Part I. Factors influencing the onset of necrosis. Part II. Dental factors; onset, duration and management of necrosis. *Int J Radiat Oncol Biol Phys* 1980; 6: 543-53.

395. Musella AE, Slater LJ. Familial florid osseous dysplasia: a case report. *J Oral Maxillofac Surg* 1989; 47: 636-40.

396. Myall RWT, Morton ThH, Worthington Ph. Melanoma metastatic to the mandible. Report of a case. *Int J Oral Maxillofac Surg* 1983; 12: 56-9.

397. Nagao T, Nakajima T, Fukushima M, et al. Calcifying odontogenic cyst: a survey of 23 cases in the Japanese literature. *J Maxillofac Surg* 1983; 11: 174-9.

398. Nandakumar H, Shankaramba KB. Hydatid cyst of the mandible: a case report. *J Oral Maxillofac Surg* 1989; 47: 759-61.

399. Nardi P, Ficarra G. Mandibular metastasis of angiosarcoma. *Int J Oral Maxillofac Surg* 1988; 17: 386-7.

400. Naylor GD, Auclair PL, Rathbun WA, et al. Metastatic adenocarcinoma of the colon presenting as periradicular periodontal disease: a case report. *Oral Surg, Oral Med, Oral Pathol* 1989; 67: 162-6.

401. Neville BW, Albenesius RJ. The prevalence of benign fibro-osseous lesions of periodontal ligament origin in black women: A radiographic survey. *Oral Surg, Oral Med, Oral Pathol* 1986; 62: 340-4.

402. Nikai H, Ijuhin N, Yamasaki A, et al. Ultrastructural evidence for neural crest origin of the melanotic neuroectodermal tumor of infancy. *J Oral Pathol* 1977; 6: 221-7.

403. Nishi M, Mimura T, Senba I. Leiomyosarcoma of the maxilla. *J Oral Maxillofac Surg* 1987; 45: 64-8.

404. Nishimura Y, Nakajima T, Yakata H, et al. Metastatic thyroid carcinoma of the mandible. *J Oral Maxillofac Surg* 1982; 40: 221-5.

405. Nishizawa S, Hayashida T, Horiguchi S, et al. Malignant fibrous histiocytoma of maxilla following radiotherapy for bilateral retinoblastoma. *J Laryngol Otol* 1985; 99: 501-4.

406. Norman JE de B, Stevenson ARL, Painter DM, et al. Synovial osteochondromatosis of the temporomandibular joint. An historical review with presentation of 3 cases. *J Cranio-Max-Fac Surg* 1988; 16: 212-20.

407. Nortjé CJ, Farman AG, Grotepass FW, et al. Chondrosarcoma of the mandibular condyle. Report of a case with special reference to radiographic features. *Br J Oral Maxillofac Surg* 1976; 14: 101-11.

408. Nortjé CJ, Wood RE, Grotepass F. Periostitis ossificans versus Garré's osteomyelitis. Part II: Radiologic analysis of 93 cases in the jaws. *Oral Surg, Oral Med, Oral Pathol* 1988; 66: 249-60.

409. Obisesan AA, Lagundoye SB, Daramola JO, et al. The radiologic features of fibrous dysplasia of the craniofacial bones. *Oral Surg, Oral Med, Oral Pathol* 1977; 44: 949-59.

410. O'Brien CJ, Carter RL, Soo K-C, et al. Invasion of the mandible by squamous carcinomas of the oral cavity and oropharynx. *Head & Neck Surg* 1986; 8: 247-56.

411. Obwegeser HL, Makek MS. Benign lipoblastoma in the mandible. *Head & Neck Surg* 1983; 5: 251-6.

412. Ohkubo T, Hernandez JC, Ooya K, et al. "Agressive" osteoblastoma of the maxilla. *Oral Surg, Oral Med, Oral Pathol* 1989; 68: 69-73.

413. Ohtake K, Yokobayashi Y, Shingaki S, et al. Central carcinoma of the jaw. A survey of 28 cases in the Japanese literature. *J Cranio-Max-Fac Surg* 1989; 17: 155-61.

414. Ohya T, Takeda Y, Yoshida H, et al. A rare case of simultaneous malignant tumors: osteosarcoma of the mandible and lung cancer. *J Oral Maxillofac Surg* 1987; 45: 261-4.

415. Okada Y, Sugimura M, Ishida T. Ameloblastoma accompanied by prominent bone formation. *J Oral Maxillofac Surg* 1986; 44: 555-7.

416. Or S. An analysis of 367 cases of temporomandibular joint dysfunction. *Int J Oral Maxillofac Surg* 1982; 11: 232-5.

417. Ord RA, El-Attar A. Osteomyelitis of the mandible in children - clinical presentations and review of management. *Br J Oral Maxillofac Surg* 1987; 25: 204-17.

418. Ord RA, Rennie JS. Central neurilemmoma of the maxilla. Report of a case and review of the literature. *Int J Oral Maxillofac Surg* 1981; 10: 137-9.

419. Ord RA, Rennie JS, McDonald DG, et al. Cancellous osteoma of the coronoid process: report of a case. *Br J Oral Maxillofac Surg* 1983; 21: 49-55.

420. Osguthorpe JD, Hungerford GD. Benign osteoblastoma of the maxillary sinus. *Head & Neck Surg* 1983; 6: 605-9.

421. Otis LL, Terezhalmy GT, Glass BJ. Paget's disease of bone: etiological theories and report of a case. *J Oral Med* 1986; 41: 214-9.

422. Padayachee A, Van Wyk CW. Two cystic lesions with features of both the botryoid odontogenic cyst and the central mucoepidermoid tumor: Sialo-odontogenic cyst? *J Oral Pathol Med* 1987; 16: 499-504.

423. Papadimitriou JM, Bruggen Van Y. Evidence that multinucleate giant cells are examples of mononuclear phagocytic differentiation. *J Oral Pathol* 1986; 148: 149-57.

424. Papageorge MB, Cataldo E, Nghiem FTM. Cementoblastoma involving multiple deciduous teeth. *Oral Surg, Oral Med, Oral Pathol* 1987; 63: 602-5.

425. Peacock TR, Fleet JD. Condylar metastasis from a bronchogenic carcinoma. *Br J Oral Maxillofac Surg* 1982; 20: 39-44.

426. Peckitt NS, Wood GA. Eosinophilic granuloma of the mandibular condyle. *Br J Maxillofac Surg* 1988; 26: 306-10.

427. Perriman AO, Figures KH. Metastatic retinoblastoma of the mandible. *Oral Surg, Oral Med, Oral Pathol* 1978; 45: 741-8.

428. Peters E, Cohen M, Altini M, et al. Rhabdomyosarcoma of the oral and paraoral region. *Cancer* 1989; 63: 963-6.

429. Peters RA, Schock RK. Oral cysts in newborn infants. *Oral Surg, Oral Med, Oral Pathol* 1971; 32: 10-4.

430. Peters WJN. Cherubism: a study of twenty cases from one family. *Oral Surg, Oral Med, Oral Pathol* 1979; 47: 307-11.

431. Petri WH. Agressive fibromatosis of the mandible. *J Oral Maxillofac Surg* 1982; 40: 663-7.

432. Phelan JA, Kritchman D, Fusco-Ramer M, et al. Recurrent botryoid odontogenic cyst (lateral periodontal cyst). *Oral Surg, Oral Med, Oral Pathol* 1988; 66: 345-8.

433. Philipsen HP. Om keratocyster (Kolesteatomer) og kaeberne. *Tandlaegebladet* 1956; 60: 963-71.

434. Phillips VM, Grotepass FW, Hendricks R. Ameloblastic odontosarcoma with epithelial atypia; a case report. *Br J Oral Maxillofac Surg* 1988; 26: 45-51.

435. Picci P, Baldini N, Sudanese A, et al. Giant cell reparative granuloma and other giant cell lesions of the bones of the hand and feet. *Skeletal Radiol* 1986; 15: 415-21.

436. Pierce AM, Wilson DF, Goss AN. Inherited craniofacial fibrous dysplasia. *Oral Surg, Oral Med, Oral Pathol* 1985; 60: 403-9.

437. Pindborg JJ, Kramer IRH, Torloni H. *Histological typing of odontogenic tumors, jaw cysts, and allied lesions. International histological classification of tumors, no. 5.* World Health Organization, Geneva, 1971.

438. Pogrel MA. Unilateral osteolysis in the mandibular angle and coronoid process in scleroderma. *Int J Oral Maxillofac Surg* 1988; 17: 155-6.

439. Polak M, Polak G, Brocheriou CL, et al. Solitary neurofibroma of the mandible: case report and review of the literature. *J Oral Maxillofac Surg* 1989; 47: 65-88.

440. Pöllmann L. Zur altersabhängigen Entwicklung von Exostosen. *Dtsch Z Mund-Kiefer-Gesichts Chir* 1988; 12: 281-2.

441. Poswillo D. The pathogenesis of the Treacher Collins syndrome (mandibulofacial dysostosis). *Br J Oral Maxillofac Surg* 1975; 13: 1-26.

442. Poyton HG, Davey KW. Thalassemia. Changes visible in radiographs used in dentistry. *Oral Surg, Oral Med, Oral Pathol* 1968; 25: 564-76.

443. Praetorius F, Hjörting-Hansen E, Gorlin RJ, et al. Calcifying odontogenic cyst; range, variations and neoplastic potential. *Acta Odontol Scand* 1981; 39: 227-40.

444. Precious DS, McFadden LR. Treatment of traumatic bone cyst of mandible by injection of autogeneic blood. *Oral Surg, Oral Med, Oral Pathol* 1984; 58: 137-40.

445. Prein J, Remagen W, Spiessl B, et al. *Atlas der Tumoren des Gesichtsschädels.* Springer-Verlag, Berlin-Tokyo. 1985.

446. Present D, Bertoni F, Enneking WF. Osteosarcoma of the mandible arising in fibrous dysplasia; a case report. *Clin Orthop, Related Res* 1986; 240: 238-44.

447. Pullon PA, Shafer WG, Elzay RP, et al. Squamous odontogenic tumor. *Oral Surg, Oral Med, Oral Pathol* 1975; 40: 616-30.

448. Punniamoorthy A. Gigantiform cementoma: review of the literature and a case report. *Br J Oral Maxillofac Surg* 1980; 18: 211-29.

449. Ragab MA, Mathog RH. Surgery of massive fibrous dysplasia and osteoma of the midface. *Head & Neck Surg* 1987; 9: 202-10.

450. Rahn R, Schneider M. Periosteale Fasziitis im Kieferbereich. *Dtsch Z Mund-Kiefer-Gesichts Chir* 1988; 12: 195-200.

451. Ramon Y, Engelberg IS. An unusually extensive case of cherubism. *J Oral Maxillofac Surg* 1986; 44: 325-8.

452. Ramon Y, Oberman M, Horowitz I, et al. Osteomyelitis of the maxilla in the newborn. *Int J Oral Maxillofac Surg* 1977; 6: 90-4.

453. Ramon Y, Samra H, Oberman M. Mandibular condylosis and apertognathia in progressive systemic sclerosis (scleroderma). *Oral Surg, Oral Med, Oral Pathol* 1987; 63: 269-74.

454. Ramzy I, Aufdemorte TB, Duncan DL. Diagnosis of radiolucent lesions of the jaws by fine needle aspiration biopsy. *Acta Cytol* 1985; 29: 419-24.

455. Rasmussen OC, Bakke M. Psoriatic arthritis of the temporomandibular joint. *Oral Surg, Oral Med, Oral Pathol* 1982; 53: 351-7.

456. Raubenheimer EJ, Dauth J, van Wilpe E. Multiple myeloma: a study of 10 cases. *J Oral Pathol* 1987; 16: 383-8.

457. Raubenheimer E, Lello GE, Dauth J, et al. Multiple myeloma presenting as localized expansile jaw tumour. *Int J Oral Maxillofac Surg* 1988; 17: 382-5.

458. Reade PC, McKellar GM, Radden BG. Unilateral mandibular cherubism: brief review and case report. *Br J Oral Maxillofac Surg* 1984; 22: 189-94.

459. Reaume CE, Schmid RW, Wesley RK. Aggressive ossifying fibroma of the mandible. *J Oral Maxillofac Surg* 1985; 43: 631-5.

460. Rebel A, Pouplard A, Filmon R, et al. Viral antigens in osteoclasts from Paget's disease of bone. *Lancet* 1980; 2: 344-6.

461. Reddick RL, Michelith HJ, Levine AM, et al. Osteogenic sarcoma. A study of the ultrastructure. *Cancer* 1980; 45: 64-71.

462. Redman RS, Behrens AS, Calhoun NR. Carcinoma of the lung presenting as a mandibular metastasis. *J Oral Maxillofac Surg* 1983; 41: 747-50.

463. Regezi JA, Zarbo RJ, Lloyd RV. HLA-DR antigen detection in giant cell lesions. *J Oral Pathol* 1986; 15: 434-8.

464. Regezi JA, Zarbo RJ, McClatchey KD, et al. Osteosarcomas and chondrosarcomas of the jaws: Immunohistochemical correlations. *Oral Surg, Oral Med, Oral Pathol* 1987; 64: 302-7.

465. Regezi JA, Zarbo RJ, Tomich CE, et al. Immunoprofile of benign and malignant fibrohistiocytic tumors. *J Oral Pathol* 1987; 16: 260-5.

466. Reichart PA, van Roemeling R, Krech R. Mandibular myelosarcoma (chloroma): primary oral manifestation of promyelocytic leukemia. *Oral Surg, Oral Med, Oral Pathol* 1984; 58: 424-7.

467. Reichart PA, Zobl H. Transformation of ameloblastic fibroma to fibrosarcoma. Report of a case. *Int J Oral Maxillofac Surg* 1978; 7: 503-7.

468. Rennie JS, Critchlow HA. Dentinoma of the maxilla. *Br J Oral Maxillofac Surg* 1981; 19: 138-41.

469. Reychler H. Les tumeurs cartilagineuses des maxillaires. *Rev Stomatol Chir Maxillofac* 1988; 89: 321-9.

470. Reychler H. Les tumeurs osseuses des maxillaires. *Rev Stomatol Chir Maxillofac* 1988; 89: 330-8.

471. Richards LC, Gurner IA. An assessment of radiographic methods for the investigation of temporomandibular joint morphology and pathology. *Austr Dent J* 1985; 30: 323-32.

472. Richards LC, Lau E, Wilson DF. Histopathology of the mandibular condyle. *J Oral Pathol* 1984; 14: 624-30.

473. Richardson J, Feldman M, Davis R. Small round cell neoplasm of jaw in a patient with medulloblastoma. *J Oral Maxillofac Surg* 1989; 47: 408-10.

474. Robbins KT, Fuller LM, Manning J, et al. Primary lymphoma of the mandible. *Head & Neck Surg* 1986; 8: 192-9.

475. Rohlin M, Akerman S, Kopp S. Tomography as an aid to detect macroscopic changes of the temporomandibular joint. An autopsy study of the aged. *Acta Odontol Scand* 1986; 44: 131-40.

476. Rohlin M, Petersson A. Rheumatoid arthritis of the temporomandibular joint: Radiologic evaluation based on standard reference films. *Oral Surg, Oral Med, Oral Pathol* 1989; 67: 594-9.

477. Rood JP, Murgatroyd J. Metronidazole in the prevention of 'dry socket'. *Br J Oral Maxillofac Surg* 1979; 17: 62-70.

478. Rosenberg SW, Lepley JB. Mucormycosis in leukemia. *Oral Surg, Oral Med, Oral Pathol* 1982; 54: 26-32.

479. Ruckert EW, Caudill RJ, McCready PJ. Surgical treatment of Van Buchem's Disease. *J Oral Maxillofac Surg* 1985; 43: 801-5.

480. Rudy HN, Scheingold SS. Solitary xanthogranuloma of the mandible: report of a case. *Oral Surg, Oral Med, Oral Pathol* 1964; 18: 262-71.

481. Ruprecht A, Wagner H, Engel H. Osteopetrosis; report of a case and discussion on the differential diagnosis. *Oral Surg, Oral Med, Oral Pathol* 1988; 66: 674-9.

482. Ruskin JD, Cohen DM, Davis LF. Primary intraosseous carcinoma: report of two cases. *J Oral Maxillofac Surg* 1988; 46: 425-32.

483. Russ JE, Jesse RH. Management of osteosarcoma of the maxilla and mandible. *Am J Surg* 1980; 140: 572-6.

484. Sadowsky D, Rosenberg RD, Kaufman J, et al. Central hemangioma of the mandible; literature review, case report, and discussion. *Oral Surg, Oral Med, Oral Pathol* 1981; 52: 471-7.

485. Sailer HF, Makek MS. Blutbildende Knochenherde als Ursache zystoider Kieferlasionen. *Schweiz Mschr Zahnmed* 1985; 95: 183-93.

486. Saleh MS, Rodu B, Prchal JT, et al. Acute myelofibrosis and multiple chloromas of the mandible and skin. *Int J Oral Maxillofac Surg* 1987; 16: 108-11.

487. Salman L, Leffler M, Reddi T, et al. Stafne's bone defect simulating dentigerous cyst of the mandible. *J Oral Med* 1986; 41: 239-41.

488. Salmo NAM, Shukur ST, Abulkhail A. Bilateral aneurysmal bone cysts of the maxilla. *J Oral Maxillofac Surg* 1981; 39: 137-9.

489. Salmo NAM, Shukur ST, Abulkhail A. Mesenchymal chondrosarcoma of the maxilla: report of a case. *J Oral Maxillofac Surg* 1988; 46: 887-9.

490. Samson J, Kuffer R, Bernard J-P, et al. Ostéoblastome des maxillaires. Deux observations et revue de la littérature. *Rev Stomatol Chir Maxillofac* 1985; 86: 285-93.

491. Sandy JR, Williams DM. Anterior salivary gland inclusion in the mandible: Pathological entity or anatomical variant? *Br J Oral Maxillofac Surg* 1981; 19: 223-9.

492. Sanerkin NG. Definitions of osteosarcoma, chondrosarcoma and fibrosarcoma of bone. *Cancer* 1980; 46: 178-85.

493. Sanner JR, Ramin JE. Osteoporotic, hematopoietic mandibular marrow defect: an osseous manifestation of sickle-cell anemia. *J Oral Maxillofac Surg* 1977; 35: 986-8.

494. Santos De LA, Jing B-S. Radiographic findings of Ewing's sarcoma of the jaws. *Br J Radiol* 1978; 51: 682-7.

495. Sariban E, Donahue A, Magrath IT. Jaw involvement in American Burkitt's lymphoma. *Cancer* 1984; 53: 1777-82.

496. Sartoris DJ, Arkoff RS, Parker BR. Aggressive fibromatosis of the mandible in childhood. *Skeletal Radiol* 1983; 10: 154-6.

497. Satterfield SD, Elzay RP, Mercuri L. Mandibular central Schwannoma: report of case. *J Oral Maxillofac Surg* 1981; 39: 776-7.

498. Saw D. Fibrosarcoma of maxilla. *Oral Surg, Oral Med, Oral Pathol* 1979; 47: 164-8.

499. Scaglietti O, Marchetti PG, Bartolozzi P. Final results obtained in treatment of bone cysts with methyl-prednisolone aceta (DEPO-Medrol) and a discussion of results achieved in other bone lesions. *Clin Orthop* 1982; 165: 33-42.

500. Schajowicz F, Ackerman LV, Sissons HA, et al. *Histological typing of bone tumours*. World Health Organization, Geneva. 1972.

501. Schneider LC, Dolinsky HB, Grodjesk JE. Solitary peripheral osteoma of the jaws: report of case and review of the literature. *J Oral Maxillofac Surg* 1980; 38: 452-5.

502. Schneider LC, Mesa ML, Fraenkel D. Osteoporotic bone marrow defect: radiographic features and pathogenic factors. *Oral Surg, Oral Med, Oral Pathol* 1988; 65: 127-9.

503. Schubert J, Grimm G und Schneider D. Die synoviale Chondromatose des Kiefergelenkes. *Dtsch Z Mund-Kiefer-Gesichts Chir* 1984; 8: 35-7.

504. Schulz A, Maerker R, Delling G. Ultrastructural study of tumor cell differentiation in osteosarcoma of jaw bones. *J Oral Pathol* 1978; 7: 69-84.

505. Schwartz HC. Sarcoid temporomandibular arthritis. *Oral Surg, Oral Med, Oral Pathol* 1981; 52: 588-90.

506. Schwartz S, Tsipouras P. Oral findings in osteogenesis imperfecta. *Oral Surg, Oral Med, Oral Pathol* 1984; 57: 161-7.

507. Sciubba JJ, Sachs SA. Schwannoma of the inferior alveolar nerve in association with the organ of Chievitz. *J Oral Pathol* 1980; 9: 16-28.

508. Sciubba JJ, Younai F. Ossifying fibroma of the mandible and maxilla: review of 18 cases. *J Oral Pathol Med* 1989; 18: 315-21.

509. Scott J, Wood GD. Aggressive calcifying odontogenic cyst - a possible variant of ameloblastoma. *Br J Oral Maxillofac Surg* 1989; 27: 53-9.

510. Seifert MH, Steigerwald JC, Cliff MM. Bone resorption of the mandible in progressive systemic sclerosis. *Arth Rheum* 1975; 18: 507-11.

511. Sengün D, Tuncer I, Ertem N, et al. Metastatic hemangioendotheliosarcoma of the mandible: report of case. *J Oral Maxillofac Surg* 1986; 44: 806-10.

512. Sepheriadou-Mavropoulou T, Patrikiou A, Sotiriadou S. Central odontogenic fibroma. *Int J Oral Maxillofac Surg* 1985; 14: 550-5.

513. Severson GS, Ruskin JD, Tu HK, et al. Malignant fibrous histiocytoma presenting in the right mandibular alveolar ridge and left lung: report of a case. *J Oral Maxillofac Surg* 1987; 45: 955-8.

514. Seward MH. Eruption cyst: an analysis of its clinical features. *J Oral Maxillofac Surg* 1973; 31: 31-5.

515. Shamaskin RG, Svirsky JA, Kaugars GE. Intraosseous and extraosseous calcifying odontogenic cyst (Gorlin cyst). *J Oral Maxillofac Surg* 1989; 47: 562-5.

516. Shapiro SD, Abramovitch K, Dis Van ML, et al. Neurofibromatosis: oral and radiographic manifestations. *Oral Surg, Oral Med, Oral Pathol* 1984; 58: 493-8.

517. Sharma JN. Hemorrhagic cyst of the mandible in relation to horizontally impacted third molar. *Oral Surg, Oral Med, Oral Pathol* 1983; 55: 17-8.

518. Shear M. *Cysts of the oral regions*, 2nd edn. John Wright & Sons, Ltd, Bristol. 1983.

519. Shiba R, Sakoda S, Yamada K. Einseitige Hypertrophie des Kiefergelenkfortsatzes mit Verschluss des aüsseren Gehörgangs. *Dtsch Z Mund-Kiefer-Gesichts Chir* 1982; 6: 320-3.

520. Shiratsuchi Y, Tashiro H, Kurihara K. Hemorrhagic cyst of the mandible associated with a retained root apex of the lower third molar. *Oral Surg, Oral Med, Oral Pathol* 1987; 63: 661-3.

521. Shiratsuchi Y, Tashiro H, Yuasa K, et al. Posterior lingual mandibular bone depression. *Int J Oral Maxillofac Surg* 1986; 15: 98-101.

522. Shiro BC, Jacoway JR, Mirmiran SA, et al. Central odontogenic fibroma, granular cell variant. A case report with S-100 immunohistochemistry and a review of the litetature. *Oral Surg, Oral Med, Oral Pathol* 1989; 67: 725-30.

523. Shteyer A, Markitziu A. Lymphosarcoma of the mandible associated with macroglobulinemia of Waldenström. *Int J Oral Maxillofac Surg* 1978; 7: 585-9.

524. Shultz RE, Richardson DD, Kempf KK, et al. Treatment of a central arteriovenous malformation of the mandible with cyanoacrylate: A 4-year follow-up. *Oral Surg, Oral Med, Oral Pathol* 1988; 65: 267-71.

525. Shultz RE, Theisen FC. Bilateral coronoid hyperplasia. Report of a case. *Oral Surg, Oral Med, Oral Pathol* 1989; 68: 23-6.

526. Siar CH, Ng KH. Squamous cell carcinoma in an orthokeratinized odontogenic keratocyst. *Int J Oral Maxillofac Surg* 1987; 16: 95-8.

527. Siegal GP, Oliver WR, Reinus WR, et al. Primary Ewing's sarcoma involving the bones of the head and neck. *Cancer* 1987; 60: 2829-40.

528. Simon MA, Bartucci EJ. The search for the primary tumor in patients with skeletal metastases of unknown primary. *Cancer* 1986; 58: 1088-95.

529. Singh S. The central giant cell granuloma; a case of recurrence after 22 years. *Br J Oral Maxillofac Surg* 1982; 20: 109-16.

530. Slee RW, Al-Hilli F, Abdul-Wahab AW. Secondary chordoma of the mandible. *Br J Oral Maxillofac Surg* 1989; 27: 346-9.

531. Slootweg PJ. Clear-cell chondrosarcoma of the maxilla. Report of a case. *Oral Surg, Oral Med, Oral Pathol* 1980; 50: 223-37.

532. Slootweg PJ. Epithelio-mesenchymal morphology in ameloblastic fibro-odontoma; a light and electronmicroscopic study. *J Oral Pathol* 1980; 9: 29-40.

533. Slootweg PJ. An analysis of the interrelationship of the mixed odontogenic tumors - ameloblastic fibroma, ameloblastic fibro-odontoma, and the odontomas. *Oral Surg, Oral Med, Oral Pathol* 1981; 51: 266-76.

534. Slootweg PJ, Müller H. Central fibroma of the jaw, odontogenic or desmoplastic. A report of five cases with reference to differential diagnosis. *Oral Surg, Oral Med, Oral Pathol* 1983; 56: 61-70.

535. Slootweg PJ, Müller H. Osteosarcoma of the jaw bones. Analysis of 18 cases. *J Maxillofac Surg* 1985; 13: 158-66.

536. Slootweg PJ, Müller H. Mandibular invasion by oral squamous cell carcinoma. *J Cranio-Max-Fac Surg* 1989; 17: 69-74.

537. Slootweg PJ, Straks W, Noorman van der Dussen MF. Primitive neuroectodermal tumor of the maxilla. *J Maxillofac Surg* 1983; 11: 54-7.

538. Slootweg PJ, de Wilde PCM. Condylar pathology in jaw dysfunction: a semi-quantitative study. *J Oral Pathol* 1985; 14: 690-7.

539. Sly WS, Whyte MP, Sundaram V, et al. Carbonic anhydrase II deficiency in 12 families with the autosomal recessive syndrome of osteopetrosis with renal tubular acidosis and cerebral calcification. *N Engl J Med* 1985; 313: 139-45.

540. Smith BJ, Eveson JW. Paget's disease of bone with particular reference to dentistry. *J Oral Pathol* 1981; 10: 233-47.

541. Smith G, Smith AJ, Basu MK, et al. The analysis of fluid aspirate glycosaminoglycans in diagnosis of the postoperative maxillary cyst. *Oral Surg, Oral Med, Oral Pathol* 1988; 65: 222-4.

542. Smith NHH. Monostotic Paget's disease of the mandible presenting with progressive resorption of the teeth. *Oral Surg, Oral Med, Oral Pathol* 1978; 46: 246-53.

543. Smith RA, Hansen LS, Resnick D, et al. Comparison of the osteoblastoma in gnathic and extragnathic sites. *Oral Surg, Oral Med, Oral Pathol* 1982; 54: 285-98.

544. Sokolosky M, Bouquot JE, Graves RW. Esophageal carcinoma metastatic to the oral cavity. *J Oral Maxillofac Surg* 1986; 44: 825-7.

545. Sones AD, Wolinsky LE, Kratochvil FJ. Osteoporosis and mandibular bone resorption: a prosthodontic perspective. *J Prosthet Dent* 1986; 56: 732-6.

546. Spahr J, Elzay RP, Kay S, et al. Chondroblastoma of the temporomandibular joint arising from articular cartilage: a previously unreported presentation of an uncommon neoplasm. *Oral Surg, Oral Med, Oral Pathol* 1982; 54: 430-5.

547. Stajcic Z, Paljm A. Keratinization of radicular cyst epithelial lining or occurrence of odontogenic keratocyst in the periapical region? *Int J Oral Maxillofac Surg* 1987; 16: 593-5.

548. Steinberg B, Shuler C, Wilson S. Melanotic neuroectodermal tumor of infancy. Evidence for multicentricity. *Oral Surg, Oral Med, Oral Pathol* 1988; 66: 666-9.

549. Steiner M, Gould AR, Rasmussen J, et al. Parosteal lipoma of the mandible. *Oral Surg, Oral Med, Oral Pathol* 1981; 52: 61-5.

550. Stern K, Nersasian RR, O'Keefe P, et al. Eikenella osteomyelitis of the mandible associated with anemia of chronic disease. *J Oral Maxillofac Surg* 1978; 36: 285-9.

551. Stewart JCB, Regezi JA, Lloyd RV, et al. Immunohistochemical study of idiopathic histiocytosis of the mandible and maxilla. *Oral Surg, Oral Med, Oral Pathol* 1986; 61: 48-53.

552. Stimson CW, Leban SG. Recurrent ankylosis of the temporomandibular joint in a patient with chronic psoriasis. *J Oral Maxillofac Surg* 1982; 40: 678-80.

553. Stoelinga PJW, Bronkhorst FB. The incidence, multiple presentation and recurrence of aggressive cysts of the jaws. *J Cranio-Max-Fac Surg* 1988; 16: 184-95.

554. Storch H, Löwicke G, Stiehl P, et al. Solitäre Plasmozytome im Kopfbereich. Diagnostische und therapeutische Erwägungen. *Dtsch Z Mund-Kiefer-Gesichts Chir* 1989; 13: 174-7.

555. Strauss M, Kaufman RA, Baum S. Osteomyelitis of the head and neck: sequential radionuclide scanning in diagnosis and therapy. *Laryngoscope* 1985; 95: 81-4.

556. Stroncek GG, Dahl EC, Fonseca RJ, et al. Multiosseous osteosarcoma involving the mandible: metastatic or multicentric? *Oral Surg, Oral Med, Oral Pathol* 1981; 52: 271-6.

557. Struthers PJ, Shear M. Aneurysmal bone cyst of the jaws. Clinicopathological Features (I). Pathogenesis (II). *Int J Oral Maxillofac Surg* 1984; 13: 85-100.

558. Sturrock BD, Marks RB, Gross BD, et al. Giant cell tumor of the mandible. *J Oral Maxillofac Surg* 1984; 42: 262-7.

559. Stypulkowska J, Bartkowski S, Panas M, et al. Metastatic tumors to the jaws and oral cavity. *J Oral Maxillofac Surg* 1979; 37: 805-8.

560. Sugimura M, Okunaga T, Yoneda T, et al. Cementifying fibroma of the maxilla. *Int J Oral Maxillofac Surg* 1981; 10: 298-303.

561. Swart JGN, Netelenbos JC, van Zanten TEG, et al. Die polyostotische fibröse Dysplasie des Kiefers. *Dtsch Z Zahn-Mund-Kiefer-Gesichts Chir* 1978; 2: 45-50.

562. Swartz JD, Vanderslice RB, Korsvik H, et al. High resolution computed tomography: part VI, craniofacial Paget's disease and fibrous dysplasia. *Head & Neck Surg* 1985; 8: 40-7.

563. Tagawe T, Ohse S, Hirano Y, et al. Aggressive infantile fibromatosis of the submandibular region. *Int J Oral Maxillofac Surg* 1989; 18: 264-5.

564. Takeda Y, Fujioka Y. Multiple cemento-ossifying fibroma. *Int J Oral Maxillofac Surg* 1987; 16: 368-71.

565. Talacko AA, Radden BG. The pathogenesis of oral pulse granuloma: an animal model. *J Oral Pathol* 1988; 17: 99-105.

566. Tanaka H, Yoshimoto A, Toyama Y, et al. Periapical cemental dysplasia with multiple lesions. *Int J Oral Maxillofac Surg* 1987; 16: 757-63.

567. Tang JSH, Gold RH, Mirra JM, et al. Hemangiopericytoma of bone. *Cancer* 1988; 62: 848-59.

568. Tanimoto K, Tomita S, Aoyama M, et al. Radiographic characteristics of the calcifying odontogenic cyst. *Int J Oral Maxillofac Surg* 1988; 17: 29-32.

569. Tant L, Dourov N, Vanatoru P, et al. Le granulome eosinophile (histiocytose X); a propos d'un cas de localisation au niveau du condyle mandibulaire. *Acta Stomatologica Belgica* 1984; 81: 181-204.

570. Tetsch P, Hauser I. Die Alveolarkammresorption nach Zahnverlust. *Dtsch Zahnärztl Z* 1982; 37: 102-6.

571. Thibault JCl, Harel J, Lepoivre M. A propos d'un cas d'ostéo-arthrite tuberculeuse primitive de l'articulation temporo-mandibulaire. *Revue Stomat (Paris)* 1972; 73: 162-6.

572. Thiébaud D, Jaeger P, Gobelet C, et al. A single infusion of the biphosphanate AHPrBP (APD) as treatment of Paget's disease of bone. *Am J Med* 1988; 85: 207-12.

573. Thieme V, Müller E-I, Mägdefessel U, et al. Zur Füllung zystischer Knochendefekte mit oberflächenmodifiziertem a-Trikalziumphosphat. Eine klinische, röntgenologische und histologische Studie. *Dtsch Z Mund-Kiefer-Gesichts Chir* 1988; 12: 18-24.

574. Thompson K, Schwartz HC, Miles JW. Synovial chondromatosis of the temporomandibular joint presenting as a parotid mass. Possibility of confusion with benign mixed tumor. *Oral Surg, Oral Med, Oral Pathol* 1986; 62: 377-80.

575. Thompson SH, Shear M. Fibrous histiocytoma of the oral and maxillofacial regions. *J Oral Pathol* 1984; 13: 282-94.

576. Tideman H, Arvier JF, Bosanquet AG, et al. Esophageal adenocarcinoma metastatic to the maxilla. *Oral Surg, Oral Med, Oral Pathol* 1986; 62: 564-8.

577. Timmis DP, Schwartz JG, Nishioka G, et al. Granulocytic sarcoma of the mandible. *J Oral Maxillofac Surg* 1986; 44: 814-8.

578. Toljanic JA, Lechewski E, Huvos AG, et al. Aneurysmal bone cysts of the jaws: a case study and review of the literature. *Oral Surg, Oral Med, Oral Pathol* 1987; 64: 72-7.

579. Tolvanen M, Oikarinen VJ, Wolf J. A 30-year follow-up study of temporomandibular joint meniscectomies: a report of five patients. *Br J Oral Maxillofac Surg* 1988; 26: 311-6.

580. Tomich CE. Chondroma of the anterior nasal spine. *J Oral Maxillofac Surg* 1976; 34: 911-5.

581. Tovi F, Zirkin H, Sidi J. Trismus resulting from a parotid hemangioma. *J Oral Maxillofac Surg* 1983; 41: 468-9.

582. Ueno S, Mushimoto K, Shirasu R. Prognostic evaluation of ameloblastoma based on histologic and radiographic typing. *J Oral Maxillofac Surg* 1989; 47: 11-5.

583. Ueno S, Nakamura S, Mushimoto K, et al. A clinicopathologic study of ameloblastoma. *J Oral Maxillofac Surg* 1986; 44: 361-5.

584. Vaillant JM, Romain P, Divaris M. Cherubism. Findings in three cases in the same family. *J Cranio-Max-Fac Surg* 1989; 17: 345-9.

585. Vally IM, Altini M. Fibromatoses of the oral and paraoral soft tissues and jaws. Review of the literature and report of 12 new cases. *Oral Surg, Oral Med, Oral Pathol* 1990; 69: 191-8.

586. Vedtofte P, Praetorius F. The inflammatory paradental cyst. *Oral Surg, Oral Med, Oral Pathol* 1989; 68: 182-8.

587. Verheijen-Breemhaar L, Man De K, Zondervan PE, et al. Sarcoidosis with maxillary involvement. *Int J Oral Maxillofac Surg* 1987; 16: 104-7.

588. Vigneul JC, Nouel O, Klap P, et al. Metastatic hepatocellular carcinoma of the mandible. *J Oral Maxillofac Surg* 1982; 40: 745-9.

589. Vincent SD, Williams TP. Mandibular abnormalities in neurofibromatosis. *Oral Surg, Oral Med, Oral Pathol* 1983; 55: 253-8.

590. Vogel von C, Reichart P, Schnaidt U. Zentrales Neurofibrom des Unterkiefers bei generalisierter Neurofibromatose von Recklinghausen. *Dtsch Z Mund-Kiefer-Gesichts Chir* 1980; 4: 31-4.

591. Vollmer E, Roessner A, Lipecki KH, et al. Biologic characterization of human bone tumors. VI. The aneurysmal bone cyst: an enzyme histochemical, electron microscopical, and immunohistological study. *Virchows Arch (B)* 1987; 53: 58-65.

592. Von Arx DP, Simpson MT, Batman P. Synovial chondromatosis of the temporomandibular joint. *Br J Oral Maxillofac Surg* 1988; 26: 297-305.

593. Voorsmit RACA, Stoelinga PJW, van Haelst UJGM. The management of keratocysts. *J Maxillofac Surg* 1981; 9: 228-36.

594. Vos de RAI, Brants J, Kusen GJ, et al. Calcium pyrophosphate dihydrate arthropathy of the temporomandibular joint. *Oral Surg, Oral Med, Oral Pathol* 1981; 51: 497-502.

595. Waal van der I, Rauhamaa R, van der Kwast WAM, et al. Squamous cell carcinoma arising in the lining of odontogenic cysts: report of 5 cases. *Int J Oral Maxillofac Surg* 1985; 14: 146-52.

596. Wagner DK, Varkey B, Head MD. Blastomycotic osteomyelitis of the mandible: succesful treatment with ketoconazole. *Oral Surg, Oral Med, Oral Pathol* 1985; 60: 370-1.

597. Waldron CA. Fibro-osseous lesions of the jaws. *J Oral Maxillofac Surg* 1985; 43: 249-62.

598. Waldron CA, El-Mofty SK. A histopathologic study of 116 ameloblastomas with special reference to the desmoplastic variant. *Oral Surg, Oral Med, Oral Pathol* 1987; 63: 441-51.

599. Waldron CA, Giansanti JS. Benign fibro-osseous lesions of the jaws: a clinical-radiologic-histologic review of sixty-five cases. Part I. Fibrous dysplasia of the jaws. *Oral Surg, Oral Med, Oral Pathol* 1973; 35: 190-201.

600. Waldron CA, Giansanti JS. Benign fibro-osseous lesions of the jaws: a clinical-radiologic-histologic review of sixty-five cases. Part II. Benign fibro-osseous lesions of periodontal ligament origin. *Oral Surg, Oral Med, Oral Pathol* 1973; 35: 340-50.

601. Waldron CA, Giansanti JS, Browand BC. Sclerotic cemental masses of the jaws (so-called chronic sclerosing osteomyelitis, sclerosing osteitis, multiple enostosis and gigantiform cementoma). *Oral Surg, Oral Med, Oral Pathol* 1975; 39: 590-604.

602. Waldron CA, Mustoe TA. Primary intraosseous carcinoma of the mandible with probable origin in an odontgenic cyst. *Oral Surg, Oral Med, Oral Pathol* 1989; 67: 716-24.

603. Wannfors K, Hammarstrom L. Infectious foci in chronic osteomyelitis of the jaws. *Int J Oral Maxillofac Surg* 1985; 14: 493-503.

604. Wannfors K, Lindskog S, Olander KJ, et al. Fibrous dysplasia of bone and concomitant dysplastic changes in the dentin. *Oral Surg, Oral Med, Oral Pathol* 1985; 59: 394-398.

605. Watt-Smith SR, El-Laban NG, Tinkler SM. Central odontogenic fibroma. *Int J Oral Maxillofac Surg* 1988; 17: 87-91.

606. Wei-Yung Y, Guang-Sheng M, Merrill RG, et al. Central hemangiomas of the jaws. *J Oral Maxillofac Surg* 1989; 47: 1154-60.

607. Weinberg S, Katsikeris N, Pharoah M. Osteoblastoma of the mandibular condyle; review of the literature and report of a case. *J Oral Maxillofac Surg* 1987; 45: 350-5.

608. Westesson P-L. Double-contrast arthrotomography of the temporomandibular joint: introduction of an arthrographic technique for visualization of the disc and articular surfaces. *J Oral Maxillofac Surg* 1983; 41: 163-72.

609. Whitcher BL, Beirne OR, Smith RA. Beta-lactamase-producing Bacteroides melaninogenicus and osteomyelitis of the mandible. *J Oral Med* 1983; 38: 17-20.

610. White DK, Makar J. Xanthofibroma of the mandible. *J Oral Maxillofac Surg* 1986; 44: 1010-4.

611. White DK, Selinger LR, Miller AS, et al. Primary angioleiomyoma of the mandible. *J Oral Maxillofac Surg* 1985; 43: 640-4.

612. Widmark G, Sagne S, Heikel P. Osteoradionecrosis of the jaws. *Int J Oral Maxillofac Surg* 1989; 18: 302-6.

613. Wilkes CH. Internal derangements of the temporomandibular joint. Pathological variations. *Arch Otolaryngol Head Neck Surg* 1989; 115: 469-77.

614. Wite SC, Forsythe AB, Joseph LP. Patient-selection criteria for panoramic radiography. *Oral Surg, Oral Med, Oral Pathol* 1984; 57: 681-90.

615. Williams HK, Edwards MB, Adekeye EO. Mesenchymal chondrosarcoma. *Int J Oral Maxillofac Surg* 1987; 16: 119-24.

616. Williams SA, Duggan MB, Bailey CC. Jaw involvement in acute lymphoblastic leukaemia. *Br Dent J* 1983; 155: 164-6.

617. Williams Th, Vincent SD. Embryonal rhabdomyosarcoma of the mandible. *J Oral Maxillofac Surg* 1987; 45: 441-3.

618. Wilson DF, D'Rozario R, Bosanquet A. Focal osteoporotic bone marrow defect. *Austr Dent J* 1985; 30: 77-80.

619. Winer RA, Doku HC. Traumatic bone cyst in the maxilla. *Oral Surg, Oral Med, Oral Pathol* 1978; 46: 367-70.

620. Wold LE, Dobyns JH, Swee RG, et al. Giant cell reaction (giant cell reparative granuloma) of the small bones of the hands and feet. *Am J Surg Pathol* 1986; 10: 491-6.

621. Wolf J, Hietanen J, Sane J. Florid cemento-osseous dysplasia (gigantiform cementoma) in a Caucasian woman. *Br J Oral Maxillofac Surg* 1989; 27: 46-52.

622. Wolf J, Järvinen HJ, Hietanen J. Gardner's dento-maxillary stigmas in patients with familial adenomatosis coli. *Br J Oral Maxillofac Surg* 1986; 24: 410-6.

623. Wolf J, Mattila K, Ankkuriniemi O. Development of a Stafne mandibular bone cavity. Report of a case. *Oral Surg, Oral Med, Oral Pathol* 1986; 61: 519-21.

624. Wood RE, Nortjé CJ, Grotepass F, et al. Periostitis ossificans versus Garré's osteomyelitis. Part I. What did Garré really say? *Oral Surg, Oral Med, Oral Pathol* 1988; 65: 773-7.

625. Wood RM, Markle TL, Barker BF, et al. Ameloblastic fibrosarcoma. *Oral Surg, Oral Med, Oral Pathol* 1988; 66: 74-7.

626. Woolgar JA, Rippin JW, Browne RM. The odontogenic keratocyst and its occurrence in the nevoid basal cell carcinoma syndrome. *Oral Surg, Oral Med, Oral Pathol* 1987; 64: 727-30.

627. Woolgar JA, Rippin JW, Browne RM. A comparative histological study of odontogenic keratocysts in basal cell naevus syndrome and control patients. *J Oral Pathol* 1987; 16: 75-80.

628. Woolgar JA, Rippin JW, Browne RM. A comparative study of the clinical and histologic features of recurrent and non-recurrent odontogenic keratocysts. *J Oral Pathol* 1987; 16: 124-8.

629. Worsaae N, Reibel J, Rechnitzer C. Tuberculous osteomyelitis of the mandible. *Br J Oral Maxillofac Surg* 1984; 22: 93-8.

630. Wovern Von N, Hjörting-Hansen E, Edeling C-J. Bone scintigraphy of benign jaw lesions. *Int J Oral Maxillofac Surg* 1978; 7: 528-33.

631. Wovern Von N, Stoltze K. Pattern of age related bone loss in the mandible. *Scand J Dent Res* 1980; 88: 134-46.

632. Wright BA, Jackson D. Neural tumors of the oral cavity. A review of the spectrum of benign and malignant oral tumors of the oral cavity and jaws. *Oral Surg, Oral Med, Oral Pathol* 1980; 49: 509-22.

633. Wright BA, Wysocki GP, Bannerjee D. Diagnostic use of immunoperoxidase techniques for plasma cell lesions of the jaws. *Oral Surg, Oral Med, Oral Pathol* 1981; 52: 615-22.

634. Wu P-C, Leung PKY, Ma KM. Recurrent cementifying fibroma. *J Oral Maxillofac Surg* 1986; 44: 229-34.

635. Wyk Van CW, Padayachee A, Nortjé CJ, et al. Primary intraosseous carcinoma involving the anterior mandible. *Br J Oral Maxillofac Surg* 1987; 25: 427-32.

636. Wysocki GP, Brannon RB, Gardner DG, et al. Histogenesis of the lateral periodontal cyst and the gingival cyst of the adult. *Oral Surg, Oral Med, Oral Pathol* 1980; 50: 327-34.

637. Wysocki GP. The differential diagnosis of globulomaxillary radiolucencies. *Oral Surg, Oral Med, Oral Pathol* 1981; 51: 281-6.

638. Yaacob H, Tirmzi H, Ismail K. The prevalence of oral tori in Malaysians. *J Oral Med* 1983; 38: 40-2.

639. Yagan R, Bellon EM, Radivoyevitch M. Breast carcinoma metastatic to the mandible mimicking ameloblastoma. *Oral Surg, Oral Med, Oral Pathol* 1984; 57: 189-94.

640. Yagan R, Radivoyevitch M, Bellon EM. Involvement of the mandibular canal: early sign of osteogenic sarcoma of the mandible. *Oral Surg, Oral Med, Oral Pathol* 1985; 60: 56-60.

641. Yamamoto G, Yoshitake K, Tada K, et al. Granular cell ameloblastoma. A rare variant. *Int J Oral Maxillofac Surg* 1989; 18: 140-1.

642. Yamamoto H, Caselitz J, Kozawa Y. Ameloblastic fibrosarcoma of the right mandible: immunohistochemical and electronmicroscopical investigations on one case, and a review of the literature. *J Oral Pathol* 1987; 16: 450-5.

643. Yamamoto H, Sakae T, Davies JE. Cleidocranial dysplasia: A light microscope, electron microscope, and crystallographic study. *Oral Surg, Oral Med, Oral Pathol* 1989; 68: 195-200.

644. Yamamoto H, Takagi M. Clinicopathologic study of the postoperative maxillary cyst. *Oral Surg, Oral Med, Oral Pathol* 1986; 62: 544-8.

645. Yamane H, Tanaka Y, Shimono M, et al. Nodular fasciitis of the mandible in a child. *Int J Oral Maxillofac Surg* 1986; 15: 499-502.

646. Yamashiro M, Komori A. Osteosarcoma mimicking fibrous dysplasia of the jaw. *Int J Oral Maxillofac Surg* 1987; 16: 112-5.

647. Yeoman CM. Management of haemangioma involving facial, mandibular and pharyngeal structures. *Br J Oral Maxillofac Surg* 1987; 25: 195-203.

648. Yih W-Y, Pederson GT, Bartley MH. Multiple familial ossifying fibromas: Relationship to other osseous lesions of the jaws. *Oral Surg, Oral Med, Oral Pathol* 1989; 68: 754-8.

649. York BV, Cockerham S. Bilateral hyperplasia of the coronoid process in siblings. *Oral Surg, Oral Med, Oral Pathol* 1983; 56: 584-5.

650. Yoshida T, Shingaki S, Nakajima T, et al. Odontogenic carcinoma with sarcomatous proliferation. A case report. *J Cranio-Max-Fac Surg* 1989; 17: 139-42.

651. Yoshikawa Y, Nokajima T, Kaneshiro S, et al. Effective treatment of the postoperative maxillary cyst by marsupialization. *J Oral Maxillofac Surg* 1982; 40: 487-91.

652. Yosue T, Brooks SL. The appearance of mental foramina on panoramic radiographs. I. Evaluation of patients. *Oral Surg, Oral Med, Oral Pathol* 1989; 68: 360-4.

653. Younai F, Eisenbud L, Sciubba JJ. Osteopetrosis: a case report including gross and microscopic findings in the mandible at autopsy. *Oral Surg, Oral Med, Oral Pathol* 1988; 65: 214-21.

654. Young SK, Markowitz NR, Sullivan S, et al: Familial gigantiform cementoma: Classification and presentation of a large pedigree. *Oral Surg, Oral Med, Oral Pathol* 1989; 68: 740-7.

655. Yusuf H, Battacharya MN. Syphilitic osteomyelitis of the mandible. *Br J Oral Maxillofac Surg* 1982; 20: 122-8.

656. Zachariades N. Gardner's syndrome; report of a family. *J Oral Maxillofac Surg* 1987; 45: 438-40.

657. Zachariades N, Anastasea-Vlachou K, Xypolyta A, et al. Uncommon manifestations of histiocytosis X. *J Oral Maxillofac Surg* 1987; 16: 355-62.

658. Zachariades N, Economopoulou P. Maxillary angiosarcoma. *Int J Oral Maxillofac Surg* 1986; 15: 357-60.

659. Zachariades N, Mezitis M, Vairaktaris E, et al. Benign neurogenic tumors of the oral cavity. *Int J Oral Maxillofac Surg* 1987; 16: 70-6.

660. Zachariades N, Papanicolaou S. The median palatal cyst: does it exist? Report of three cases with oro-medical implications. *J Oral Med* 1984; 39: 173-6.

661. Zachariades N, Papanicolaou S, Papavassiliou D, et al. Plasma cell myeloma of the jaws. *Int J Oral Maxillofac Surg* 1987; 16: 510-5.

662. Zachariades N, Papanicolaou S, Xypolyta A, et al. Albright syndrome. *Int J Oral Maxillofac Surg* 1984; 13: 53-8.

663. Zachariades N, Patrinou C, Benetos S, et al. Post-irradiation osteogenic sarcoma. *J Oral Maxillofac Surg* 1985; 43: 297-9.

664. Zachariades N, Skordalaki A, Papanicolaou S, et al. Infantile cortical hyperostosis: report of two cases. *J Oral Maxillofac Surg* 1986; 44: 644-8.

665. Zachariades N, Vairaktaris E, Papanicolaou S, et al. Ossifying fibroma of the jaws. Review of the literature and report of 16 cases. *Int J Oral Maxillofac Surg* 1984; 13: 1-6.

666. Zakrzewska JM. Angiosarcoma of the maxilla - a case report and review of the literature including angiosarcoma of maxillary sinus. *Br J Maxillofac Surg* 1986; 24: 286-92.

667. Zarbo RJ, Regezi JA, Baker SR. Periosteal osteogenic sarcoma of the mandible. *Oral Surg, Oral Med, Oral Pathol* 1984; 57: 643-7.

668. Zhao-ju Z, Yun-tang W, Guan-xi S, et al. Clinical application of angiography of oral and maxillofacial hemangioma. *Oral Surg, Oral Med, Oral Pathol* 1983; 55: 437-47.

669. Zohär Y, Grausbord R, Shabtai F, et al. Fibrous dysplasia and cherubism as an hereditary familial disease. Follow-up of four generations. *J Cranio-Max-Fac Surg* 1989; 17: 340-4.

670. Zuendel MT, Bowers DF, Kramer RN. Recurrent histiocytosis X with mandibular lesions. *Oral Surg, Oral Med, Oral Pathol* 1984; 58: 420-3.

671. Zuniga JR, Holmes HI, Page HL. Myelofibrosis of the facial bones. *Oral Surg, Oral Med, Oral Pathol* 1983; 56: 32-8.

Index

A
adenomatoid odontogenic tumor *194*
African jaw tumor *160*
agnathia *17*
Albers-Schönberg disease *241*
alveolitis *29*
ameloblastic carcinoma *230*
ameloblastic fibro-dentinoma *192*
ameloblastic fibroma *190*
ameloblastic fibro-odontoma *193*
ameloblastic fibrosarcoma *234*
ameloblastic odontosarcoma *234*
ameloblastic sarcoma *234*
ameloblastic, benign *178*
  - , malignant *230*
ameloblastoma, odonto- *194*
aneurysmal bone cyst *71*
angiosarcoma *154*
ankylosis *266*
arthrogryposis *266*
arthrosis deformans *269*
atrophy of alveolar ridge *253*

B
bifid mandibular condyle *268*
Birbeck granules *240*
botryoid odontogenic cyst *104*
botryomycosis *30*
"brown tumor" *56*
Burkitt's tumor *160*

C
Caffey's disease *26*
Caffey-Silverman syndrome *26*
calcifying epithelial odontogenic tumor *188*
calcifying odontogenic cyst *196*
carcinoma
    - ameloblastic *230*
    - clear cell odontogenic *232*
    - intraosseous *232*
    - odontogenic *230*
    - squamous cell *263*
Camurati-Engelmann's disease *243*
cementoblastoma *206*
cementoma *206*
  - , gigantiform *210*
chemodectoma *139*
cherubism *51*
chloroma *165*
cholesterol granuloma *30*
chondroblastoma *134*
chondroma *133*
chondromatosis *267*
chondromyxoid fibroma *140*
chondrosarcoma *135*
  - , mesenchymal *138*
clear cell odontogenic tumor/carcinoma *232*
cleidocranial dysostosis *18*
closed lock *269*
Codman's tumor *134*
Cooley's anemia *249*
craniofacial dysostosis *20*
Crowzon's disease *20*
cysts
   - aneurysmal bone *271*
   - botryoid odontogenic *104*
   - calcifying odontogenic *196*
   - dental lamina *86*
   - dentigerous *88*
   - dermal *73*
   - eruption *92*
   - follicular *88*
   - gingival *95*
   - glandular odontogenic *106*
   - globulomaxillary *74*
   - Gorlin *196*
   - hemorrhagic bone *82*
   - hydatid *80*
   - idiopathic bone *82*

cysts (cont'd)
- kerato- *96*
- lateral periodontal *104*
- lingual mandibular salivary gland depression *74*
- mandibular infected *112*
- median palatal *77*
- median mandibular *76*
- nasolabial *77*
- nasopalatine duct *78*
- paradental *107*
- parasitic *80*
- postoperative maxillary *80*
- primordial *106*
- radicular *108*
- residual *110*
- sialo-odontogenic *106*
- simple bone *82*
- solitary bone *82*
- Stafne's *74*
- surgical ciliated *80*

D

dental lamina cyst of the newborn *86*
dentigerous cyst *88*
dentinoma *192*
dermoid cyst *73*
desmoplastic fibroma *142*
"dry socket" *29*

E

Engelmann's disease *243*
eosinophilic granuloma *238*
eruption cyst *92*
Ewing's sarcoma *129*
exostoses *20*
- multiple *24*

F

fibroma
- ameloblastic *190*
- central *202*
- chondromyxoid *139*
- desmoplastic *142*

fibroma (cont'd)
- non-ossifying *144*
- odontogenic *202*
- ossifying and cementifying *225*
- peripheral *202*
fibromatosis *146*
fibrosarcoma *148*
- , ameloblastic *234*
fibrous dysplasia *61*
- monostotic *61*
- polyostotic *70*
fibrous healing *254*
fibrous histiocytoma *149*
florid osseous dysplasia *210*
focal osteoporotic bone marrow defect *255*
follicular cyst *88*

G

ganglioneuroma *172*
Gardner's syndrome *113*
Garré's osteomyelitis *33*
Gaucher's disease *235*
giant cell granuloma, central *55*
giant cell hyalin angiopathy *38*
giant cell tumor *60*
gigantiform cementoma *210*
gingival cyst *95*
glandular odontogenic cyst *106*
globulomaxillary cyst *74*
Gorlin cyst *196*
granulocytic sarcoma *165*

H

Hand-Schüller-Christian disease *236*
hemangio-endothelioma *154*
hemangio-endotheliosarcoma *154*
hemangioma *150*
hemangiopericytoma *154*
hemimaxillofacial dysplasia *24*
hemophilic pseudotumor *258*
hemorrhagic bone cyst *82*
histiocytosis X *236*
Hodgkin's lymphoma *156*
hydatid cyst *80*

hyperostosis corticalis generalisata
  familiaris *25*
hyperparathyroidism *56*
hyperplasia
    - of the condyles *268*
    - of the coronoid process *268*
hypoplasia, of the condyles *268*

I
idiopathic bone cyst *82*
infantile cortical hyperostosis *26*
intraosseous carcinoma *232*

K
Kahler's disease *163*
keratocyst *96*

L
Langerhans' cell granulomatosis *236*
lateral periodontal cyst *104*
leiomyoma *155*
leiomyosarcoma *155*
Letterer-Siwe disease *237*
leukemia *156*
lingual cortical defect of the mandible *74*
lingual mandibular salivary gland
  depression cyst *74*
lipoblastoma *155*
liposarcoma *155*
luxation, of TMJ *272*
lymphangioma *155*

M
macrognathia *18*
macrostomia *27*
malignant lymphoma *156*
mandibular infected buccal cyst *112*
mandibulofacial dysostosis *27*
marble bone disease *241*
massive osteolysis *258*
median mandibular cyst *76*
median palatal cyst *77*
melanotic neuroectodermal tumor *166*

metastatic tumors *168*
micrognathia *17*
mucormycosis *30*
myelofibrosis *165*
myelomatosis *163*
myelosarcoma *165*
myospherulosis *40*
myxoma, odontogenic *204*

N
nasolabial cyst *77*
nasopalatine duct cyst *78*
neurilemmoma *171*
neuroblastoma *171*
neurofibroma *171*
neurofibromatosis *171*
neurogenic sarcoma *172*
nevoid basal cell carcinoma syndrome *96*
non-Hodgkin's lymphoma *156*
non-ossifying fibroma *144*
Noonan syndrome *51*

O
odontoameloblastoma *194*
odontogenic carcino-sarcoma *234*
odontoma *199*
"osseous keloid" *67*
ossifying and cementifying fibroma *225*
osteitis, condensing *33*
osteitis deformans *245*
osteoarthrosis *269*
osteoblastoma *117*
ostogenesis imperfecta *27*
osteoid osteoma *117*
osteoma *113*
  - osteoid *117*
osteomyelitis *31*
osteopetrosis *241*
osteoporosis *243*
osteoporotic bone marrow defect *255*
osteoradionecrosis *41*
osteosarcoma *119*

P

Paget's disease *245*
pain dysfunction syndrome *269*
paradental cyst *107*
parasitic cyst *80*
periapical granuloma *45*
periapical cemental dysplasia *210*
periodontal disease *48*
periostitis ossificans *33*
phantom bone disease *258*
phycomycosis *30*
Pierre Robin syndrome *17*
Pindborg tumor *188*
plasma cell myeloma, multiple *163*
  - , solitary *162*
plasmacytoma *162*
postoperative maxillary cyst *80*
primary intraosseous carcinoma *232*
primordial cyst *106*
progonoma *166*
progressive resorption of bone *258*
"pulse granuloma" *38*
pychnodysostosis *28*

R

radicular cyst *108*
Recklinghausen's disease *171*
renal osteodystrophy *248*
residual cyst *110*
rhabdomyosarcoma *173*

S

salivary gland tumor, intraosseous *174*
sarcoidosis *249*
sarcoma
  - ameloblastic *234*
  - ameloblastic fibro- *234*
  - ameloblastic odonto- *234*
  - angio- *154*
  - chondro- *135*

sarcoma (cont'd)
  - Ewing's *129*
  - fibro- *148*
  - granulocytic *165*
  - leiomyo- *188*
  - lipo- *188*
  - myelo- *165*
  - neurogenic *172*
  - odontogenic carcino- *234*
  - osteo- *119*
  - rhabdomyo *173*
Schwannoma *171*
scleroderma *249*
sclerotic healing *254*
sclerotic cemental masses *210*
sialo-odontogenic cyst *106*
simple bone cyst *82*
solitary bone cyst *82*
squamous odontogenic tumor *187*
Stafne's cyst *74*
subluxation, of TMJ *272*
surgical ciliated cyst *80*

T

teratoma *176*
thalassemia *249*
torus palatinus *20*
torus mandibularis *22*
traumatic bone cyst *82*
Treacher Collins syndrome *27*
trismus *273*

V W

Van Buchem's disease *25*
Waldenström's macroglobulinemia *165*

X

xanthofibroma *144*
xanthogranuloma *144*
xanthoma *144*

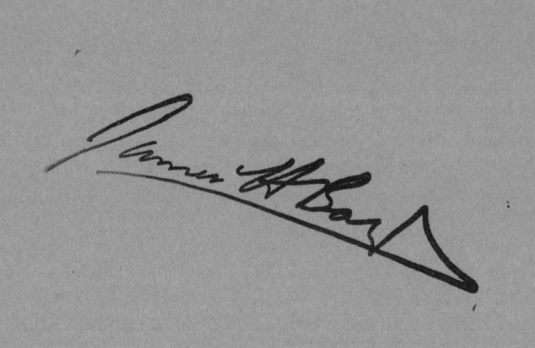